CARDIAC REHABILITATION

CARDIAC REHABILITATION

Edited by

Dee Jones
*Director of Research Team for the Care of Elderly People,
University of Wales College of Medicine, Cardiff*

and

Robert West
*Reader in Epidemiology, University of Wales College of
Medicine, Cardiff*

BMJ
Publishing
Group

First published in 1995
by the BMJ Publishing Group, BMA House, Tavistock Square, London WC1H 9JR

British Library Cataloguing in Publication Data

A catalogue record for this book is available from the British Library

ISBN 0-7279-0852-9

Typeset in Great Britain by Apek Typesetters Ltd., Nailsea, Avon.
printed and bound in Great Britain by Latimer Trend, Plymouth

Contents

List of contributors

Editors

Dee Jones BSc PhD MFPHM
Director, Research Team for the Care of Elderly People
University of Wales College of Medicine
Cardiff Royal Infirmary
Cardiff

Robert West MA PhD MFPHM
Reader in Epidemiology
University of Wales College of Medicine
Cardiff

Contributors

Hugh JN Bethell MB BChir MRCP FRCGP DObs RCOG
General Practitioner
Alton Health Centre
Alton
Hampshire
Also: Hospital Practitioner (Cardiac Rehabilitation), Basingstoke District
Hospital

Jean-Paul Broustet MD
Professor of Cardiology
University of Bordeaux II
Chief, Department of Exercise Testing and Clinical Cardiology
Hôpital Cardiologique Haut Leveque
Pessac
France

Elizabeth Lorna Cay MD FRCP FRC Psych DPM
Consultant in Medical Rehabilitation
Astley Ainslie Hospital
113 Grange Loan
Edinburgh
Also: Honorary Senior Lecturer in Rehabilitation Studies
University of Edinburgh

Christopher Davidson MB BChir FRCP FESC
Consultant Cardiologist
Royal Sussex County Hospital
Brighton

Hervé Douard MD
Hospital Practitioner

Department of Exercise Testing and Clinical Cardiology
Hôpital Cardiologique Haut Levêque
Pessac
France

John Horgan MD FRCPI FACC FESC
Associate Professor of Medicine and Consultant Cardiologist
Department of Cardiology
Beaumont Hospital
Dublin 9
Ireland

Desmond G Julian CBE MD FRCP FACC
Formerly Consultant Medical Director
British Heart Foundation
London
Emeritus Professor of Cardiology, University of Newcastle Upon Tyne

Veikko Kallio MD PhD
Professor and Rehabilitation Physician
Research Centre
Social Insurance Institution
Turku
Finland

Terence Kavanagh MD FRCPC FACC FCCP
Medical Director and Chief Executive Officer
Toronto Rehabilitation Centre
Toronto
Ontario
Canada
Also: Associate Professor, Department of Medicine, University of Toronto, and Honorary Advisor to the Heart Transplant Unit, Harefield Hospital, Middlesex

Bob Lewin MA M.Phil
Director, British Heart Foundation Rehabilitation Research Unit
Department of Health Psychology
Astley Ainslie Hospital
Edinburgh

Hannah M McGee PhD FPsSI
Senior Lecturer in Psychology and Health Psychologist
Department of Cardiology
Beaumont Hospital
Dublin 9
Ireland

Introduction: objectives and definition of cardiac rehabilitation

Heart disease is the leading cause of death in most of the developed world. In the United Kingdom, for example, coronary heart disease was the underlying cause of nearly 170 000 deaths in 1992—26% of all deaths. Similar numbers of patients are admitted to hospital with acute myocardial infarction so that by the age of 65 in men and 75 in women more than 10% have experienced myocardial infarction. Estimates of the prevalence of chronic stable angina range between 2 and 8% of middle-aged men and women, depending on how angina is defined, and many of these are referred to cardiologists and in turn to cardiac surgeons. Nearly 17 000 coronary artery bypass graft operations (equivalent to 290 per million total population) and nearly 10 000 percutaneous transluminal coronary angioplasties (170 per million) were performed in the United Kingdom in 1991. Higher operation or intervention rates have been recorded in many other Western countries. These figures illustrate the burden of heart disease on the populations of developed countries. Many patients experience some chronic morbidity from persistent disease; many are rushed to hospital following an acute event; and many are admitted to hospital electively for major open-heart surgery. While there may be numerous opportunities for rehabilitation among these large numbers of patients with heart disease, the primary need is for active treatment, and this is the main focus of the health services provision in primary care, the district hospital, or the regional specialist centre.

Cardiac rehabilitation programmes have developed in a number of countries over the past twenty years. Initially most programmes concentrated on patients following acute myocardial infarction. While these patients remain the largest group, programmes have developed more recently to include patients discharged after elective procedures (coronary artery bypass graft and percutaneous transluminal coronary angioplasty) and for patients with chronic stable angina. While the overall objectives of rehabilitation, to facilitate the patient's own return to as near normal as possible, are common to all three patient groups, the specific needs of these patient groups differ.

Rehabilitation is understood by most practitioners as the process enabling, encouraging, and assisting patients to make the transition from a state of illness back to a state of health, as near as possible to normal. In practice although it may begin earlier and end later, most cardiac rehabilitation is concentrated primarily in outpatients departments, bridging the transition from dependence in the coronary care unit or intensive care unit to independence in the community. It is useful in a discussion of cardiac rehabilitation to identify its boundaries but to appreciate that such boundaries are not absolute: health care outside these boundaries undertaken by health care professionals other than rehabilitation therapists may overlap with and contribute significantly to rehabilitation. For the purposes of this book treatment, including medication in acute care and in longterm maintenance, is not regarded as rehabilitation. A full discussion of treatment clearly lies outside the scope of this book. Similarly, although some opportunistic "secondary prevention" is often included in programmes, this is regarded as prevention. Rehabilitation therapists will appreciate the relevance of both treatment and prevention to rehabilitation in so far as they impinge on rehabilitation practice, and both are included, but readers who seek more detail on these subjects should refer to the relevant specialist texts. This book focuses on the need for and rationale, development, and evaluation of rehabilitation centred on exercise training and psychological support and counselling.

In the first chapter Julian sets the scene by summarising the medical management of cardiac disease. Most rehabilitation programmes, whether predominantly exercise-based, predominantly psychologically-based, or comprehensive, include some patient education on the heart, heart disease, risk factors, treatment, and management in hospital. Rehabilitation therapists should have some knowledge of the condition and experiences of patients referred to their care. Cay discusses the goals of rehabilitation, including the changing emphasis away from mortality and return to work towards quality of life (chapter 2). Kavanagh presents the rationale for physical training and describes many of the benefits of exercise training programmes (chapter 3). The Toronto rehabilitation centre is renowned for its success in improving exercise performance in many cardiac patients including training some to run marathons. Lewin describes the background for psychological therapy (chapter 4). Both acute and chronic disease may affect patients psychologically and in some patients can induce clinical anxiety or depression, or both, which requires specialist clinical management. Kallio develops the idea of tailoring rehabilitation round individual patient needs (chapter 5). Comprehensive rehabilitation offers physical training and psychological therapy as well as health education, social support, and assistance with, for example, return to work, but individual patient needs for constituent elements of the total programme vary widely. Broustet and Douard consider the rather different needs of patients following coronary artery bypass graft, percutaneous transluminal coronary angioplasty, and treatment of other less common cardiac conditions (chapter 6). The natural history of the acute phase in these planned procedures and hospital admissions differ considerably from the unexpected crisis of myocardial infarction.

Historically cardiac rehabilitation in the United Kingdom has lagged behind America, Canada, and most of Northern Europe. Davidson outlines the development of cardiac rehabilitation in Britain, centred on the district general hospital. Bethell presents the case for siting rehabilitation more firmly in the community to encourage patients away from the hospital and enable self-care (chapter 8). One of us (West) reviews the evolution of health care evaluation and the evidence for effectiveness of exercise based, psychologically based, and comprehensive rehabilitation (chapter 9). The case for a major multicentre trial of psychologically based rehabilitation with patients of both sexes and of all ages is outlined in chapter 10. The principal findings of this trial are compared with those of previous trials in the context of pragmatic health care evaluation. The other (Jones) discusses both the effect of illness on spouses and the importance of the spouse's role in rehabilitation. Since much of the research on rehabilitation has included only male patients, much of the literature on spouses has included only wives. The trial described in chapter 10 includes 623 women and 377 husbands. In the closing chapter Horgan and Magee consider the future of cardiac rehabilitation and focus particularly on the need to develop and recognise a formal training programme.

The book is not intended as a text or prescriptive guide, and a uniform structure was not imposed on contributing authors. Individual chapters reflect individual views. Some overlap in a multi-author book allows each chapter to be complete in itself within the overall theme. Some differences in interpretation of evidence, in what to include in rehabilitation programmes, in patient selection, and in detail of rehabilitation protocols will be apparent, but these may be interpreted as a sign of academic health in a developing field such as cardiac rehabilitation. We trust that this book will prove useful to many health professionals involved in this developing subspeciality.

DEE JONES
ROBERT WEST

1 Medical background to cardiac rehabilitation

DESMOND G JULIAN

The causes and prevalence of heart disease

Heart diseases predominate as causes of death and disability in the Western World and are of increasing importance in the developing countries. In the United Kingdom, disorders of the heart and circulation are responsible for about half of all deaths, with coronary disease being the cause in about 60% of these (some 170 000 deaths a year).[1] Rheumatic heart disease, a major problem in this and other advanced countries 50 years ago, has largely disappeared except in immigrants, whereas in the overcrowded cities of the Indian subcontinent and South America it remains a common disabling illness. Although prevention and treatment will greatly reduce the incidence and the impact of nearly all forms of heart disease, there will continue to be large numbers of individuals who will suffer from their effects. There are some 240 000 hospital admissions a year in England for myocardial infarction. For these people, rehabilitation will have an important role.

Coronary heart disease

Nature and causes

Coronary heart disease is the consequence of atherosclerotic changes in the larger coronary arteries. These probably start as fatty streaks in the arterial wall in youth, but then progress with the progressive deposition of lipid and fibrous tissue in the succeeding years. The lesions occur as plaques, which are most commonly located at the bends and bifurcations of the vessels. The plaques vary in their characteristics. Some are largely composed of fatty tissue; if these are covered by a thin cap, as they may be, they are liable to rupture. Rupturing or fissuring is likely to lead to platelet and then fibrin deposition. The clot so formed may completely occlude the affected artery and result in myocardial infarction. In other cases, the lesions are predominantly fibrous. Plaques may gradually encroach upon the lumen of the artery. When the lumen is reduced by 50% or more, the blood supply to the muscle beyond the obstruction is limited, leading to ischaemia when the demand increases on exercise.

The causes of coronary disease have not, as yet, been fully established, but several risk factors have been identified. It seems probable that the prevention or modification of these factors will reduce the risk or mitigate the effects of the disease.

Risk factors and the primary prevention of coronary heart disease

Cigarette smoking

The risk of coronary disease in smokers is two or three times that in non-smokers, and is related to the number of cigarettes smoked.[2] The smoking of pipes and cigars may not be so harmful, at least in those who have never smoked cigarettes, but it does not seem to reduce the risk in those who convert to one of these forms of smoking from cigarettes. After stopping smoking cigarettes, the risk of coronary disease is progressively reduced but it may take up to 10 or 20 years for it to fall to that of a non-smoker.[3]

Hyperlipidaemia

There is a clearly established relationship between total blood cholesterol levels and the risk of coronary disease.[2,4] Lipid factors other than cholesterol also play a part. The main risk of coronary disease relates to high levels of low density lipoprotein (LDL); by contrast, high density lipoprotein (HDL) appears to be protective. Triglycerides are a weak risk factor when only they are raised, but they are a more potent risk factor when associated with high LDL or low HDL.[5]

In men with a blood cholesterol level below 5·0 mmol/l, coronary disease is relatively uncommon. A moderate increase in risk is seen with levels above this, up to about 6·5 mmol/l, above which there is a steep rise in risk. Women tolerate a high cholesterol level better than men, probably because of the protection afforded by female hormones. Even quite high levels of blood cholesterol are associated with a good prognosis provided there are no other risk factors, such as cigarette smoking and hypertension.

The level of blood cholesterol is determined by both genetic and dietary factors. Thus, those who inherit a particular defective gene may develop familial hyperlipidaemia, a condition with a high risk of coronary disease at an early age. There are a number of other less clearly defined inherited disorders of lipid metabolism.

5

The most important dietary component leading to hypercholesterolaemia is saturated fat, which is converted into cholesterol after absorption. Monounsaturated fats, such as olive oil, and polyunsaturated fats, as in some margarines, lower cholesterol levels, particularly if they are used to replace saturated fats. Fish oils also seem to have a valuable protective effect.

While high blood cholesterol is undoubtedly associated with a greater risk of coronary disease, it is less certain to what extent lowering cholesterol (by diet or drugs) is beneficial in those without manifest coronary heart disease. Lipid lowering drugs should, at present, probably be reserved for those with very high levels that do not respond to diet.

Lack of physical exercise

The evidence is increasing that lack of physical exercise is a contributory factor to coronary disease. Studies on Harvard graduates have shown that lifelong exercise protects against coronary events, independently of smoking, obesity, hypertension, or parental death from heart disease.[6] Although earlier studies had suggested that exercise had to be vigorous in order to be effective, more recent studies have suggested that only moderate exercise is needed to achieve a benefit. It has been found that it is necessary to undertake at least 20–30 minutes of exercise sufficient to cause slight breathlessness three times a week for this purpose.[7]

Can physical exercise trigger a heart attack? Convincing evidence that it can has been provided by two recent studies[8,9] that showed that strenuous physical exercise at least doubled the risk of a heart attack. This increased risk, however, was confined to those who did not exercise regularly. In those who did, strenuous exercise did not appear to precipitate heart attacks.

Hypertension

The higher the blood pressure, systolic or diastolic, the greater the chance of developing coronary disease. The risk doubles with a systolic blood pressure over 160 mm Hg and diastolic over 96 mm Hg.[2] Lowering blood pressure decreases the risk of a myocardial infarction to a modest extent,[10] but care must be taken not to produce hypotension.

Family history

It is common for coronary disease to occur in several members of the same family. To some extent this can be attributed to the genetic inheritance of hyperlipidaemia and hypertension, but shared habits (for example, cigarette smoking) may play a part. When coronary disease occurs in an individual under the age of 50–55, consideration should be given to investigating other members of the family for risk factors.

Mental stress

It is widely believed that stress leads to coronary disease but good scientific evidence that it does so is lacking. However, stress can precipitate and/or aggravate angina in patients with coronary disease and, occasionally, seems to be a triggering factor in a myocardial infarction. Stress management is, therefore, an important component of the care of patients with coronary disease.

Coronary disease has been linked by some to certain personality types, notably the type A described by Rosenman *et al*[11] and Friedman.[12] Type A individuals are highly competitive, hard driving and obsessed by completing things on time. Other observers have failed to confirm these findings, but there may well be certainly personality traits, such as hostility and suppressed anger, that are associated with the disease.

Alcohol and coffee

There is now good evidence that the moderate consumption of alcohol is associated with a lower risk of coronary disease than either teetotalism or heavy drinking.[13] However, the evidence is not such as to encourage non-drinkers to take up drinking.

The evidence against coffee is not strong,[14] but some individuals develop sinus tachycardia or even arrhythmias with strong coffee, so too much strong coffee is to be avoided.

Other dietary factors

So-called antioxidants appear to exert a protective effect. The most common of these are vitamins C and E, which are mainly found in fruit and vegetables.

Sex hormones

Men are much more likely to develop coronary disease at a young age, and it is uncommon in women until after the menopause. Thereafter, coronary disease becomes more common in women, so that by the late 60s there is little difference in incidence. These facts must be largely explained by hormonal factors; it has been found that hormonal replacement therapy reduces the risk of coronary disease in the post-menopausal woman.[15]

Myocardial infarction—the heart attack

Definition

Myocardial infarction is a pathological term used to describe death (necrosis) of a portion of heart muscle. It is, however, now the most common term used by health professionals to describe the clinical condition that results from it. Myocardial infarction is nearly always due to a clot blocking a coronary artery previously narrowed by athero-sclerosis; thus the terms *coronary thrombosis* and *coronary occlusion* are often used synonymously with myocardial infarction. The expression *heart attack* covers both myocardial infarction and sudden coronary death, which can occur in patients with coronary disease in the absence of a fresh myocardial infarction.

Presentation

The typical heart attack starts with a severe pain in the central chest which radiates to one or both arms, especially the left. It may start very abruptly or increase progressively, or be intermittent, coming and going over a number of hours. The pain is described as tight, crushing, or heavy, and is not relieved by glyceryl trinitrate; opiates are usually required for its relief. The pain may be accompanied by weakness, breathlessness, sweating, and nausea. It usually lasts at least half an hour and may persist for many hours. While this is the classical and, perhaps, the most common mode of presentation, there are great variations. In some cases, the dominant feature is syncope, and in others breathlessness; pain may be slight or absent. Myocardial infarction in elderly patients is often atypical, with weakness, collapse, or breathlessness often being more prominent than pain.

In many cases, the patient dies very suddenly from ventricular fibrillation—instantaneously or after a few minutes before any profes-sional help is available.

Some myocardial infarctions are truly "silent", that is asymptomatic, the patient being recognised as having sustained an infarction only by ECG abnormalities found some time later.

Diagnosis

The symptoms are often strongly suggestive of myocardial infarction, but the diagnosis cannot be confirmed with certainty without evidence provided by the electrocardiogram (ECG) and cardiac enzymes. The ECG usually shows abnormalities within minutes of the onset of the attack, but the definitive changes may take hours to develop. In some cases, the changes on the ECG never become diagnostic, although it is rare for the record to remain entirely normal. The diagnosis is also supported by the detection in the blood of enzymes predominantly found in the heart and only released into the circulation in large quantities when heart muscle cells die. The enzyme most commonly measured today is creatine kinase or, more specifically, creatine kinase MB. Usually, these enzymes are found in only small amounts in the blood; in myocardial infarction their blood level starts to rise within a few hours of the onset and reaches a peak in the first day or two before falling back to the normal level.

Because both the ECG and enzymes may not show diagnostic changes within the first few hours, it is not always possible to be sure of the diagnosis at this time. Treatment in myocardial infarction is, however, urgent; thus it must often be started on the basis of suspicion rather than certainty.

Complications

In a substantial proportion of patients, once the pain has subsided, the subsequent course is uncomplicated. However, even in those who are apparently doing well, ventricular fibrillation may supervene, especially in the first six hours.

Cardiac failure is a common complication, producing dyspnoea in perhaps 20% of patients. On radiographs, pulmonary congestion is seen to be a more common complication, however. Shock, with hypotension, cold extremities, and mental dulling or confusion occurs in about 5% of patients and carries a very high mortality. Arrhythmias other than ventricular fibrillation are common but usually not important. However, atrial fibrillation, which occurs as a transient arrhythmia in 10-15% of patients, is associated with the provocation of heart failure and a risk of emboli to the brain and elsewhere. Heart block also is usually transient and is particularly a complication of inferior myocardial infarction. It may require the use of a temporary external pacemaker, but permanent pacing after infarction is seldom needed.

Mortality and prognosis

The mortality in the month following myocardial infarction is in the region of 40–50%, but a high proportion of these deaths occur outside hospital almost immediately after the onset.[16] In-hospital mortality used to be about 25–30%, but the advent of coronary care and the successful treatment of ventricular fibrillation and other complications reduced this to some 15–20%. Today, the overall one month mortality is in the region of 10–18% but is very dependent upon the age of the patient.

An overview of 36 studies undertaken before the advent of thrombolysis (1960-87) reported that the one month mortality figures in hospitalised patients were 31% in the '60s, 21% in the '70s and 18% in the '80s.[17] A recent British survey reported a mortality of 16% at 30 days, 22% at one year and 30% at three years.[18] Mortality is higher in the elderly, those with diabetes, and those who have experienced heart failure during the acute event.

The introduction of thrombolytic drugs and aspirin has reduced the in-hospital mortality of those who receive these drugs by some 40%, but there remain a substantial proportion of patients—perhaps 30–50%—for whom there are contraindications to their use.

Most deaths occur within the first two days after the onset; deaths at this time are due usually to arrhythmias or shock. Those who survive this period progress well if they have not developed heart failure or serious arrhythmias.

Treatment of the acute attack

Usually, the most urgent need is to relieve pain with opiates. In the United Kingdom, this is most commonly with diamorphine (heroin) but in all other countries, where this is banned, morphine is given.

Also urgent is the intravenous administration of a thrombolytic drug such as streptokinase or tissue plasminogen activator (alteplase). Clinical trials have shown that the earlier this is given after the onset of the attack, the more effective it is.[19] Not all patients are suitable for thrombolytic therapy; it is contraindicated in those liable to bleed, for example from recent surgery or an active peptic ulcer.

Aspirin is routinely prescribed for nearly all patients with myocardial infarction, usually in a dosage of 160 mg daily.[19] This is subsequently continued into the convalescent period and beyond.

Heparin may also be administered, usually intravenously in the first place and subcutaneously thereafter for patients thought to be at high risk of thrombotic complications.

β blockers are given routinely by some cardiologists;[20] others reserve their use in the acute stage for patients who have persistent tachycardia, high blood pressure, or continuing pain.

Other drugs may be given for specific purposes. Thus, diuretics and angiotensin converting enzyme (ACE) inhibitors may be needed for cardiac failure, and antiarrhythmic drugs for the management of serious arrhythmias. In a small number of cases, temporary pacing may be needed for heart block; it is most unusual for permanent pacing to be required after a myocardial infarction.

Bed rest versus early ambulation

The heart certainly needs to be rested in the immediate period after a heart attack. In previous years, it was usual to keep patients in bed for several weeks; this practice was based on postmortem findings that it might take six weeks for the necrotic area of the infarction to be transformed into scar tissue. In the '30s and '40s, physicians followed the advice of Sir Thomas Lewis, the most celebrated cardiologist of the day, who recommended a minimum six to eight weeks in bed.[21] In 1959, Paul Wood in the leading British textbook,[22] advised three to six weeks' strict bed rest. However, years before this Levine (in Boston) had recognised the dangers of prolonged immobilisation and encouraged patients to get up into a chair on the second day.[23] Gradually over the succeeding years, the time spent in bed and in hospital has been reduced, as it has been realised that prolonged immobilisation leads to deep vein thrombosis and pulmonary embolism, deconditioning, anxiety, and depression. Yet, even in the '70s, a trial was conducted in Glasgow comparing "early" (15th day) mobilisation with 25th day mobilisation, with hospital discharge on the 22nd and 35th day, respectively.[24]

In the United Kingdom today, it is common for the patient who has no complications to sit out of bed on the second day and leave hospital on the fifth to ninth day. In some other countries, longer average stays, such as two weeks, are common. To some extent this is due to a more cautious approach, but it also relates to the more frequent and fuller investigation of patients prior to hospital discharge. In these countries, assessment of left ventricular function by echocardiography or nuclear imaging, ambulatory ECG monitoring, and coronary angiography are often undertaken at this time, and patients often undergo angioplasty or coronary artery bypass surgery in the weeks after infarction.

While early ambulation is to be encouraged in those without complications, it is important to recognise that more prolonged rest may be needed in those who have suffered from shock, heart failure, or serious arrhythmias in the acute phase. Such patients may have to stay in bed for several days and may not be fit for discharge for two or three weeks.

The coronary (or cardiac) care unit (CCU)

Coronary care units were first created in the early '60s following the development of external cardiopulmonary resuscitation.[25] It was shown that only if patients with myocardial infarction were cared for and monitored by highly trained nursing and medical staff could good results be achieved from the treatment of cardiac arrest due to ventricular fibrillation.[26] The coronary care unit environment also allows the prompt correction of the other complications of myocardial infarction, but it was found that patients who have had an uncomplicated first day or two seldom have serious problems during the rest of their hospital stay. It is, therefore, usual practice to transfer such patients to a general or post-acute ward after 24–48 hours. By contrast, those who have experienced shock or cardiac failure at an early stage quite often have a stormy later period, being liable to further cardiac failure or serious arrhythmias during convalescence. These patients warrant a more prolonged period in the unit and careful follow up.

The psychological impact of myocardial infarction

The severe pain that is usual in myocardial infarction and the fear engendered by the idea of a heart attack inevitably cause anxiety in patients and their relatives. This may be compounded by the drama that an acute medical crisis can cause, the ambulance journey, the arrival in a busy casualty department, and the ultimate admission to the unfamiliar environment of the coronary care unit. This anxiety usually subsides quickly when the pain is relieved and patients are reassured by the individual attention and high standard of care they receive. The "high-tech" atmosphere may alarm some initially and it is essential that staff make clear that this is all part of a routine. The process of psychological rehabilitation must start at this time with adequate but simple and brief explanations of what has happened. Some people respond to the situation by denial—apparently refusing to believe that they could possibly have had a heart attack. This may help them to cope with the immediate crisis but it causes problems later when the true nature of their illness becomes undeniable.

The transition to an ordinary ward may be accompanied by the recurrence of anxiety, as patients move to a new unfamiliar environment with less privacy and a less close relationship with the staff.[27] It is important that patients and their relatives realise that the move is a sign that the risk of further problems is considered to be low and that there is good reason for optimism.

Anxiety may occur again on going home, but often gives way to depression. Mild degrees of depression are common but it may become severe and prolonged in some cases.[28] The depth of depression is not related to the extent of coronary disease, more to preceding psychological problems and medical illnesses.[29]

Post-infarction treatment and secondary prevention

The period between leaving the coronary care unit and discharge from hospital is a crucial one in the rehabilitation of the patient. Although the rehabilitatory programme should start in the unit, there are many aspects that must be left until the acute medical emergency is over. Unfortunately, when patients are discharged to a general medical ward, there is a risk that the importance of some of the issues that need to be tackled at this time will be overlooked. These issues include progressive mobilisation, treatment of any complications, the assessment of prognosis, the initiation of secondary preventive measures, counselling on lifestyle, and discussion of individual social and psychological problems.

Progressive mobilisation

By the time patients are transferred from the coronary care unit, they will normally be walking about in the ward. Over the succeeding days, unless there are complications, they should be walking further distances and walking up and down a few stairs.

Treatment of complications

The complications that are most likely to be troublesome at this time are heart failure, arrhythmias, and recurrent angina. Heart failure is usually treated with a combination of a diuretic and an ACE inhibitor; if the heart failure disappears, it is probably wise to continue with the ACE inhibitor indefinitely[30] (see below). If it continues, the cause of the heart failure must be determined to find out whether there is a remediable cause, such as a ventricular aneurysm. When serious ventricular arrhythmias, such as ventricular fibrillation or sustained ventricular tachycardia, occur during the convalescent phase, they are usually associated with extensive myocardial damage. The risk of recurrence is considerable and the patient may need further investigation by ambulatory monitoring or invasive physiological testing in addition to assessment of myocardial function.

Some patients experience a recurrence of angina or develop the symptom on slight exertion during the late hospital phase. It may be possible to control this readily by conventional antianginal measures but, if it is occurring frequently or getting worse, there is a danger of further infarction. Full investigation should be undertaken with a view to early angioplasty or surgery.

Assessment of prognosis

An essential component of the aftercare of myocardial infarction is an assessment of prognosis so that a suitable programme of prophylactic measures can be designed. One of the best guides to medium and long term outcome is the history of pulmonary congestion during the acute event.[31] A substantial proportion of patients develop widespread bilateral rales or radiological evidence of pulmonary congestion during the first two days in hospital. Such patients have a much worse prognosis than those who do not have these features, even though in many cases the evidence of congestion disappears quite quickly. Other simple observations that indicate a poor prognosis are a history of previous infarction or heart failure, diabetes, and advanced age.[32]

Prognosis is closely related to the extent of myocardial damage. A variety of different methods have been used to measure this, the most popular being the estimation of left ventricular ejection fraction by nuclear imaging or echocardiography. Widely employed in the United States and parts of Europe, these are not routinely practised in many United Kingdom hospitals because of the additional expenditure in time and money, the sometimes unreliable results, and the delay in discharge that may result from undertaking such tests. However, they should undoubtedly be arranged for patients who are continuing to experience heart failure or serious arrhythmias, as they may reveal a ventricular aneurysm that merits surgical therapy.

Debate continues about the value of an exercise test undertaken prior to hospital discharge. Several studies have shown that the inability to undertake an exercise test or failure to complete 8-10 minutes of a low level exercise test (for example 8 minutes of the modified Bruce protocol) is associated with a poor prognosis.[33] On the other hand, completion of the test without incurring angina, severe breathlessness, or ST changes on the ECG provides reassurance to the patient and serves as a guide to those involved in rehabilitation as to the speed with which exercise can be increased. Some cardiologists argue that a much better guide to prognosis is provided by a full symptom-limited exercise test, but often this can not be performed until four to six weeks have elapsed, by which time the most high risk post-infarction period has passed.

Ambulatory ECG monitoring may be undertaken in the pre-discharge period for two distinct reasons: to determine whether there are serious arrhythmias and to find out whether there is evidence of "silent ischaemia"—that is, ST segment depression in the absence of angina. Both major arrhythmias and silent ischaemia are associated with a worse prognosis, but it is not yet established whether the treatment of these complications is effective.

Coronary angiography is clearly indicated in the early post-infarction period if there is troublesome angina, but some cardiologists, especially in the United States, recommend this investigation in every patient who has had an infarction. This leads to a high rate of angioplasty and surgery; whether this policy is justified by the results has yet to be domonstrated.

Secondary prevention

This term is used to describe measures that are designed to prevent reinfarction and death due to coronary disease.

Cigarette smoking. Those who continue to smoke after myocardial infarction have a high risk of reinfarction and death, which can be considerably reduced by giving up the habit. A long term study from Sweden reported that the mortality rate at five years was 14% in former smokers who gave up the habit compared with 29% in those who continued; the rates at seven and a half years were 16% and 49%, respectively.[34] Although it has not proved possible to conduct a randomised controlled trial of the cessation of smoking, it can be regarded as the single most preventable risk factor for coronary events.[35] Every assistance should be given to patients to help them quit the habit.

Exercise. It has proved difficult to establish whether an exercise programme improves prognosis, but overviews of clinical trials have shown a trend towards a reduction in overall mortality.[36] This subject is discussed at length elsewhere in this book.

Reduction of lipid levels. An overview of the studies of the effectiveness of lipid lowering after infarction showed that reducing cholesterol in those with hyperlipidaemia reduced the risk of myocardial infarction, although there was not a significant reduction in mortality.[37] It is, therefore, important to establish the lipid status of those with myocardial infarction. Unfortunately, the infarction has the effect of lowering the cholesterol level for up to 12 weeks. Thus blood should preferably be drawn for cholesterol measurement on the first day of the infarction, before these changes have taken place; if not done then, estimation of lipids should be delayed for three months.

Hyperlipidaemia should first be treated by diet and only if the lipid levels remain high after three months' adherence to a lipid lowering diet should drugs be considered.[37] A recent trial has shown that administration of the lipid lowering drug, Simvastatin, taken for five years, reduces total mortality by 30 per cent in patients with previous myocardial infarction or angina.[38] Other aspects of the diet should also be considered, and all patients should be encouraged to eat at least five items of fruit or vegetables a day.

Hypertension. Blood pressure should be controlled, by controlling weight, diet, salt and alcohol and, if persistent, by antihypertensive drugs. Treatment of hypertension following myocardial infarction has shown reduced mortality.[39]

Overweight. Overweight is closely related to other risk factors, such as hyperlipidaemia, hypertension, and diabetes, and it has been difficult to identify obesity as an independent risk factor. None the less, it is clearly disadvantageous for the heart to carry around an unnecessary burden, and weight loss can play an important part in lowering blood lipid levels and blood pressure, and in the control of diabetes.

Diabetes. Diabetics who have sustained a myocardial infarction have an increased short term and long term risk of recurrent infarction and death. Good control of the diabetes is important in preventing further complications.

Anticoagulants and aspirin. It has been established in a number of clinical trials that both anticoagulants[40](such as warfarin) and aspirin[41] are effective in reducing the risk of recurrent myocardial infarction. Because of the greater risk of bleeding and the problems of anticoagulant control, aspirin is regarded by most physicians as the preferred option and is indicated in all post-infarction patients for whom there are no contraindications. The usual dosage is 160 mg daily, but 75 mg may be sufficient. If there have been major thromboembolic events, such as pulmonary embolism, an anticoagulant should be administered.

β blockers. Randomised controlled clinical trails have established that β blockers reduce mortality and reinfarction rates by 20–25% in the months and years following myocardial infarction.[20] The most convincing results have been seen with timolol, propranolol, and metoprolol, but there is probably little difference between the various preparations available. Some physicians recommend β blockers for all patients for whom they are not contraindicated. Others, basing their reasoning on the finding that β blockade has virtually no effect on the prognosis of those who are at low risk,[42] reserve the use of these drugs to those who have had a complicated course or who have readily induced myocardial ischaemia. It is important to appreciate that β blockers may interfere with the assessment of patients after myocardial infarction, as they affect the pulse rate and blood pressure response to exercise. Furthermore, they may cause tiredness, fatigue, and sexual dysfunction (impotence and loss of libido), which may erroneously be attributed to the disease or to depression rather than to the drugs.

Calcium antagonists and nitrates. Although these drugs have an important place in the treatment of angina, there is no evidence that they reduce mortality after infarction.[43] Some studies have shown, however, that verapamil[44] and diltiazem[45], may reduce the risk of recurrence of infarction, although they may aggravate heart failure in those with poor left ventricular function.[46] They may, therefore, be prescribed to those with small infarctions if β blockers are contra-indicated.

Angiotensin converting enzyme inhibitors. These reduce mortality in patients who have suffered from heart failure during the acute event[30] or who have a reduced ejection fraction.[47] These agents should certainly be used long term in those who are in heart failure in the convalescent period, but they are probably also of value in those whose heart failure has been brought under control.

Hormone replacement therapy. Hormone replacement therapy has been recommended for primary prevention in post-menopausal women with risk factors.[15] While there is little specific guidance for its use in secondary prevention, this may be revised in the future.

The role of rehabilitation

There is an increasing appreciation of the value of a rehabilitation programme in helping patients back to a normal or near normal life after myocardial infarction. As discussed in detail in later chapters, it is essential for a number of different aspects to be addressed because of the many different types of problems that may arise.

As stated above, the psychological effect of sustaining a myocardial infarction is great. The fact that the possibility of death has had to be faced, perhaps for the first time, the potential for prolonged invalidity or loss of employment, concern about the return to sexual activity, and the impact of the illness upon the spouse and other members of the family are all issues that need discussion and counselling by personnel who are trained in this specialty. Lifestyle modification, for example stopping smoking, and the adoption of a healthier diet can be achieved with professional advice and help. Learning how to cope with stress may be of considerable value in preventing angina. Finally, an exercise programme tailored to the individual ensures that physical activity can be returned to as rapidly as is desirable in the context of the severity of the coronary disease.

16

Traditionally, cardiac rehabilitation has concentrated on patients who have made a good physical recovery from the infarction. Such patients are at relatively low risk and may be limited more by anxiety and depression than by physical incapacity. Rehabilitation does, however, have a place in the management of patients with heart failure and angina, provided that these are not severe. The risks of physical rehabilitation are greater in such patients but are acceptable if medical facilities for dealing with any complications are available. Many of these more disabled patients are, at present, being denied the help with psychosocial and lifestyle problems that is available to less seriously affected individuals.

ANGINA PECTORIS

Nature and causes

Angina pectoris is a symptom complex of which the most characteristic feature is a discomfort in the chest, which is provoked by exercise or emotion and relieved by rest. Angina results from ischaemia—a transiently inadequate supply of blood to the heart muscle. The overwhelming majority of cases of angina can be attributed to coronary atherosclerosis but a small proportion are due to such conditions as aortic stenosis and cardiomyopathies. Spasm of the coronary arteries causes a rare form of angina: Prinzmetal's or variant angina. In this condition, angina usually occurs at rest in the early morning and is accompanied by ST elevation in the ECG in contrast to the ST depression usual in other forms of angina.

Presentation and course

Mortality and prognosis

It is difficult to predict with confidence the prognosis in the individual either with regard to symptoms or life expectancy. Symptoms may wax and wane over long periods, apparently spontaneously, and severe symptoms do not necessarily mean a poor prognosis. Life expectancy is largely determined by the extent of the coronary artery lesions and the severity of left ventricular damage sustained as a consequence of myocardial infarction. If the left main artery is involved, few patients survive more than one to two years; the prognosis is generally very good in those with disease of only one coronary artery. The outlook is intermediate in those with two or three vessels involved. The prognosis may be poor in the latter case if the proximal parts of the arteries are affected, especially if this is accompanied by severe ischaemia or impaired left ventricular function.

17

Unstable angina

This term is used to describe angina of sudden onset or pre-existing angina that worsens abruptly for no apparent reason. It is probably due to plaque rupture, upon which platelet deposition is superimposed. There is a high risk of progression to myocardial infarction within the succeeding days or weeks.

General management

It is essential in the management of angina that all aspects of the life of the affected individual are addressed. It is, of course, vital that the diagnosis is first established, as many patients have been wrongly labelled as angina sufferers because the necessary steps have not been undertaken to confirm the diagnosis. It is also obligatory to find out whether it is due to some remediable cause, such as aortic stenosis.

If the cause of the angina appears to be coronary atherosclerosis, it is necessary to consider what risk factors might have been responsible. Smokers should be given every encouragement and assistance to overcome the habit. Those who have been cigarette smokers should be discouraged from changing to cigars or a pipe, as such a change does not appear to reduce the risk.

Blood lipid levels should be measured in all patients and appropriate dietary changes advised. If the blood cholesterol level remains high in spite of dietary modification, consideration needs to be given to the use of lipid lowering drugs. Some authorities have recommended that an attempt should be made to lower the total blood cholesterol level to 5·2 mmol/l or less; many would agree that drugs should be considered if it remains above 5·5 mmol/l.[38] In addition to reducing the fat, and especially saturated fat, content of the diet, patients should be encouraged to eat more fish, vegetables, and fruit. A weight reducing diet should be prescribed for the overweight.

Blood pressure should be controlled, first by attention to the control of obesity and a reduction in the consumption of salt and alcohol if this is excessive. If the blood pressure remains high, antihypertensive drugs should be administered, but care must be taken not to lower the blood pressure excessively.

Because physical activity is the most common precipitating factor in angina, patients (and often their health professional advisors) are very cautious about exercising. While it is inadvisable to encourage exercise to the point of pain, there is increasing evidence that regular exercise short of this level is beneficial and actually increases the threshold at which angina occurs.[48] Patients should, therefore, be encouraged to exercise within their limitations, but to avoid cold or high winds. Exercise should preferably be dynamic; patients should not undertake competitive sports such as squash.

Emotional stress often provokes angina and the patient with angina must be advised as to how to reduce the chance of this happening. The individual should be taught how best to cope with stressful situations at work or in the home, and the patient's family and associates need to be aware of the problem. On the other hand, many people thrive in what others would regard as unacceptable stress, and unnecessary restrictions should not be imposed.

Sexual intercourse commonly induces angina; patients and their partners may become so concerned about this that intercourse is completely avoided. Others, however, learn that angina during intercourse may be avoided if it is gentle; drugs, especially, glyceryl trinitrate taken beforehand may prevent the onset of the symptom.

Medical treatment

Most patients with angina are helped by the use of antianginal drugs. There are three main categories of drugs used in this context: nitrates, β blockers, and calcium antagonists.

Nitrates

Nitrates relieve angina by relaxing the walls of arteries (including the coronary arteries) and veins. In doing this, they reduce the work of the heart and improve its blood supply.

The most commonly used nitrate preparation is glyceryl trinitrate (trinitrin or nitroglycerin) administered sublingually. This relieves angina promptly in most patients, but it is most effective when used prophylactically to prevent an anticipated attack. It can cause a severe throbbing headache, especially when first tried, but this effect diminishes with continued use. It may also cause syncope; until the patient is familiar with its side effects, it is wise to sit down when taking the tablet. Other preparations of nitrates include a spray, a buccal form (which is retained between the gum and upper lip), oral mono- and dinitrates, and skin patches. These are all effective, but there is a risk of the patient becoming tolerant to the drug if an attempt is made to provide 24 hour nitrate cover.

β Blockers

These drugs work by blocking the effect of hormones such as adrenaline on the heart. They limit the increase in heart rate and blood pressure that occurs on exercise and emotion. They must be used with caution in those whose pulse rate or blood pressure is already low. They may aggravate heart failure and can induce bronchospasm in those prone to asthma, although this effect is less with those β blockers known as "selective".

β Blockers have become standard prophylactic therapy in anginal patients but are usually not prescribed for those with heart failure or asthma. They may prevent the symptoms of hypoglycaemia and therefore need to be used cautiously in those with insulin dependent diabetes. There is not a great deal to choose between the many different β blockers available, although it is preferable to use a "selective" one such as atenolol or metoprolol in those with asthma or diabetes. Compliance is likely to be higher if a preparation is used that needs to be taken only once or twice a day.

Side effects are seldom serious but frequent ones include tiredness, fatigue, and cold extremities. Less commonly there may be nausea, nightmares, sexual disorders including impotence, and pins and needles in the fingers.

Calcium antagonists

These drugs relax the arteries, including the coronary arteries. Broadly they fall into two groups: those that increase the heart rate (for example, nifedipine) and those that slow it (verapamil and diltiazem). Both are effective in preventing angina, but the combination of nifedipine and a β blocker is particularly so. Calcium antagonists that slow the heart rate should not, in general, be combined with a β blocker.

Combination therapy

All three types of antianginal drug may be combined, but it is usual to start with one or two. Indeed, in those whose angina is infrequent, only prophylactic glyceryl trinitrate may be prescribed. If more prolonged prophylactic treatment is needed, a β blocker may be added and, if this is insufficient, a calcium antagonist or a long acting nitrate or both may be given.

Aspirin

It is becoming standard practice to advise the use of aspirin in a dosage of 75-160 mg a day, as this reduces the risk of a myocardial infarction.[41]

Management and follow up of unstable angina

As mentioned above, unstable angina is a condition in which there is a rapid escalation of angina and a high risk of progression to myocardial infarction. It should be considered as an emergency and the patient admitted to a coronary care unit. Usually, with rest, and the administration of antianginal drugs, aspirin and, often, heparin the symptoms subside quickly. When they do not, coronary angiography is usually carried out with a view to early angioplasty or surgery.

Patients who respond well to medical treatment should be investigated in the convalescent period to determine the severity of the underlying disease. This often includes an exercise test and, perhaps, angiography.

The role of rehabilitation

Traditionally, patients with angina pectoris have not been included in rehabilitation programmes, unless they have recently had a myocardial infarction or undergone surgery. There is, however, now good evidence that the methods used in cardiac rehabilitation, such as exercise programmes and stress control techniques, may alleviate the symptoms in angina and may even reduce the need for drugs and cardiac interventional procedures.

Patients who have recently suffered from unstable angina pose a special problem with regard to rehabilitation. Because of what may be continuing instability, care must be taken with the exercise programme and advice may be more difficult to give than when an apparently stable situation has been achieved after myocardial infarction. On the other hand, angina patients benefit from the counselling and lifestyle advice given to post-infarction patients; it is unfortunate that these patients are often not offered a rehabilitation programme.

Angioplasty and coronary artery bypass surgery

Angioplasty and coronary bypass surgery are both highly effective methods of treating angina, but they are usually resorted to when medical treatment has failed to control symptoms adequately. However, surgery may be undertaken even in the absence of severe symptoms if the findings on coronary angiography suggest that it may improve prognosis.[49]

Percutaneous Transluminal Coronary Angioplasty[50]

The term angioplasty is used to describe a technique in which a catheter with a balloon at its tip is introduced into the area of narrowing in an artery. The balloon is inflated in the affected area, as a result of which the artery is stretched and the lumen of the artery increased.

A major drawback of angioplasty is that in up to 30% of cases re-stenosis recurs within the succeeding six months; this does not necessarily result in a recurrence of symptoms, but in a substantial proportion of patients a further procedure—either a second angioplasty or surgery—is required within months.[51]

Effect on symptoms and prognosis. Angioplasty is successful in relieving angina in most patients, either abolishing it completely or reducing it greatly. It is probably somewhat less effective in this regard than bypass surgery, but it avoids the considerable discomfort and prolonged convalescence of bypass surgery. Most patients with angioplasty can be discharged from hospital within a day or two and can start walking straight away, unless there have been complications.

Although angioplasty is, as far as the patient is concerned, a relatively simple procedure, the rate and speed of return to work has been found to be disappointing. This may be because of the attitude of employers but is also due to the patients' perception of their fitness.

The role of rehabilitation. Few cardiologists arrange for their patients to participate in a formal rehabilitation programme, but it is likely that many patients would benefit from it. This is particularly relevant for those who wish to return to work. There is a danger that angioplasty patients, because of their brief hospital admission, will miss out on the lifestyle advice, counselling, and exercise prescription.

Coronary Artery Bypass Surgery

The procedure and its complications. Coronary artery bypass grafting is now the commonest major surgical procedure of any kind undertaken in most Western countries, some 250 000 being undertaken each year in the United States and 15 000 in the United Kingdom. There is a great variation in the number of operations undertaken per head of the population in different countries, reflecting both the availability of resources and the criteria used by physicians in the selection of cases for surgery. Thus in the United Kingdom, less than 300 operations are performed each year per million people, compared with more than 1000 in the United States. A target of about 500 per million is now regarded as appropriate in the United Kingdom, but it is likely that it will be some years before this figure is reached. This would represent some 200 patients undergoing coronary bypass surgery every year in each health service district.

The purpose of coronary bypass surgery is to provide heart muscle beyond an area of narrowing in a coronary artery with an adequate new blood supply. Since 1967, the most commonly used conduit has been a segment of saphenous vein removed at the beginning of the operation from the subject's leg.

The mortality of coronary artery bypass surgery is very dependent on myocardial function prior to the procedure. In good risk cases, which constitute the majority, the mortality is in the region of 1–3%, but this can rise sharply if there has been severe myocardial damage from previous infarctions. The risks are also enhanced in the presence of concomitant disease in other organ systems (for example, renal or hepatic impairment). Coronary surgery is well tolerated by the elderly, provided the patient is in good general condition. In a small percentage of patients, the postoperative course is impaired by one or more complications, which can include a myocardial infarction, a variety of arrhythmias, sepsis in a wound, bleeding, or pulmonary infection.

The operation itself takes some one to three hours. After this procedure, the patient is returned to the intensive care unit, where ventilation through an endotracheal tube is maintained until the patient is breathing satisfactorily without support. In low risk cases, this may be within very few hours, but in those with poor cardiopulmonary function ventilatory support may need to be continued for many hours or days.

From the patient's standpoint, the main problems in the immediate postoperative period are the discomfort of an endotracheal tube and the pain in the sternal region (made much worse by movement, and especially by coughing or sneezing). If a vein has been removed from the leg, this may be painful or swollen; if there has been an internal mammary artery graft there may be pain and numbness in the region of the sternum. Other complaints include tiredness, breathlessness, loss of concentration and memory, and difficulty with micturition and defecation. Many of these problems can be overcome, for example by the adequate use of analgesia, by the early removal of the endotracheal tube, by supporting the sternum with a pillow or a hand when coughing, and by allowing the patient to use a commode as soon as possible. It is often possible for the patient to sit out of bed on the second day, but if the leg has been used for a graft an elastic stocking should be applied before this is allowed because swelling can otherwise be troublesome.

The neuropsychiatric complications of surgery have not been sufficiently appreciated in the past; these may seriously impede recovery from the procedure. Some 1–3% of patients may have obvious features of cerebral injury, such as a stroke, after surgery, but subtler abnormalities are common and often go unrecognised. These include loss of concentration and memory, and depression. In most cases, these problems will resolve with time but in a few cases they are long lasting or permanent.

In the majority of cases, it is possible for the patient to be discharged from hospital about 1 week after the operation, but when the procedure had been complicated it may be considerably longer.

When patients leave hospital, they have often been walking short distances. They should progressively increase this in the succeeding days and weeks, until they are able to walk several miles, if they are physically capable of doing so. Some will be limited still by angina or discomfort in the operated leg and others by other problems such as arthritis.

In the month following discharge from hospital, life should gradually return towards normal. There is no reason why sexual activity should not be resumed within two or three weeks of discharge, provided it does not provoke discomfort. Often discomfort is due to the sternal wound and there may be some difficulty in finding a comfortable position.

Effect on symptoms and prognosis. Coronary artery bypass surgery is effective in abolishing angina completely in at least 50–60% of cases; in a further 20–30% of patients, residual angina is mild and can be controlled by medical treatment. There is, however, a small proportion of patients for whom the operation is unsuccessful and whose subsequent management can be very difficult.

Randomised controlled clinical trials have shown that the coronary artery bypass surgery can improve prognosis in certain categories of patients.[49] These include those whose disease affects the left main coronary artery and those who have involvement of all three main coronary arteries, particularly if this is accompanied by easily induced myocardial ischaemia.

Although the results of surgery are often remarkably good as regards symptoms and life expectancy, other aspects of the quality of life may be disappointing. Thus, many patients do not return to work even though, on purely medical grounds, they appear fit to do so. This is due to a whole variety of reasons, including the psychological effects of surgery, the reluctance of employers to re-employ those who have often been off work for a considerable time prior to the operation, and the opportunity that the operation may give to take early retirement.

Postoperative medical management

Medical management of the postoperative case includes measures designed to preserve graft function, attention to the risk factors for coronary disease, and the treatment of symptoms which have not been relieved by surgery.

Several trials have shown that graft patency is enhanced by the use of aspirin; it is now customary to prescribe this drug in dosages which vary from 75 to 300 mg daily.[41] There is also good evidence that high lipid levels are associated with the development of atherosclerotic lesions in the grafts. If these cannot be reduced by diet, lipid lowering drugs should be administered.

Other risk factors also need to be addressed, as after a myocardial infarction. These include cessation of smoking, taking adequate exercise, avoidance of overweight, and attention to such disorders as diabetes and hypertension, which are common in patients undergoing coronary surgery. After surgery many patients can discontinue the drugs, such as nitrates, β blockers, and calcium antagonists, that they have previously used, but some still need antianginal medication.

The role of rehabilitation

The return to a normal or near normal life after coronary artery bypass surgery is often impeded by a number of factors that can be mitigated by a rehabilitation programme. Patients are naturally hesitant after such a major operation to increase the amount of exercise they do and need reassurance they are not doing harm to themselves. In particular, because they have discomfort in the sternal and sometimes in the shoulder area, they are uncertain whether the pain is due to angina or whether they will adversely affect wound healing by activity. The supervision of increasing activity by health professionals is a valuable way of providing reassurance on this matter.

As after myocardial infarction, but more often starting at an earlier time, depression can be a major impediment to recovery; it is important to determine to what extent this is associated with other evidence of neuropsychiatric disturbance. Usually these problems can be adequately addressed by the members of a rehabilitation team, but specialised psychiatric help is needed sometimes.

Valvar heart disease

Nature and causes

Disorders of the heart valves are due to several causes, including congenital heart disease, rheumatic heart disease, and degenerative changes. Until 20–30 years ago, valve damage as a consequence of rheumatic heart disease was much the most common cause, the major problems being mitral and aortic stenosis and regurgitation. These affected young and middle aged people and were unusual at a later age. While these valve lesions remain an important cause of disability and death in immigrants from African and Asian countries, they are now rare in those born in Western Europe and when they are seen it is more often at a greater age. In contrast, degenerative aortic stenosis is being seen with increasing frequency as the population ages.

Natural history

Mitral stenosis, almost invariably a complication of rheumatic heart disease, usually starts causing breathlessness in the third or fourth decade of life and may progress rapidly to early death unless treated by valvoplasty or surgery. Some mild cases may not produce symptoms until late in life. Apart from heart failure, risks include atrial fibrillation and emboli, often causing stroke. Mitral regurgitation may accompany mitral stenosis, in which case the outlook is similar. Sometimes, however, it is a condition of unknown cause associated with prolapse of the mitral cusps; in this case, the prognosis is very variable and depends largely on the severity of the regurgitation. Usually, the course is benign, but heart failure may ensue as may arrhythmias and emboli.

Aortic stenosis and regurgitation often complicate mitral valve disease and may contribute to heart failure in youth or middle age. Pure aortic stenosis is nowadays most often due to degenerative changes, sometimes on the basis of a valve that is congenitally bicuspid rather than having the usual three cusps. This is mainly a disease of the elderly and is liable to lead to angina, heart failure, syncope, and sudden death. Unless surgery or valvoplasty are carried out in those with severe stenosis, early death is likely.

Medical management

Medical treatment plays little part in the management of valve disorders, except for the control of arrhythmias (especially atrial fibrillation), the prevention of emboli (by anticoagulants in high risk cases), the treatment of heart failure, and prophylaxis against infective endocarditis.

The role of surgery

Surgery plays an important role in the management of severe valve disorders. Mitral valve disease may require the repair or replacement of the mitral valve. Severe aortic disease almost always necessitates replacement of the valve. In the United Kingdom, there are some 4000–5000 valve operations undertaken each year, with a mortality of about 5%. The risk of the operation depends largely on the status of the myocardium. Valves may be replaced by biological or mechanical prostheses. Biological valves may be taken from humans (homografts) or from animals such as the pig (xenografts). These function satisfactorily initially, but are apt to deteriorate or become calcified after about seven years, particularly in the young. Prosthetic valves made from artificial materials also function well, but they are subject to thrombosis, with a risk of embolism. It is therefore usual for patients receiving these valves to be given permanent anticoagulant therapy, with its attendant risks and inconvenience. Prosthetic valves are also prone to act as a focus for infective endocarditis, and prophylaxis against this is important.

In the immediate postoperative period, patients encounter many of the same problems as those who have undergone coronary bypass surgery. Elderly patients subjected to aortic valve replacement may require no therapy beyond anticoagulation, if this is thought necessary. Patients with rheumatic valve disease often require additional medication for arrhythmias. Furthermore, operations are not always totally successful in abolishing symptoms and drugs may be needed to prevent or control heart failure.

The role of rehabilitation

Rehabilitation in patients with valvar heart disease is largely concerned with the care of those who have undergone heart surgery. (Rehabilitation after rheumatic fever is a special problem beyond the scope of this chapter.) Patients have often been limited in their exercise capacity prior to surgery and may be seriously deconditioned; a suitable exercise programme can be invaluable in helping patients to restore themselves to a more normal life.

Congenital heart disease

Nature and causes

Congenital heart disease is, by definition, present from birth, but it may not be detected until many years later. It affects about eight in every 1000 babies born. Some defects are at present incurable, but most either need correction in infancy or childhood, or are so minor that no action is needed. A small number of cases with conditions such as atrial septal defect and coarctation of the aorta may not be recognised until adolescence or adult life and may require surgery at this time.

The role of rehabilitation

In many children with congenital disease, the lesion is effectively treated early in life and they have no further problems. Some, however, have not had a complete correction and may need careful medical follow up in case further surgery or medical treatment is necessary. Serious difficulties may be encountered even in those who have been successfully treated, in relation to such matters as training, employment, insurance, marriage, and pregnancy. Skilled counselling is of immense value to such individuals.

Arrhythmias and conduction disturbances

Disorders of cardiac rhythm and conduction are common but are very often associated with coronary or rheumatic heart disease, and their management is an integral part of the care of these diseases.

When arrhythmias occur without concomitant heart disease, they can usually be controlled by medical treatment or by techniques such as ablation. Some patients may, however, have continuing problems. This applies particularly to patients with pacemakers or implantable defibrillators. Usually, patients with these devices are under the care of specialised clinics that provide good advice and follow up, but some may require rehabilitation.

Heart failure

Traditionally, patients with heart failure have been considered as unsuitable for rehabilitation programmes but this attitude is changing — partly because it is now appreciated that affected patients have not been receiving the professional counselling and advice on lifestyle modification that are available to the less seriously ill. It also has been shown that an exercise programme tailored to the individual needs can relieve substantially the symptoms of heart failure.[52] It is important to recognise, however, that these patients are at greater risk of complications, and an exercise programme should be undertaken only with adequate medical supervision.

Summary of the role of cardiac rehabilitation

- Early mobilisation is now considered essential after myocardial infarction; the rehabilitation programme should begin as soon as the patient leaves the coronary care unit

- Increasing importance is being given to psychological counselling, lifestyle modification, stress management, and exercise programmes following myocardial infarction

- Traditionally, patients with angina pectoris have not been included in rehabilitation programmes, but exercise and stress control may alleviate symptoms and reduce the need for drugs

- After angioplasty, patients are not usually entered into rehabilitation programmes, but it is likely that many would benefit

- Depression can be a major problem after coronary artery bypass surgery and should be addressed by a rehabilitation and/or specialised psychiatry team

- Prior to surgery for valvar heart disease, patients may become seriously deconditioned and benefit from a suitable postoperative exercise programme

- Although congenital heart defects are usually corrected in childhood, later counselling on training, employment, pregnancy, etc, is of great value

- Heart failure patients have traditionally been considered unsuitable for rehabilitation programmes, but lifestyle modification is important and tailored exercise programmes can be of benefit

---

References

1 *British Heart Foundation.* Coronary heart disease statistics. BHF, London 1994.
2 Shaper AG, Pocock SJ, Walker M, Phillips AM, Whitehead TP, Macfarlane PW. Risk factors for ischaemic heart disease: prospective phase of the British Regional Heart Study. *Br J Epidemiol Community Health* 1985; **39**: 197–209.
3 Cook DG, Shaper AG, Pocock SJ, Kussick SJ. Giving up smoking and the risk of heart attacks. *Lancet* 1986; ii: 1376–80.
4 Kannel WB, Neaton JD, Wentworth D, *et al.* Overall and coronary heart disease mortality rates in relation to major risk factors in 325 348 men screened for the MRFIT. *Am Heart J* 1986; **112**: 825–36.
5 Castelli WP. The triglyceride issue: a view from Framingham. *Am Heart J* 1986; **112**: 432–7.
6 Paffenberger RS, Wing AL, Hyde RT. Physical activity as an index of heart attack risk in college alumni. *Am J Epidemiol* 1978; **108**: 161–7.
7 Harris SS, Caspersen CJ, de Friese GH, Estes EH. Physical activity counseling for healthy adults as a primary preventive intervention in the clinical setting: report for the US preventive services task force. *JAMA* 1989; **261**: 3590–8.
8 Mittleman MA, Maclure M, Tofler GH, Sherwood JB, Goldberg RJ, Muller JE. Triggering of acute myocardial infarction by heavy physical exertion-protection against triggering by regular exertion. *N Engl J Med* 1993; **329**: 1677–83.

9 Willich SN, Lewis M, Löwel H, Arntz H-R, Schubert F, Schröder R. Physical exertion as a trigger of acute myocardial infarction. *N Engl J Med* 1993; **329**: 1684–90.

10 Collins R, Peto R, MacMahon S. Blood pressure, stroke and coronary heart disease. Part 2. Short-term reductions in blood pressure: overview of randomised drug trials in their epidemiological context. *Lancet* 1990; **335**: 827–38.

11 Rosenman RH, Friedman M, Straus R, *et al*. A predictive study of coronary heart disease. The Western Collaborative Group Study. *JAMA* 1964; **189**: 15–21.

12 Friedman M. Type A behaviour: its diagnosis, cardiovascular relation and effect of its modification on the recurrence of coronary artery disease. *Am J Cardiol* 1989; **64**: 12c–19c.

13 Steinberg D, Pearson TA, Kuller LH. Alcohol and atherosclerosis. *Ann Intern Med* 1991; **114**: 967–76.

14 Wilson PW, Garrison RJ, Kannel WB, *et al*. Is coffee consumption a contribution to cardiovascular disease? Insights from the Framingham Study. *Arch Intern Med* 1989; **149**: 1169–72.

15 Jacobs HS, Loeffler FE. Post-menopausal hormone replacement therapy. *BMJ* 1992; **305**: 1403–8.

16 Löwel H, Dobson A, Keil U, *et al*. Coronary heart disease fatality in four countries. *Circulation* 1993; **88**: 2524–31.

17 de Vreede JJM, Gorgels APM, Verstaaten GMP, Vermeer F, Dassen WRM, Wellens HJJ. Did prognosis after acute myocardial infarction change during the past 30 years? A meta-analysis. *J Am Coll Cardiol* 1991; **18**: 698–706.

18 Stevenson R, Ranjadayalan K, Wilkinson P, Roberts R, Timmis AD. Short and long-term prognosis of acute myocardial infarction since the introduction of thrombolysis. BMJ 1993; **307**: 349–53.

19 ISIS-2 (Second International Study of Infarct Survival) Collaborative Group. Randomised trial of intravenous streptokinase, oral aspirin, both, or neither among 17 187 cases of suspected acute myocardial infarction: ISIS-2 *Lancet* 1988; **ii**: 349–60.

20 Yusuf S, Peto R, Lewis J, Collins R, Sleight P. Beta-blockade during and after myocardial infarction: an overview of the randomized trials. *Prog Cardiovasc Dis* 1985; **27**: 335–71.

21 Lewis T. *Diseases of the Heart*. New York: Macmillan, 1933: 49.

22 Wood P. *Diseases of the Heart and Circulation*. London: Eyre and Spottiswoode, 1959: 746.

23 Levine SA. Some harmful effects of recumbency in the treatment of heart disease. *JAMA* 1940; **126**: 80–3.

24 Groden BM. The management of myocardial infarction. A controlled study of the effects of early mobilization. *Cardiac Rehabil* 1971; **1**: 13–17.

25 Julian DG. Treatment of cardiac arrest in acute myocardial ischaemia and infarction. *Lancet* 1961; **ii**: 840–4.

26 Julian DG. The history of coronary care units. *Br Heart J* 1987; **57**: 497–502.

27 Wallace AG. Catecholamine metabolism in patients with acute myocardial infarction. In: Julian DG, Oliver MF, eds. *Acute Myocardial Infarction*. Edinburgh, Livingstone 1968: 237–42.

28 Leng GC. Depression following myocardial infarction. *Lancet* 1994; **343**: 2–3.

29 Cay EL, Vetter N, Philip AE, Dugard P. Psychological status during recovery from an acute heart attack. *J Psychosom Res* 1972; **16**: 425–35.

30 AIRE (Acute Infarction Ramipril Efficacy) Investigators. Effect of ramipril on mortality and morbidity of survivors of acute myocardial infarction with clinical evidence of heart failure. *Lancet* 1993; **342**: 821–8.

31 The Multicenter Postinfarction Research Group. Risk stratification and survival after myocardial infarction *N Engl J Med* 1983; **309**: 331–6.

32 Norris RM, Caughey OE, Mercer CJ, Scott PJ. Prognosis after myocardial infarction. Six year follow-up. *Br Heart J* 1974; **36**: 786–90.

33 Gunnar RM, Bourdillon PDV, Dixon DW, *et al*. Guidelines for the early management of patients with acute myocardial infarction. *J Am Coll Cardiol* 1990; **16**: 249–92.

34 Åberg A, Bergstrand R, Johansson S, *et al*. Cessation of smoking after myocardial infarction. Effects on mortality after 10 years. *Br Heart J* 1983; **49**: 416–22.

35 Working Group on Cardiac Rehabilitation of the European Society of Cardiology. Long-term comprehensive care of cardiac patients. *Eur Heart J* 1992; **13** (suppl C): 1–45.

36 O'Connor GT, Buring JE, Yusuf S, *et al.* An overview of randomized trials of rehabilitation with exercise after myocardial infarction. *Circulation* 1989; **80**: 234–44.

37 Roussouw JE, Lewis B, Rifkind BM. The value of lowering cholesterol after myocardial infarction. *N Engl Med J* 1990; **323**: 1112–9.

38 Scandinavian Simvastatin survival study group. Randomised trial of cholesterol lowering in 4444 patients with coronary heart disease: the Scandinavian Simvastatin Survival Study (45). *Lancet* 1994; **344**: 1383–9.

39 Browner W, Hulley S. Effect of risk status on treatment criteria: complications of hypertension trials. *Hypertension* 1989; **13** (suppl 1): 51–6.

40 Smith P, Arnesen H, Holme I. The effect of warfarin on mortality and reinfarction after myocardial infarction. *N Engl J Med* 1990; **323**: 147–52.

41 Antiplatelet Trialists' Collaboration. Collaborative overview of randomised trials of antiplatelet therapy. I. Prevention of death, myocardial infarction, and stroke by therapy in various categories of patients. *BMJ* 1994; **308**: 81–106.

42 Furberg CD, Hawkins CM, Lichstein F. Effect of propranolol in postinfarction patients with mechanical and electrical complications. *Circulation* 1983; **69**: 761–5.

43 Yusuf S, Held P, Furberg C. Update of effects of calcium antagonists in myocardial infarction or angina in light of the second Danish Verapamil Infarction Trials (DAVIT-II) and other recent studies. *Am J Cardiol* 1991; **67**: 1295–7.

44 The Danish Study Group on Verapamil in Myocardial Infarction. Effect of verapamil on mortality and major events after myocardial infarction (the Danish Verapamil Infarction Trial II-DAVIT II). *Am J Cardiol* 1990; **66**: 779–85.

45 Gibson RS, Boden WE, Theroux P, *et al.* Diltiazem and reinfarction in patients with non-Q wave infarction. *N Engl J Med* 1986; **315**: 423–9.

46 The Multicenter Diltiazem Postinfarction Trial Research Group. The effect of diltiazem on mortality and reinfarction after myocardial infarction. *N Engl J Med* 1988; **319**: 385–92.

47 Pfeffer MA, Braunwald E, Moyé LA, *et al.* Effect of captopril on mortality and morbidity in patients with left ventricular dysfunction after myocardial infarction. *N Engl J Med* 1992; **327**: 669–77.

48 Todd IC, Ballantyne D. Antianginal efficacy of exercise training: a comparison with β blockade. *Br Heart J* 1990; **64**: 14–19.

49 Julian DG. The practical implications of the coronary artery surgery trials. *Br Heart J* 1985; **54**: 343–50.

50 Ryan TJ, Bauman WB, Kennedy JW, *et al.* Guidelines for percutaneous transluminal coronary angioplasty. *J Am Coll Cardiol* 1993; **23**: 2033–54.

51 RITA Trial Participants. Coronary angioplasty versus coronary artery bypass surgery. *Lancet* 1993; **341**: 573–80.

52 Coats AJS, Adamopoulos S, Meyer TE, *et al.* Effects of physical training in chronic heart failure. *Lancet* 1990; **335**: 63–6.

2 Goals of rehabilitation

ELIZABETH LORNA CAY

Introduction

Long term care of the patient with coronary artery disease, modern comprehensive cardiac rehabilitation, has as its overall aim improvement in function, relief of symptoms, and enhancement of the patient's quality of life. Recently, as knowledge of the value of secondary prevention has grown and it has become possible to investigate progression of the underlying disease and thus reduce rates of re-infarction, graft closure, and cardiac mortality, cardiac rehabilitation programmes have been extended to include secondary preventive measures. However, within this framework, the defined goals of cardiac rehabilitation remain the same; this chapter is confined to these, while secondary prevention is discussed in other chapters.

Historical background

In the early 1960s, cardiovascular disease was the leading cause of death and morbidity in the majority of industrialised countries. After a myocardial infarction, many patients led miserable unproductive lives; they were frightened to return to work and unnecessarily became cardiac invalids.[1] There were obvious discrepancies between the physical results of treatment and functional outcome. Recognising that many patients after a myocardial infarction require active intervention if they are to return to "normal", a few cardiologists pioneered the idea of cardiac rehabilitation for this group of patients. As early as 1964, a World Health Organization (WHO) expert committee published its first important report on cardiac rehabilitation[2] and in 1969 the Regional Office for Europe, in its first report, defined cardiac rehabilitation as "the sum of the activities to ensure them (the patients) the best possible physical, mental and social conditions so that they may, by their own efforts, resume as normal a place as possible in the life of the community".[3] It was not claimed that cardiac rehabilitation was a secondary preventive measure, but, during the '70s, largely because little was known of the psychological sequelae of myocardial infarction and the measuring instruments for these were in their infancy, cardiac rehabilitation became synonymous with physical training. The end points of secondary prevention, reduction in mortality, and rates of re-infarction, with assessment of return to work (factors that were relatively easy to measure), were used as the indicators of successful rehabilitation.

Physical training

Physical training was deemed suitable for selected groups of patients (younger male patients and those with uncomplicated infarction) and the result was an upsurge in knowledge of the effects of training in those who had had an uncomplicated myocardial infarction: increase in functional capacity with a decrease in heart rate and systolic blood pressure at a submaximal workload,[4] on average a 25% increase in submaximal oxygen uptake,[5] and an increase in ischaemic threshold.[6] Controlled trials of exercise training failed to demonstrate reduction in cardiac mortality and rates of re-infarction.[7,8] The effect of cardiac rehabilitation on return to work was unconvincing. While some studies revealed higher rates of return to work among those attending an exercise programme,[9] others did not. It was suggested that such programmes delayed or prevented the patient from going back to his job. As a result, apart from a few specialist centres, there was little general interest in cardiac rehabilitation, and medical opinion was that it had not been shown to be effective.

Comprehensive cardiac rehabilitation

About this time, attention was directed to the failures of treatment. Non-cardiac causes appeared just as important as physical ones for failure to return to work.[10] It was apparent that 20–30% were left clinically anxious or depressed following a myocardial infarction.[11] If this was unresolved, these patients had a poor treatment outcome which was not due to the severity of the underlying disease.[12] They lacked confidence in resuming an active life, were afraid of even minor physical symptoms, felt uncertain of the safety of undertaking any physical exertion, and worried that, as a result, they could not go back to work. Wives were likely to be more frightened than their husbands.[13] An important indicator of successful rehabilitation thus became the absence of maladjustment.

It appeared that, if outcome was to be improved, cardiac rehabilitation had to become comprehensive. Its components could be defined as:

• Physical training

- Education about the disease, its treatment, and prognosis
- Promotion of psychological adjustment
- Help with social problems (return to work, leisure activities, sexual life).

These conclusions, arrived at through research, were echoed by the patients themselves. When 221 individuals were asked four weeks after a first myocardial infarction what was of concern to them at that stage, it was obvious that their expectations of treatment extended far beyond mere survival or relief of anxiety (see box). They wanted a good quality of life.[13]

When rehabilitation became comprehensive, it was applicable to all post-infarction patients, not only a selected few.

Issues raised by patients four weeks after a first myocardial infarction (adapted from Cay[13])

- Uncertainty about the safe level of exercise
- Should the insurance company be informed?
- Overprotectiveness of spouse and family
- Boredom and irritability at home
- The reasons for the heart attack
- Concern over angina and/or breathlessness
- Aches and pains in the chest
- What is the safety of glyceryl trinitrate?
- Conflicting advice from the hospital and general practitioner
- Keen to return to work quickly
- When to return to strenuous work and/or leisure activities
- Negotiations with the social security department
- Unsuitable housing
- Definite guidelines sought on: sexual intercourse, drinking, amount of weight loss, stopping smoking, driving

---

The indications for rehabilitation

As the concept of comprehensive rehabilitation gained acceptance, re-vascularisation of the myocardium by coronary artery bypass graft surgery or later by angioplasty became increasingly common. It was soon apparent that a poor functional outcome of surgery was the result of the same mixture of physical, psychological, social, and economic factors,[14] so during the '80s the indications for cardiac rehabilitation widened to include these patients. Those with stable angina,[15] following surgery for

33

valvular heart disease,[16] or after cardiac transplantation[17] were also shown to improve after rehabilitation. More recently, as evidence accumulated of its benefits in older people,[18] and in those with poor left ventricular function[19] or with a low ischaemic threshold,[20] these patients joined rehabilitation programmes. Their goal is different, usually preservation of independence, but because psychological benefits occur independently of physical ones then even these severely ill patients can be helped. Rehabilitation should be considered in patients known to have coronary heart disease but who are free of symptoms (after angioplasty, with silent ischaemia) and in those at high risk of developing the disease, but in these cases educational counselling and behaviour modification are the most important aspects.

The goals of modern cardiac rehabilitation

It is obvious that the definition of cardiac rehabilitation which was proposed by the WHO expert committee in 1969[3] fails to take into account the significant changes in cardiac rehabilitation that have taken place following recent evidence of the success of secondary preventive measures so that it now seems possible to slow down or even reverse the underlying pathological process of atherosclerosis. Recognising this, a recent WHO report, *Needs and action priorities in cardiac rehabilitation and secondary prevention*, suggested a new definition which more accurately reflects the aims of modern cardiac rehabilitation:[21]

> The rehabilitation of cardiac patients is the sum of activities required to influence favourably the underlying cause of the disease, as well as to ensure the patients the best possible physical, social and mental conditions so that they may, by their own efforts, preserve, or resume when lost, as normal a place as possible in the life of the community. Rehabilitation cannot be regarded as an isolated form of therapy, but must be integrated with the whole treatment, of which it forms only one facet.

Thus rehabilitation becomes part of total patient care. It is an active process and individuals taking part must assume responsibility for their own health, wellbeing, and quality of life. It is convenient (though artificial) to separate its goals into medical, psychological, social, and health service categories (see box).

Quality of life

Taken together, the goals reflect the patient's quality of life. Though, at a clinical level, this has been recognised for a long time, it was only during the '80s that systematic work to examine quality of life in detail and devise

---

The goals of cardiac rehabilitation

Medical goals

- Prevention of sudden death
- Decrease in cardiac morbidity, infarction, and graft closure
- Relief of symptoms: angina, breathlessness
- Increase in work capacity

Psychological goals

- Restoration of self confidence
- Relief of anxiety and depression
- Improved adaptation to stress
- Restoration of enjoyable sexual activity
- Relief of anxiety and depression in partners or carers

Social goals

- Return to work, if appropriate
- Independence in the activities of daily living in the elderly and in those with severely compromised left ventricular function

Health service goals

- Reduction in direct medical costs
- Early discharge and early rehabilitation
- Fewer drugs
- Fewer readmissions

---

ways of measuring it was undertaken. An important first step was the recognition that physician and patient do not necessarily agree on what is a good outcome; the physician is interested in improvement or cure of the disease while the patient wants a feeling of wellbeing and health and the ability to lead a normal active life. Descriptive studies of the results of cardiac rehabilitation certainly demonstrated decrease of various adverse factors but, more importantly, pointed out the positive gains of intervention: these can be summarised:

- *Medical*: increased maximal work capacity of 20%; less angina
- *Psychological*: increased energy and enthusiasm, wellbeing; decreased depression and anxiety; improved self image; improved ability to deal with stress; better relaxation and sleep; improved sexual activity; fewer tranquillisers and hypnotics

- *Social*: increased optimism, enthusiasm, and creativity; less illness or absenteeism; shorter invalidism; reduced expenses and dependence on social benefits.

As a result of these findings, quality of life, as applicable to the patient with coronary heart disease, can be easily understood, yet a precise definition remains elusive. It depends on the individual's ability to perform the tasks of daily living with the least physical and psychological restrictions and the least threat to life or health.[22]

The determinant factors of quality of life have been identified; they include functional capacity, personal functioning (activities of daily living), and symptoms and risks as a result of the disease process[23] (see box). These different variables are not independent but are interrelated and influenced by a variety of social, cultural, and environmental factors[22] (fig. 2.1).

The activities of daily living or the individual's lifestyle depend on the demands imposed on him and will be limited by any decrease in functional

---

Determinants of quality of life

Objective function: functional capacity

- Activities of daily living
- Work (job performance, satisfaction)
- Social (marital, family, leisure)
- Intellectual
- Emotional
- Economic

Subjective function

- Health status
- Life satisfaction
- Wellbeing
- Control

Symptoms

- Recurrent acute events and hospitalisation
- Pain, dyspnoea, and fatigue
- Medication
- Side effects of treatment

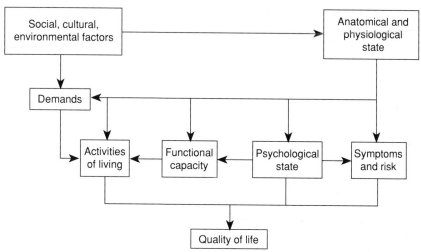

Figure 2.1   Interrelationships of factors determining quality of life (adapted from Imperial[22]).

capacity. Demands on the individual are the result of the way in which the society in which he lives expects him to behave. Functional capacity includes physical, mental, emotional, and social components; it thus depends on the underlying disease process, the patient's reactions to acute events, his perception of disease, and his expectations of the outcome of treatment. The attitudes of family, employers, and fellow workers, which contribute to his environment, have a strong influence on outcome. The presence of symptoms and risk depends on cardiac state but is modified by lifestyle and medication. Quality of life thus is the result of an interaction of a wide variety of variables; a good quality of life means different things to different people.

Outcome of cardiac rehabilitation

There are implications when quality of life is used as the outcome of rehabilitation. Assessment of outcome becomes multifactorial and can no longer be represented by a single entity. Every patient can benefit from some of the components of a rehabilitation programme. For example, psychological benefits of rehabilitation may occur quite independently of physiological improvement. This means that intervention becomes applicable to all patients; even the severely disabled can be helped. The needs of the individual must be taken into account to a far greater extent than before. For example, there has been much stress in the last 20 years on the value of educating patients about their disease, its treatment, and prognosis, but only very recently have patients' perceptions regarding the cause of their myocardial infarction and their knowledge of risk factors been studied.[24] Psychological factors (overwork, stress, and worry) were the most frequently cited perceived causes of their infarction, ahead of smoking, being overweight, and over-eating. This conflicts with medical opinion, which emphasises biological causes. Unless these specific areas of concern are addressed, patients feel that they receive little help with the most life threatening aspects of their disease, and the result is likely to be poor compliance and high psychological morbidity.

Women do less well than men after a myocardial infarction; they consult their doctors more frequently and are more likely to be readmitted to hospital with suspected unconfirmed myocardial infarction.[25] They receive little or no advice on sexual problems[26] and are not referred for rehabilitation programmes.[27] Their outcome after coronary artery bypass graft surgery is poorer; they see themselves as functionally less rehabilitated than men, as being more depressed, and as coping less well,[28] possibly because they receive less social and rehabilitative support.

Medical goals

Though prognosis after myocardial infarction is greatly determined by the extent of myocardial damage, it can be modified by lowering of risk factors even after the manifestation of coronary artery disease. Severity of disease varies from "normalised" hearts after angioplasty for single-vessel disease to severe heart failure. The medical goals of cardiac rehabilitation vary depending on severity; prevention of progression of atherosclerosis is appropriate in those with minor disease, while maintaining a reasonable level of independence is the aim of those who are seriously ill.

By far the most important factor is persistence in smoking. In this respect, stopping smoking is a prime goal of rehabilitation intervention. It is worth noting that women find it harder to stop than men.[29]

Drug treatment is concerned in the management of myocardial ischaemia, cardiac performance and long term prognosis. The indications for treatment include:

- Angina pectoris
- Rhythm disturbances
- Prevention of sudden death
- Prevention and control of chronic heart failure
- Limiting the progression of atherosclerosis.

Medication may also be indicated to control hypertension, hyperlipidaemia, diabetes mellitus, and hyperuricaemia.

Elderly patients with coronary artery disease often have multiple physical problems requiring treatment, so that potential drug interactions are important. Also aging affects the action of many drugs; particular care is necessary in these patients when prescribing treatment.

The benefits of exercise training are no longer in dispute and include:

- Improved maximal functional capacity of 11–56% in post-infarction patients and from 14 to 66% in post-surgical patients[30]
- Improved cardiovascular efficiency for submaximal efforts: a reduction in heart rate and blood pressure at a given level of physical exercise occurs so that patients can do more and are less tired by their ordinary physical activities[31]
- Reduction in risk factors: exercise training increases high density lipoprotein cholesterol levels, helps to lose weight, reduces elevated blood pressure, and improves glucose tolerance.[32,33]

Psychological goals

It has been established that 20–30% of patients are clinically anxious or depressed for many years following a myocardial infarction.[13,34] There is a similar picture after an elective myocardial revascularisation procedure.[35]

Subsequently, there is considerable psychological adjustment;[36] indeed 20% of patients report a spontaneous improvement in their quality of life following an infarction.[37] Nevertheless, poor psychological adjustment leads to undue illness behaviour and the unnecessary use of health resources.[25] For some patients, life revolves round their illness. In the weeks and months following a myocardial infarction, the patient's partner may be more upset than the patient and this may have an effect on his reaction to the acute event.[13] Poor psychological adjustment is not related to severity of illness[11] but is predictive of subsequent mortality.[38]

Cardiac rehabilitation aims to redress this problem. A variety of interventions have been shown to reduce anxiety and promote self confidence in patients after myocardial infarction or coronary artery bypass graft surgery. The benefits of comprehensive rehabilitation programmes are apparent within a few weeks, but good results can be expected in the long term; in one study, five years after the infaction there were fewer smokers and patients with uncontrolled hypertension in rehabilitated post-infarction patients, compared with controls who used more sedatives and long-acting nitroglycerin and had a lower rate of return to work.[39] Almost all clinical trials of exercise training that have measured psychological variables have showed substantial improvement in outlook and morale; of 107 patients in an exercise class, 86% reported a decreased fear of physical exertion, 77% improved physical fitness, and 65% reported the loss of a sense of invalidism.[40] Group programmes help to overcome feelings of social isolation, in as much as its members share a common experience. Peer support and encouragement are fostered.

Adding relaxation training to one post-infarction exercise programme improved the training success by 50% as well as significantly reducing ST segment abnormalities.[41] Two to three years later patients who had had relaxation training in addition to exercise had had significantly fewer cardiac events.[42] Another study of relaxation training in high risk (moderately hypertensive) patients demonstrated useful reduction in blood pressure and fewer acute cardiac events over the subsequent four years.[43] Stress management training programmes extend relaxation training by including additional techniques for dealing with stress. A controlled trial of stress management and relaxation produced significant improvements in both treated groups. Six months later patients who had received stress management training had had fewer cardiac complications than those who had had relaxation alone.[44]

There are problems in long term compliance with behaviour modification, which is after all the prime goal of cardiac rehabilitation and requires the patient to change his attitudes and lifestyle. Education can increase knowledge about heart disease, encourage short term changes in health behaviours and may help to reduce negative psychosocial consequences after infarction and coronary artery bypass graft surgery. But, in the long term, education alone does not lead to changes in smoking habit,[45] diet,[46] compliance with exercise advice,[47] or reduction in clinical levels of psychological disturbance.[48] Cognitive behavioural treatments appear to be a more promising approach to long term changes in lifestyle. They encourage patients to examine the beliefs, motivations, and environmental factors that maintain their unwanted behaviour and, at the same time, involve them in systematically practising new behaviours. Exercise programmes that have incorporated cognitive behaviour treatment methods have shown worthwhile gains in long term compliance,[49] as have weight reduction[50] and smoking cessation programmes.[51] A controlled trial of a cognitive behaviour modification programme in a symptom-free, high risk population produced an overall reduction of 41% in coronary events over the next year.[52]

Return to work

About three out of every four previously employed people return to work after a myocardial infarction yet, without rehabilitation, less than half work as effectively as before their illness.[12] Though approximately 90% of patients obtain symptomatic relief from angina after coronary artery bypass graft surgery, the numbers returning to work have often been disappointing.[53] It was hoped that percutaneous transluminal coronary angioplasty might allow previously disabled individuals to go back to work but, in general, this has not occurred. Following heart transplantation at seven centres in the United States, of 250 patients, 45% were employed, 36% were unemployed, 13% were medically disabled, and 6% had retired. Of those employed, 87% had returned to their previous employment and only 13% had secured new jobs. Of the unemployed, 16% had made job applications but no fewer than 63% had no current plan to seek employment.[54]

Return to work is considered to be an important goal of rehabilitation, though if this is accepted as the only measurement of success it is all too easy to overlook the possibility that patients may be working in jobs that are too demanding both physically and emotionally. Ideally, the individual and the job should match.

Although there is considerable variation throughout Europe, individuals with coronary heart disease may be precluded from returning to certain occupations; in the United Kingdom, all but a few cannot hold heavy goods or public service vehicle licences, and train drivers and airline pilots automatically lose their jobs. They cannot work as deep-sea divers or as scaffolders. With these exceptions there are no clear guidelines on employment, so that the patient and medical adviser may both be uncertain what level of exercise is safe and whether the patient can carry out the physical requirements of a job.

Studies on patients after myocardial infarction, coronary artery bypass graft surgery, angioplasty and, more recently, heart transplantation have revealed that the number returning to work, their rate of return and their efficiency when they do go back depends on a variety of interrelated medical, demographic, psychological and social factors[55-57] (see box).

Non-cardiac causes of invalidism are as important as cardiac ones and are the same after the unpredictable acute event, elective revascularisation of the myocardium or heart transplantation.[55-57] An adverse psychological reaction to infarction or surgery is associated with poorer levels of compliance with treatment but, in the end, the patient's subjective evaluation of his health is a greater determinant of his rehabilitation outcome and eventual return to work than his clinically assessed physical capacity.[58] Equally important are the expectations of the patient. In one study, a positive attitude to the future was important in early return to work after infarction, while over two thirds of patients who initially expected future work problems in fact reported a year later that they had encountered no difficulties.[59] Negative expectations of return to work were closely related to the patient's initial reaction to the illness, particularly if the patient was depressed and expressed hopelessness about the future. Both factors correlated highly with later work status.[60] Out of a large number of variables, the patient's preoperative expectations of return to work after surgery were found to be the best predictor of postoperative employment status.[61]

A number of studies have looked at the influence of personality traits or coping styles on return to work. Denial, health locus of control, and repression-sensitisation have been examined but, in general, they appear

---

Factors determining return to work (adapted from Cay and Walker[64])

After myocardial infarction

- Age
- Number of previous infarctions and their severity
- Other chronic diseases
- Functional capacity and symptoms related to the demands of the patient's job
- The patient's own perception of his/her health status
- Socioeconomic situation
- Psychological factors
- Attitudes of the treating physicians
- Attitudes of employers and fellow workers

After coronary artery bypass graft surgery

- Age
- Whether relief of symptoms is partial or total
- Whether the patient worked up to the time of operation
- Psychological problems
- Previous history of psychological symptoms
- Social difficulties
- Attitudes of the doctor

After angioplasty

- Age
- Relief of symptoms without complications
- Whether the patient was working before the procedure
- Social factors

After cardiac transplantation

- Length of disability prior to transplantation
- The patient's self perception of ability to work
- Potential loss of insurance/disability income

---

to exert a much weaker influence on outcome than the patient's reactions to and expectations of illness.[62,63]

A variety of vocational factors influence how the individual reacts to a coronary event; some are inherent in the patient, while others depend on the job, either aspects of the work itself or the environment as the individual perceives it.[64] Patients with a type A behaviour pattern react badly to the manifestations of heart disease, seeing the infarction and surgery as interrupting or destroying their career; they are unable to cope if promotion prospects are seriously affected. Perceived occupational stress affects the psychological response. Stress can be associated with a variety of situations, such as heavy workloads, working to deadlines, changes in technology and work groups, poor personal relationships with colleagues or management, or simply boredom. Individuals who regard their jobs as non-stressful are likely to return to work speedily after an infarction or surgery, particularly if they were working up to the time of the coronary event.[14] Individuals who feel that they make a useful contribution to the success of their industry (job satisfaction) are motivated to return, and fears and anxieties about going back to work are much less. This is enhanced where morale in the workforce is high and relationships between management and workers are good.

Shift work may be a factor; much night shift work is carried out in situations where the employee is isolated and there is less opportunity for close supervision and good first aid treatment. This increases anxiety in both patient and employer so that, unless temporary day shift working is feasible, delay in going back to work is common.

Pay structures at work are important. If productivity agreements or bonus schemes are in operation, patients feel that they will not be able to keep pace with their colleagues, who will come to resent them.

A working environment that the individual perceives as being detrimental to health, such as noisy uncomfortable situations or predominantly out of doors, will influence the decision on whether to go back to work. Travelling to and from the job and the complexity of the journey is another factor which influences the decision.

Industries vary in their policies on sickness absence. While some take a responsible attitude and look after the interests of their employees when they are off sick, others may terminate employment within a relatively short period. Fear of losing the job may prompt the employee to return to work prematurely, before being certain of the physical ability to cope with the demands of the job.

In the end, return to work may well be determined by the level of benefits received by the patient; in poorly paid jobs it may not be worthwhile financially for the patient to return to work.

The goal of rehabilitation for the patient who was previously working is return to work, taking all these factors into account. Good aftercare is an exercise in collaboration involving patient and family, general practitioner, cardiologist, cardiac surgeon, occupational physician, employer, and fellow workers. There should be close liaison between these people and respect for their various roles. The patient must not receive conflicting advice, because uncertainty increases anxiety and results in loss of confidence in the physical capacity for work. The benefits of a comprehensive cardiac rehabilitation programme, in ensuring that those capable of going back to work do so and that they remain in employment, have been demonstrated.[39]

Realistically, some patients, particularly if they are nearing retirement, will elect not to return to work after myocardial infarction or surgery; in these individuals this may well be an appropriate goal. Similarly, in those with severely compromised left ventricular function, return to work is not feasible. These patients require practical advice on retirement benefits and pensions.

Rehabilitation in older patients

Heart disease is a major cause of mortality and morbidity among adults over 65 years of age. It has been estimated that in the United States it accounts for about 18% of hospital discharges, 10% of visits to a physician, and 44% of all deaths in this age group.[65,66] In most developed countries the population is aging; the projected growth of the elderly underlines the importance of assuring that the quality of life for older persons is maintained.

In these patients, return to work is not an option; their goals include the achievement of optimal physical capacity to keep their independence, to be able to carry out their normal daily activities, and to enjoy their leisure. Psychological adjustment to coronary artery disease and reduction of risk factors are as important as in younger patients and have been shown to be just as effective.[67]

Difficulties facing older patients in rehabilitation

- Limitation of activity
- Problems in following advice from their physician and in taking medication
- Uncertainty about a safe level of exercise
- Learning new patterns of behaviour
- Fear and anxiety
- Overprotective attitudes of family members

Older people with heart disease face very similar problems to their younger counterparts. Their most troublesome management difficulties have been documented. They recognised the importance of optimism, with emphasis on retained physical capacity and taking pride in what could be done within the limitations of their disease.[68]

In the past, elderly myocardial infarction patients were not referred to rehabilitation programmes or encouraged to join them. The picture has changed as knowledge of their problems has grown and data on the benefits of cardiac rehabilitation, supervised exercise, and secondary prevention in the elderly have accumulated. Also, coronary artery bypass graft surgery is increasingly being carried out in older patients; they, too, benefit from rehabilitation.

Health service goals

It is necessary in these days of economic constraint to demonstrate that cardiac rehabilitation is effective. Before 1970 this was seldom done, but examples of this type of evaluation are beginning to appear.

In Sweden, health care is organised in such a way that *all* patients with myocardial infarction from a particular area are referred to a single hospital. Cost analysis of an unselected group of 149 patients attending the cardiac rehabilitation programme at this hospital was compard with 158 patients receiving standard care at a hospital in the neighbouring district. After five years there was a significant reduction in cardiac events, a higher rate of return to work and fewer readmissions to hospital in rehabilitated patients compared with controls.[69] After 10 years, there was a significant reduction in total mortality in the intervention group and fewer of these patients suffered a non-fatal reinfarction. All direct and indirect costs were calculated for both groups and the result was a saving of about US$10 000 for each patient who left hospital alive and took part in the rehabilitation programme.

In a randomised controlled trial of an eight week cardiac rehabilitation programme following myocardial infarction, control patients visited the hospital over the next 10 months more frequently than rehabilitated patients, with resulting increased health-care costs even after the cost of the rehabilitation programme was taken into account.[70]

Patients with continuing angina use a great many resources: re-admissions to hospital, re-investigations, and re-vascularisation procedures. A controlled trial of a seven week outpatient pain management programme for patients with angina resulted in a decrease in symptoms, increased physical activity and less dependence on medication for those who attended the programme compared with controls (unpublished data). Fifty per cent of patients on the waiting list for elective coronary artery bypass graft surgery who attended the programme have not required an operation and these beneficial results have persisted for a year.

Rehabilitation of the spouse

Adaptation to coronary heart disease is a complex phenomenon involving a process of continual adjustment for patient and family. Although the whole family is affected, the spouse is most seriously involved. The diagnosis of myocardial infarction can produce severe emotional distress in the spouse, including feelings of guilt, fear, anger, anxiety, and depression.[71] Adjustment problems within the marriage may be associated with over protectiveness by the spouse, increased dependency on the part of the patient, sexual difficulties, role reversal, financial strain, and reduced social support. Similar problems occur after coronary artery bypass graft surgery, though dependency, impaired communication, and altered effective responses are much less frequent than after an infarction.[72]

It follows that, if the patient is to attain his rehabilitation goals, the family must be involved in any intervention. Correction of the spouse's erroneous beliefs and unreal expectations is just as important as it is for the patient. Patients in a coronary care unit where families received an information booklet and who had access to a nurse counsellor were less anxious than controls.[73] Those whose wives received instructions before surgery on how to support their husbands in the immediate postoperative phase were better orientated, less confused, had fewer delusions, and slept longer than controls.[74] At a later stage of recovery, male patients taking part in a rehabilitation programme whose wives joined in group discussions adjusted more successfully than did other groups of male patients who either did not participate in the programme or, if they did participate, their wives did not.[75]

The decision to return to work rests primarily with the patient and family. If comprehensive rehabilitation is to be successful, the patient and family must appreciate the physical, psychological, and financial benefits of returning to work.[14] In a series of 413 men, all patients were advised that work rehabilitation was one of the principal purposes of surgery. Rates of return to work were much higher than those of other published series: 95% of those working before operation went back to work and 88% of those who were not working prior to surgery. The authors of the report emphasised that the patients and their families were psychologically prepared before operation to understand that rehabilitation, including vocational rehabilitation, was the immediate goal of surgery and stressed the importance of medical advice and encouragement.[61]

Measurement of outcome

Clinical events

Evaluation of rehabilitation as a secondary preventive measure is relatively straightforward because defined hard end points—for example, death, cardiac events, risk factor reduction, and angiographic evidence of atherosclerosis—are appropriate measurements. Obviously, this type of evaluation is particularly suited to research by controlled trials of rehabilitation interventions.

Quality of life

In contrast, outcome on quality of life cannot be so easily assessed if there is no firm consensus on objectives or goals. Quality of life varies with the individual so that, in theory, goals can be different for each patient. The goals depend on a contract between physician and patient; the patient's goal must be realistic within the limitations of his disease and the physician must be aware of his or her patient's beliefs, attitudes, and expectations. For a good outcome, what is perceived as feasible by the physician must match what the patient wants. Outcome is multifactorial and consists of assessment of the variables in the box on p. 36. All can be measured.

Outcome of cardiac rehabilitation depends on the stage of illness and the clinical state of the patient because the goals of treatment are not the same for patients in hospital immediately after a myocardial infarction, patients who have no symptoms or only minimal angina who are being treated as outpatients, patients for whom coronary artery bypass graft surgery or angioplasty may be an option, and patients with congestive cardiac failure. The variables that determine quality of life change depending on circumstances. Immediately after a myocardial infarction, relief of pain, stabilisation of cardiac state, reassurance about the future, and help with immediate emotional reactions are important. Later on, increasing mobilisation, education about the disease, correction of erroneous beliefs, control of risk factors, medication (and its side effects), modification of social problems, and training in stress management determine quality of life. If surgery is contemplated, the possible risks and potential benefits must be considered. Patients with congestive failure are seriously ill with a poor prognosis; quality of life in these patients and in frail elderly individuals means control of symptoms, independence in self care, comfort, freedom from financial worries, sense of optimism, and as much preservation of social life with family and friends as is compatible with their severe physical limitations.

With the variables relevant to the patient with coronary heart disease determined, there has been much interest in developing a scale to measure quality of life. The aim is to depict this complex concept by a single score or series of subscale scores. Originally, scales that could quantify and reliably describe subjective features of health status in patients with cancer,[76] rheumatoid arthritis,[77] or in community studies[78] were used, but more recently specific scales for patients with coronary heart disease have been developed: there are scales for post-infarction patients,[79,80] for those with angina pectoris,[81] and for those with severe heart failure.[82] At first, scales were lengthy and time-consuming to administer and score, but the newer scales are much shorter and simpler. Nevertheless, at present, their use is restricted to research and evaluation of programmes of intervention, and they are not suitable for use in a busy clinic or district general hospital.

A promising development, however, is the concept of "utility scales"[80] whereby patients, in response to a single question, are asked to rate on a scale of 1 to 10 various aspects of their health status. For example, post-infarction patients in a controlled trial of a self help manual of comprehensive cardiac rehabilitation had no difficulty in rating the degree to which they considered that they had made a full recovery, their confidence in making a full recovery, and their overall quality of life.[83] Replies correlated with objective measurements of various aspects of quality of life.

Assessing whether rehabilitation goals have been achieved

- Is the patient back to the normal activities of daily living?
- Are the demands of these activities within the limits of the patient's functional capacity?
- Is the patient psychologically stable?
- Were measures against risk implemented?
- Has the patient's quality of life improved?

At a clinical level, the physician should be aware of quality of life issues and, at interview with the individual patient, should routinely enquire not only about physical symptoms and their treatment, but the patient's emotional reactions, relationship with spouse, family, and friends, sexual adjustment, and leisure activity. At first, this may seem daunting and far removed from traditional medical expertise and training, but it has been shown that, with appropriate communication and interviewing skills, it is possible to acquire the information in a quite short interview.[84]

Whether the individual's rehabilitation goals have been achieved can be evaluated by consideration of a number of questions (see box).

The concept of quality of life has dramatically changed the goals of cardiac rehabilitation. We have moved from consideration of relief of symptoms, return to work, and absence of emotional upset to a situation where the aim is that rehabilitation of patients with coronary artery disease should result in positive changes in lifestyle.

The overall goal of cardiac rehabilitation

Despite a genuine decrease in mortality from cardiovascular disease in the majority of industrialised countries in the last 10 years, its place as the leading cause of death and morbidity remains unchanged. This is in spite of considerable increase since the '60s in knowledge of the disease and demonstration of the value of primary and secondary preventive measures, new improved methods of investigation and treatment of acute coronary events, and the advent of coronary artery bypass graft surgery, angioplasty, and heart transplantation. Cardiac rehabilitation and secondary preventive measures have not become part of routine total patient care, despite evidence of their effectiveness and the recommendations of numerous reports on cardiac rehabilitation that it should be available to all patients.[21,85-87]

There are understandable reasons for this; advances in the treatment of acute episodes, new investigative techniques, coronary artery bypass graft surgery, and angioplasty have greatly increased the workload of the cardiologist and have required considerable input of often scarce resources, while the rehabilitation physician has instituted expensive elaborate inpatient or outpatient programmes requiring a team of specialist staff. Too little attention has been paid to developing simple methods of rehabilitation suitable for the majority of patients attending district general hospitals or being looked after in the community by their general practitioners.

There are indications that the picture is changing as cardiologists become more aware of the benefits of cardiac rehabilitation and secondary prevention and of the fact that simple rehabilitation interventions have been shown to be effective. To this has been added an increased patient demand for rehabilitation, as patients become more knowledgeable of what they can expect of treatment. They have been encouraged to voice their own beliefs and hopes and have been subjected to intensive media coverage on the benefits of a healthier lifestyle and the avoidance of risk factors.

Every effort must be made to accelerate these changes in order to achieve the overall goal of cardiac rehabilitation: long term care, tailored to the needs of the individual, for every patient with coronary heart disease.

References

1 Goble AJ, Adey GM, Bullen JF. Rehabilitation of the cardiac patient. *Med J Aust* 1963; 2: 975–82.
2 World Health Organization. Rehabilitation of patients with cardiovascular disease: Report of a WHO expert committee. *WHO Tech Rep Ser*, 1964, 270.

3 World Health Organization. *Rehabilitation of patients with cardiovascular disease: Report on a seminar.* Copenhagen: WHO Regional Office for Europe, 1969. (Euro 0381.)

4 DeBusk RF, Houston N, Haskell W, *et al.* Exercise training soon after myocardial infarction. *Am J Cardiol* 1979; **44**: 1223–9.

5 Savin WM, Haskell WL, Houston-Miller N, DeBusk RF. Improvement in aerobic capacity soon after myocardial infarction. *J Card Rehabil* 1981; **1**: 337–42.

6 Jensen D, Atwood JE, Froelicher V, *et al.* Improvement in ventricular function during exercise studied with radionuclide ventriculography after cardiac rehabilitation. *Am J Cardiol* 1980; **46**: 770–7.

7 Wilhemsen L, Sanne H, Elmfeldt D, *et al.* A controlled trial of physical training after myocardial infarction. *Prev Med* 1975; **4**: 491–508.

8 Shaw LW. Effects of a prescribed supervised exercise programme on mortality and cardiovascular morbidity in patients after a myocardial infarction. *Am J Cardiol* 1981; **48**: 39–46.

9 Dennis C, Houston-Miller N, Schwartz RG, *et al.* Early return to work after uncomplicated myocardial infarction. Results of a randomised trial. *JAMA* 1988; **260**: 214–20.

10 Nagle R, Gangota R, Picton-Robinson I. Factors influencing return to work after myocardial infarction. *Lancet* 1971; **ii**: 454–6.

11 Cay EL, Vetter NJ, Philip AE, Dugard P. Psychological status during recovery from an acute heart attack. *J Psychosom Res* 1972; **16**: 425–35.

12 Cay EL, Vetter NJ, Philip AE, Dugard P. Return to work after a heart attack. *J Psychosom Res* 1973; **17**: 231–43.

13 Cay EL. Psychological aspects of cardiac rehabilitation. *Update* 1986; **Mar**: 377–86.

14 Oberman AL, Wayne JB, Kouchoukos NT, Charles ED, Russell ROJR, Rogers WJ. Employment status after coronary artery bypass surgery. *Circulation* 1982; **65** (suppl III): 115–19.

15 Todd IC, Ballantyne D. The anti-anginal efficacy of exercise training: a comparison with beta blockade. *Br Heart J* 1990; **64**: 14–19.

16 König K. Rehabilitation of congenital and acquired heart disease. In: *Rehabilitation of non-coronary heart disease: report of a symposium,* International Society of Cardiology, 1969.

17 Niset G, Coustry-Degré S. Psychosocial and physical rehabilitation after heart transplantation: 1 year follow up. *Cardiology* 1988; **75**: 311–17.

18 Siddiqui MA. Cardiac rehabilitation and elderly patients. *Age Ageing* 1992; **21**: 157–9.

19 Conn EH, Sanders W, Wallace AG. Exercise responses before and after physical conditioning in patients with severely depressed left ventricular function. *Am J Cardiol* 1982; **49**: 296–300.

20 Hammond HK, Kelly TL, Froelicher VF, Pewer W. Use of clinical data in predicting improvement in exercise capacity. *J Am Coll Cardiol* 1985; **6**: 19–26.

21 World Health Organization. *Needs and action priorities in cardiac rehabilitation and secondary prevention in patients with CHD: report on two consultations.* Copenhagen: WHO, 1993. (ICP/CVD/125.)

22 Imperial ES. Approach to cardiac rehabilitation. *Clin Rehabil* 1987; **1**: 203–10.

23 Wenger NK. Quality of life: concept and approach to measurement. *Adv Cardiol* 1986; **33**: 122–30.

24 Murray PJ. Rehabilitation information and health benefits in the post coronary patient: do we meet their information needs? *J Adv Nurs* 1989; **14**: 686–93.

25 Maeland JG, Mavik OE. Use of health services after a myocardial infarction. *Scand J Soc Med* 1989; **17**: 93–102.

26 Papadopoulos C, Beaumont C, Shelley SI, Larrimore P. Myocardial infarction and sexual activity of the female patient. *Arch Intern Med* 1983; **143**: 1528–30.

27 Wenger NK, Alpert JS. Rehabilitation of the coronary patient in 1989. *Arch Intern Med* 1989; **149**: 1504–6.

28 Kos-Munsen BA, Alexander LD, Culbert-Hinthorn PA, *et al. Psychosocial predictors of optimal rehabilitation post coronary artery bypass surgery. Schol Inquiry Nurs Pract Int J* 1988; **2**: 171–93.

29 Higgins C, Schweiger MJ. Smoking termination patterns in a cardiac rehabilitation population. *J Cardiac Rehabil* 1983; **3**: 55–9.

30 Monpere C. *Current principles of cardiac rehabilitation and secondary prevention in patients with coronary heart disease. Needs and action priorities in cardiac rehabilitation and secondary prevention in patients with CHD: report on two consultations (Annex 3).* Copenhagen: WHO, 1993. (ICP/CVD/125.)

31 Laslett L, Paumer L, Amsterdam EA. Exercise training in coronary artery disease. *Cardiol Clin* 1987; **5**: 211–25.

32 Ballantyne FC, Clark RS, Simpson HS, *et al.* The effects of moderate physical exercise on the plasma lipoprotein subfractions of male survivors of myocardial infarction. *Circulation* 1982; **65**: 913–18.

33 Bonanno JA, Lies JE. Effects of physical training on coronary risk factors. *Am J Cardiol* 1974; **33**: 760–4.

34 Lloyd GG. Cawley RH. Psychiatric morbidity after myocardial infarction. *Q J Med* 1982; **51**: 33–42.

35 Mayou R, Bryant B. Quality of life after coronary artery surgery. *Q J Med* 1987; **234**: 239–48.

36 Langeluddecke P, Fulcher G, Baird D, *et al.* A prospective evaluation of the psychosocial effects of coronary artery bypass surgery. *J Psychosom Res* 1989; **33**: 37–45.

37 Laerum E, Johnsen N, Smith P, Larsen S. Myocardial infarction may induce positive changes in lifestyle and in the quality of life. *Scand J Prim Health Care* 1988; **6**: 67–71.

38 Frasure-Smith N. In hospital symptoms of psychological stress as predictors of long term outcome after acute myocardial infarction in men. *Am J Cardiol* 1991; **167**: 121–7.

39 Hedback B, Perk J. Five year results of a comprehensive rehabilitation programme after myocardial infarction. *Eur Heart J* 1987; **8**: 234–42.

40 Sanne H. Selection of patients for cardiac rehabilitation. In:Amsterdam N, edit. *Coronary artery disease, exercise testing and cardiac rehabilitation.* New York: Stratton, 1977.

41 Dixhoorn Van J, Duivenvoorden HJ, Staal HA, Pool J. Physical training and relaxation therapy in cardiac rehabilitation assessed through a composite criterion for training outcome. *Am Heart J* 1989; **118**: 545–52.

42 Dixhoorn Van J, Duivenvoorden HJ, Staal HA, *et al.* Cardiac events after myocardial infarction: possible effect of relaxation therapy. *Eur Heart J* 1987; **8**: 1210–14.

43 Patel C, Marmot MG, Terry DJ, *et al.* Trial of relaxation in reducing coronary risk: four year follow up. *BMJ* 1985; **290**: 1103–6.

44 Langosch W. Behavioural interventions in cardiac rehabilitation. In: *Health care and human behaviour.* London: Academic Press, 1984: 301–24.

45 Sivarajan ES, Newton KM, Almes MJ. Limited effects of out patient teaching and counselling after myocardial infarction: a controlled study. *Heart Lung* 1983; **12**: 65–73.

46 Barbarowicz P, Nelson M, DeBusk RF, Haskell WL. A comparison of in-hospital education approaches to coronary bypass patients. *Heart Lung* 1980; **9**: 127–33.

47 Oldridge NB. Cardiac rehabilitation exercise programme compliance and compliance enhancing strategies. *Sports Med* 1985; **6**: 42–55.

48 Horlick L, Cameron R, Firor W, *et al.* The effects of education and group discussion in the post myocardial infarction patient. *J Psychosom Res* 1984; **28**: 485–92.

49 Oldridge NB, Guyatt G'H, Fischer ME, Rimm AA. Cardiac rehabilitation after myocardial infarction. Combined experience of randomised clinical trials. *JAMA* 1988; **260**: 945–50.

50 Brownell KD, Jeffery RW. Improving long term weight loss: pushing the limits of treatment. *Behav Ther* 1987; **18**: 353–74.

51 Glasgow RE, Lichtenstein E. Long term effects of behavioural smoking cessation interventions. *Behav Ther* 1987; **18**: 297–324,

52 Lovibond SH, Birrell P, Langeluddecke P. Changing coronary heart disease risk-factor status: the effects of three behavioural programs. *J Behav Med* 1986; **9**: 415–37.

53 Gundle MJ, Reeves BR, Tate S, Raft D, McLaurin LP. Psychosocial outcome after coronary artery surgery. *Am J Psychiatry* 1980; **137**: 1591–4.

54 Paris W, Woodbury A, Thompson S, *et al.* Social rehabilitation and return to work after cardiac transplantation: a multi centre survey. *Transplantation* 1992; **2**: 433–8.

55 Stewart MJ, Gregor FM. Early discharge and return to work following myocardial infarction. *Soc Sci Med* 1984; **18**: 1027–36.
56 Russell RO, Abi-Mansour P, Wenger NK. Return to work after coronary artery bypass surgery and percutaneous transluminal angioplasty: issues and potential solutions. *Cardiology* 1986; **73**: 306–22.
57 Meister ND, McAleer MJ, Meister JS, Riley JE, Copeland JG. Returning to work after heart transplantation. *J Heart Transplant* 1986; **5**: 154–61.
58 Maeland JG, Mavik OE. Psychological predictors for return to work after a myocardial infarction. *J Psychosom Res* 1987; **31**: 471–81.
59 Crooq SH, Levine S. *The heart patient recovers.* New York: Human Sciences Press, 1977: 102–6.
60 Garrity TF. Vocational adjustment after the first myocardial infarction: comparative assessment of several variables in the literature. *Soc Sci Med* 1973; **7**: 705–7.
61 Stanton BA, Jenkins CD, Denlinger P, *et al.* Prediction of employment status after cardiac surgery. *JAMA* 1983; **249**: 907–11.
62 Stern MJ, Pascale L, McLoone JB. Psychosocial adaptation following an acute myocardial infarction. *J Chronic Dis* 1976; **29**: 513–26.
63 Shaw RE, Cohen F, Doyle B, Paleshy J. The impact of denial and repressive style on information gain and rehabilitation outcomes in myocardial infarction patients. *Psychosom Med* 1985; **47**: 262–73.
64 Cay EL, Walker DD. Psychological factors and return to work. *Eur Heart J* 1988; **9** (suppl L): 74–81.
65 US Department of Health and Human Services. *Expenditures for the medical care of elderly people living in the community throughout 1980.* Washington: *US Department of Health and Human Services, 1983. (Health Care Financing Administration Data Report No 4.)*
66 US Department of Health and Human Services. *1982 Summary: national hospital discharge survey, Advance data No. 95 (PHS).* Washington: US Government Printing Office, 1983 (Publication No. 84–1205.)
67 Lavie CJ, Milani RV, Littman AB. Benefits of cardiac rehabilitation and exercise training in secondary coronary prevention in the elderly. *J Am Coll Cardiol* 1993; **22**: 678–83.
68 Clark NM, Rakowski W, Wheeler JRC, Ostrander LD, Oden S, Keteyian MA. Development of self-management education for elderly heart patients. *Gerontologist* 1988; **28**: 491–4.
69 Levin L-A, Perk J, Hedback B. Cardiac rehabilitation—a cost analysis. *J Intern Med* 1991; **230**: 427–34.
70 Ades PA, Huang D, Weaver MS. Cardiac rehabilitation participation predicts lower hospitalisation costs. *Am Heart J* 1992; **123**: 917–21.
71 Mayou R, Foster A, Williamson B. The psychological and social effects of myocardial infarction on wives. *Br Med J* 1978; **1**: 699–701.
72 Benson-Stanley MJ, Franz RA. Adjustment problems of spouses of patients undergoing coronary artery bypass graft surgery during early convalescence. *Heart Lung* 1988; **17**: 677–82.
73 Duerr BC, Jones JW. Effect on family preparation on the state anxiety of the CCU patient. *Nurse Res* 1979; **28**: 315–19.
74 Chatham MA. The effect of family involvement in patients manifestations of post cardiotomy psychosis. *Heart Lung* 1978; **7**: 995–1001.
75 Dracup KA. The effect of a role supplementation program for cardiac patients and spouses of the at-risk male [Doctoral Dissertation, University of California, San Francisco]. *Dissertation Abstr Int* 1982; **43**: 3534–5B.
76 Prestman TJ, Baum M. Evaluation of quality of life in patients receiving treatment for advanced breast cancer. *Lancet* 1976; **ii**: 899–902.
77 Chambers LW, MacDonald LA, Tugwell P, *et al.* The McMaster Health Index Questionnaire as a measure of the quality of life for patients with rheumatoid disease. *J Rheumatol* 1982; **9**: 780–4.
78 Ware JE, Davies-Avery A, Donald CA. *Conceptualisation and measurement of health for adults in the health insurance study. Vol V: general health perceptions. R-1987/5–HEW.* Santa Monica: Rand Corp, 1978.

79 Waltz M. Marital context and post infarction quality of life: is it social support or something more? *Soc Sci Med* 1986; **22**: 791–805.

80 Oldridge N, Guyatt G, Jones N, *et al.* Effects on quality of life with comprehensive rehabilitation after acute myocardial infarction. *Am J Cardiol* 1991; **67**: 1084–9.

81 Taylor SH. Drug therapy and quality of life in angina pectoris. *Am Heart J* 1987; **114**: 234–40.

82 Wiklund I, Lindvall K, Swedberg K, Zupkis RV. Self assessment of quality of life in severe heart failure: an instrument for clinical use. *Scand J Psychol* 1987; **28**: 220–25.

83 Lewin B, Robertson IH, Cay EL, Irving JB, Campbell M. Effects of self-help post myocardial infarction rehabilitation on psychological adjustment and use of health services. *Lancet* 1992; **339**: 1036–40.

84 Cohen-Cole SA. Interviewing the cardiac patient, I—a practical guide for assessing quality of life. *Qual Life Cardiovasc Care* 1985; **2**: 7–12.

85 *Guidelines for cardiac rehabilitation programmes by the American Association of Cardiovascular and Pulmonary Rehabilitation and the American College of Cardiology.* Champaign, Ill: Human Kinetics Books 1991.

86 Long term comprehensive care of cardiac patients. Recommendations by the working group in rehabilitation of the European Society of Cardiology. *Eur Heart J* 1992; **13** (suppl C).

87 Horgan J, Bethell H, Carson P, *et al.* British Cardiac Society working party report on cardiac rehabilitation. *Br Heart J* 1992; **67**: 412–18.

3 The role of exercise training in cardiac rehabilitation

TERENCE KAVANAGH

Historical background

The concept of exercise training as a therapy for patients suffering from coronary heart disease is not entirely a twentieth century phenomenon. The eighteenth century English physician, William Heberden, who was the first to describe the classical picture of effort-induced angina pectoris, also recorded the case of a patient "who set himself the task of sawing wood every day and was nearly cured".

Almost a century later, in 1854, the Irish physician William Stokes published his classic work *The Diseases of the Heart and Aorta*, in which he wrote, "the symptoms of debility of the heart are often removable by a regulated course of gymnastics, or by pedestrian exercise." Essentially, his "pedestrian cure" consisted of comfortable walking on level ground, the distance being extended as tolerance improved—always, however, cautioning against excessive fatigue, breathlessness, or chest pain.

After Stokes' death in 1878, and over the ensuing years, his exercise training regimen was largely forgotten, obscured by the teaching of the London surgeon, John Hilton, who advised that strict bed rest was an essential component of medical treatment. Unfortunately Hilton's precept was carried to extremes. Prolonged immobilisation in bed became the mainstay of medical care for close to a century, and seldom was it practised more assiduously than after an acute myocardial infarction. Constantly haunted by the spectre of cardiac rupture, the physician insisted that the heart attack survivor be nursed in bed for eight weeks or more, washed and fed, and not even allowed up to use the bedside commode. Small wonder that by the time of hospital discharge, often three to four months after the acute event, the patient was severely deconditioned, weakened, demoralised, and permanently unemployable.

Early mobilisation

The annual meeting of the American Medical Association, held in Chicago in 1944 included a symposium on "The abuse of rest in the treatment of disease", at which for the first time physicians collectively questioned the wisdom of prolonged immobilisation.[1] Ultimately it would be recognised that enforced bed rest, even in healthy individuals, and for as short a period as 21 days, could cause muscle wasting, increased calcium excretion and bone demineralisation, reduction in blood volume, decrease in heart size, stroke volume and cardiac output, tachycardia, orthostatic hypertension, and an overall decline in the efficiency of the body's oxygen transportation system.[2]

In 1952, Levine and Lown introduced their innovative "armchair treatment", in which they progressed their patients to sitting up in a chair by the bed a few days after admission.[3] Despite dire predictions to the contrary, none of the patients came to any harm. Indeed, their morale was higher, their physical status better, and their recovery more rapid than those treated in the orthodox fashion. Shortly thereafter, Chapman and Fraser catheterised uncomplicated post-myocardial infarction patients during exercise, and demonstrated that their cardiovascular responses were thoroughly normal.[4]

Throughout the '50s and '60s there were increasing reports of the beneficial effects of early ambulation and progressive graded activity.[5,6] Deconditioning was avoided and complications such as pulmonary embolism dramatically reduced, without an increase in post-discharge morbidity or mortality.

Inpatient exercise programmes

From early mobilisation to a formal inpatient exercise regimen was a natural progression. Pioneers in this area were Wenger[7] and Zohman[8]. Low level self care activities were commenced in the coronary care unit followed, after transfer to the general ward, by more strenuous activities of daily living and monitored upper and lower limb strengthening exercises. These inpatient, or phase I, programmes were conceived when the average hospital stay after myocardial infarction was three to four weeks. However, as early as 1975 McNeer and coworkers were recommending that uncomplicated myocardial infarction patients needed to be hospitalised for only seven days.[9] Subsequent investigators confirmed their findings, and this is the current practice. At the same time, this reduction in the length of the phase I programme led to greater emphasis on outpatient training regimens.

Outpatient exercise programmes

Gottheiner of Israel was the first to embark upon a large scale post-coronary outpatient exercise training programme. Under his guidance some 1100 patients completed five years of endurance training, which included activities such as walking, jogging, and cycling.[10] Over a five year period the average annual fatal recurrence rate was 0·88%, compared with 4·8% per year for non-exercised patients. These results attested to the safety of supervised physical training for patients recovering from an uncomplicated myocardial infarction.

Other exercise proponents from Israel were Kellerman *et al*,[11] who reported a 25% increase in physical work capacity and a lower recurrence rate in their trained patients, and Brunner and Manelis,[12] who documented a two- to threefold higher recurrence rate in controls than in exercisers over a one year period.

In North America, Hellerstein of Cleveland was one of the early supporters of exercise in post-coronary rehabilitation. In 1968 he described the results of a three year exercise programme involving 254 patients. Over that period the fatal recurrence rate was 2% per annum, which compared very favourably with the 4·5% figure considered to be usual in the Cleveland area.[13] As with Gottheiner's group, the safety of such an approach was all too evident. In Canada, Rechnitzer and his associates from London, Ontario, first reported in 1967 on the short term benefits of a six month training programme, and in 1972 published a five year follow up that compared data with results from patients treated at other hospitals in the London area.[14] Both fatal and non-fatal recurrence rates were significantly higher in the conservatively treated groups.

At the Toronto Rehabilitation Centre, we investigated the risk factors influencing fatal and non-fatal recurrences in a group of 610 post-myocardial infarction patients who had participated in our outpatient walking/jogging training programme over the period of 1968-75.[15] While many of the risk factors for recurrence were similar to those identified in sedentary heart attack survivors, even after adjusting for these, compliance with the exercise regimen conferred a fivefold benefit in both fatal or non-fatal recurrence over the non-compliers, and thus a reduction in hospital readmissions.

A major problem during those early years was the perception of the post-myocardial infarction patient as a chronic invalid, a legacy of the era of prolonged bed rest. It was partly to offset this situation, and partly to demonstrate the high level of fitness that could be achieved by supervised training, that we entered seven post-coronary patients from the Toronto Programme in the 1973 Boston Marathon.[16] Their completion of the run without mishap was a medical first. It focused considerable attention on cardiac rehabilitation, and did much to convince patients and public alike that most heart attack survivors could lead a full and active life.[17,18]

Tertiary prevention studies

Nowadays the favourable impact of thrombolytic therapy, angioplasty, and coronary bypass surgery on coronary heart disease mortality is so pervasive that it is well nigh impossible to isolate the possible additional benefit that exercise training might have on post-infarction survival. Nevertheless, throughout the '70s and '80s this quest for exercise-related improvement in fatal and non-fatal recurrence assumed paramount importance, and led to a series of randomised control trials in Europe,[19-23] and North America.[24,25] Only one of these showed a significant benefit in favour of exercise, although the majority indicated a strong trend in that direction. The methodological problems encountered included inadequate sample size, difficulty in "teasing out" the effect of other interventions such as smoking cessation and β blocker therapy, poor compliance and high drop-out rate, and an overall incidence of recurrent myocardial infarction lower than had been anticipated and allowed for. In an attempt to overcome these difficulties, the data were subjected to a series of meta-analyses. May et al[26] compared the effect of β blockers, aspirins, antiarrhythmics, lipid-lowering drugs, long term anticoagulants, and exercise rehabilitation (six trials). They calculated that β blockers conferred a reduction in mortality of 20-25%, with exercise 19%, and aspirin 10%. The remaining treatments were apparently ineffectual. More recently, O'Connor and colleagues pooled the results of 22 studies involving some 4500 patients and showed that exercise conferred a significant reduction in total mortality, cardiovascular mortality, and re-infarction mortality of 20, 22, and 25%, respectively. In their overview, O'Connor and colleagues, while admitting to the problems inherent in the meta-analysis approach, stressed that their choice of inclusion criteria, the careful manner in which they reviewed the data (contacting investigators personally if need be), and the large number of patients randomised and end points recorded, all strongly supported the plausibility of their findings.[27]

By the '80s, the demonstrable benefits of exercise rehabilitation training were sufficiently convincing that the various national and international heart associations were urging acceptance. In 1981 the Council on Scientific Affairs of the American Heart Association recommended that "cardiac rehabilitation should be considered one of the treatments for coronary heart disease complementary to drug therapy or surgery."[28] The following year the World Health Organization concurred, recommending "regular dynamic exercise as a rehabilitative measure in view of its effects on symptoms and work capacity, and risk factors."[29]

Today it is accepted that the major component of a cardiac rehabilitation programme must be exercise training.

Influence of space medicine

Rarely does a medical strategy develop in isolation, and this short history would be incomplete without mentioning two other closely related areas of investigation. The '60s saw man's first venture into outer space, and with it the realisation that weightlessness produced a deconditioning effect that had many of the hallmarks of prolonged bed rest. This was a potent incentive to investigate all aspects of cardiovascular fitness—and by an agency that could afford more time and money than most medical grant-aiding bodies. The net result was an even greater appreciation of the ill effects of deconditioning and the benefits of physical fitness.

Influence of epidemiology

With the ascendency of coronary heart disease as the leading cause of death in the twentieth century, came a series of epidemiological studies that suggested that a sedentary lifestyle might be a risk factor. Most consistently reported a two- to threefold greater incidence of CHD in sedentary as compared with physically active subjects. In 1987 Powell *et al*[30] from the Centers for Disease Control, Atlanta, using a set of criteria developed by the English biostatistician, Sir Bradford Hill, analysed all 43 studies purporting to show the beneficial effects of physical activity. They concluded that "the observations reported in the literature support the inference that physical activity is inversely and causally related to the incidence of CHD" and that "the relative risk of inactivity appears to be similar in magnitude to that of hypertension, hypercholesterolemia, and smoking."

More recently, researchers have concentrated on the level of fitness rather than the amount of reported physical activity as a risk factor for cardiovascular disease.[31-33] Even after adjusting for the other risk factors, age, family history, and allowing for the possibility of subclinical disease at baseline measurement, it is apparent that the higher the initial level of fitness, the lower the subsequent cardiovascular mortality.

Finally, in 1992 the American Heart Association published its position paper on exercise, in which it elevated physical activity to the level of a major risk factor for the development of coronary artery disease.[34] It went on to say "exercise training increases cardiovascular functional capacity ... in apparently healthy persons as well as in most patients with cardiovascular disease," and that "results of pooled studies reveal that persons who modify their behavior after myocardial infarction to include regular exercise have improved rates of survival."

Physiological responses to exercise

It is customary to categorise physical exercise in accordance with the type of demand it places upon the body's energy transport systems. This in turn is related to the intensity and duration of the effort involved. Short term maximum intensity performance of 10 seconds or less, such as a 100 m sprint, requires an immediate source of energy, and this is provided by the active muscles' small and rapidly depleted store of adenosine triphosphate and creatine phosphate. Phosphate replenishment occurs within 60 seconds of exercise cessation. If the activity is slightly less intense, it can be continued for up to three minutes or so by the re-synthesis of adenosine triphosphate from glucose and glycogen stores, a process referred to as glycolysis. Glycolysis occurs in the absence of oxygen and results in the accumulation of lactic acid, which ultimately leads to muscle fatigue and hyperventilation. This type of activity is referred to as being anaerobic—that is, without oxygen.

If the physical effort can be continued for five minutes or more, such as in a slow jog, the adenosine triphosphate regeneration takes place in the presence of oxygen, a process in which the accumulation of lactic acid is minimal. A balance is reached between energy requirement and the rate of oxygen expenditure. This type of activity is referred to as aerobic—that is, with oxygen.

Regularly repeated bouts of exercise result in a series of bodily adaptations, or training responses. These are specific to the type of exercise training employed. In the context of this chapter, we are concerned with the aerobic type of training responses.

Adaptations to aerobic training are widespread and involve both functional and structural changes in skeletal muscle in the heart, as well as in the peripheral and central circulation. The extent to which these changes occur depend upon the intensity and duration of the training regimen and the initial fitness of the subject. Nevertheless, they are observed to varying degress in the young as well as the elderly, the healthy and the disabled, and even in cardiac patients.

In the presence of ischaemic heart disease, factors that influence training outcome include age, severity of disease, passage of time from the acute event to when training commences, and the intensity, duration, and rate of progression of the training programme itself.

Improved efficiency in the oxygen transport system

Since the circulatory system's prime function is to transport oxygen from the lungs to the active tissues, the best overall measure of cardiorespiratory performance is maximum oxygen intake ($\dot{V}O_2max$). In the healthy individual, aerobic type training results in an increase in

$\dot{V}O_2$max. The average gain over a 12-16 week training period varies from 10 to 25%.

The experience of the Toronto Programme is that peak oxygen intake is reduced by about 30% following acute myocardial infarction.[35] In post-myocardial infarction patients who also suffer from angina, the reduction can be as great as 50%. In both circumstances exercise rehabilitation is associated with gains in $\dot{V}O_2$max ranging from 10 to 60%.[36] While some of this improvement is due to the natural process of recovery, there is no doubt that physical training can not only hasten but also enhance this spontaneous gain. In the Toronto Programme, we have compared the gains made by a group of post-myocardial infarction patients randomly assigned to aerobic training with a non-exercising control group who received instructions in self hypnosis.[37] The controls increased their $\dot{V}O_2$max by an average of 17%; presumably the result of the continuing recovery process together with a low level training effect arising from day to day routine physical activity. The exercisers gained an additional 20% over the same period, with a total gain in $\dot{V}O_2$max of 37%.

Patients, unlike healthy subjects, will frequently continue to exhibit significant cardiorespiratory training responses even after 16 weeks. Improvements in $\dot{V}O_2$max may continue for up to two years, and, indeed, some of our post-coronary marathoners have experienced their most dramatic improvements two to three years after commencing training.[38] Reluctance on the part of the patient to undertake (and the medical advisor to prescribe), vigorous training during the initial months of the programme are the likely causes of the delayed response. Age also has to be taken into account. Analysis of the Toronto data shows that younger patients made a 40% greater gain in peak oxygen intake over a two year period than their older counterparts.[39] Finally, the presence of anginal pain is an additional restriction to aerobic training. However, this can be largely offset by a programme of modified interval training.[40]

The relevance for the post-myocardial infarction patient of a training-induced improvement in $\dot{V}O_2$max is not only that it permits a higher level of all-out physical effort (a rare event in everyday living), but that it enables the individual to carry out submaximal exertion at a lower percentage of $\dot{V}O_2$max. For example, an individual exercising at a rate of 1·5 l/min, and who has a $\dot{V}O_2$max of 3·0 l/min would be utilising 50% of $\dot{V}O_2$max. Increasing the $\dot{V}O_2$max to 4 l/min would now permit completion of the same task at only 37·5% of $\dot{V}O_2$max. The task would be perceived as easier, since less stress would be applied to all components of the oxygen transport chain.

A further refinement of this approach is the use of a measurement referred to as the anaerobic threshold, which is the percentage of $\dot{V}O_2$max at which lactic acid begins to accumulate in the blood. This signals the onset of anaerobic work, the stage at which the oxygen requirements of the exercising muscles cannot be completely supplied by the oxygen delivery system. The anaerobic threshold can be detected by sampling blood lactate levels during exercise, or non-invasively by analysis of expired air for oxygen and carbon dioxide levels (when it is referred to more correctly as the "ventilatory threshold").[41] It normally occurs at about 50–65% of $\dot{V}O_2$max and, in patients who suffer from angina, frequently marks the threshold for the onset of that symptom. Obviously, any increase in $\dot{V}O_2$max will enable a greater level of submaximal effort to be accomplished before the anaerobic threshold is reached. Furthermore, apart from an increase in the anaerobic threshold relative to the percentage of $\dot{V}O_2$max, training also results in an *absolute* increase, with lactate accumulating at a higher oxygen intake level.

Central versus peripheral training adaptations

The relationship of the major components in the oxygen transport system is expressed in the equation:

O_2 consumption = stroke volume × heart rate
× arteriovenous O_2 difference.

Any increase in $\dot{V}O_2$max due to training must therefore be due to an increase in some or all of these three factors. Since maximum heart rate remains unchanged (or may even be slightly reduced), the other two factors, stroke volume and arteriovenous oxygen difference, must be responsible.

Peripheral adaptations

Aerobic training results in significant changes in skeletal muscle structure and metabolism, which enable it to extract more oxygen from the circulating blood. Specifically, at the cellular level there is an increase in stored levels of adenosine triphosphate, creatine phosphate, and glycogen, an augmentation in the number and size of the mitochondria, and an intensification in the activity and/or concentration of aerobic enzymes. Additional factors that aid in this process are (a) shunting of blood from the poorer oxygen extracting tissues, such as the skin and internal organs, to the working muscles, (b) increased capillarisation, and (c) an increase in blood volume and total haemoglobin content. Indeed, there is some suggestion that for older individuals and those suffering from severe ischaemic heart disease, improvement in $\dot{V}O_2$max is mediated entirely by the increase in peripheral oxygen extraction.

Central adaptations

Stroke volume. In healthy individuals, training results in a significant improvement in stroke volume, both at rest and at all levels of exercise. This comes from a change in cardiac dimensions and performance. There is an increase in left ventricular wall thickness and volume (due, in turn, to the sustained greater pre-load from increased blood volume and enhanced venous tone) as well as heightened intrinsic myocardial contractility (due to improved adenosine triphosphatase activity). In cardiac patients, failure of such changes to occur may be due to a reduced training response from an aging and poorly perfused myocardium, or to an inadequate training programme.

Detry et al [42] were unable to find stroke volume augmentation among a group of 12 post-myocardial infarction patients exposed to a 3–12 week training programme. They ascribed the observed improvement in maximal oxygen intake and physical capacity entirely to an increased maximal arteriovenous oxygen difference. However, a randomised study carried out at the Toronto Rehabilitation Centre and involving 79 post-myocardial infarction patients demonstrated increases in stroke volume after one year of exercise training but no increase observed at the end of the first six months,[43] suggesting that a long term training period is necessary in order to obtain cardiac adaptations. Since the matched control group showed a slight decrease in stroke volume over the year of the study, the enhanced stroke volume in the exercisers can not be attributed to the process of natural recovery.

Changes in Cardiac Dimensions. The evidence favouring changes in cardiac dimensions in patients with ischaemic heart disease is inconsistent. Hindman and Wallace,[44] utilising radionuclide ventriculography, demonstrated increases in end–diastolic and end–systolic volumes in 14 patients with ischaemic heart disease following 6 months of a jogging programme. Ehsani et al,[45] employing echocardiography, recorded significant increases in left ventricular end diastolic dimensions and left ventricular posterior wall thickness in eight post-myocardial infarction patients who complied well with a 12 month jogging regime. On the other hand, Ditchey and coworkers,[46] while showing improvement in cardiac function in their patients, were unable to demonstrate either dimensional or structural changes.

Changes in cardiac function. In a number of reports, left ventricular ejection fraction has been used to measure cardiac function. DeBusk and Hung[47] were unable to show any change in either resting or exercise ejection fraction after eight weeks of training. Similar findings were reported by Sklar et al.[48] Jensen et al, however, demonstrated improvement in submaximal ejection fraction in 16 coronary heart disease patients who were trained for 6 months.[49]

In a recent experiment, the present author and colleagues investigated the time course of central and peripheral changes in a group of 32 post-coronary artery bypass patients, who were exposed to six months of a walking/jogging training programme carried out at an intensity of 65–75% of peak oxygen intake.[50] There was a 20% improvement in $\dot{V}O_2$max over the period of training. Exercise testing at three months showed that peripheral blood flow had increased by 25%, with only small changes in ejection fraction. At six months there was an 11% increase in ejection fraction. This substantiates our previous findings that in cardiac patients peripheral training responses occur early, with longer and more vigorous exercise required for central change.[43]

Circulatory changes

A characteristic of endurance training is a reduced heart rate at rest and at all submaximal levels of work. This training bradycardia occurs in cardiac patients as well as in healthy subjects. The cardiovascular centre in the medulla controls heart rate through the autonomic nervous system, and physical conditioning appears to increase vagal tone at rest, and decrease sympathetic drive during exercise. There is some evidence that the stimulus for this arises in the periphery, since arm training does not produce a bradycardia when the subject is subsequently tested with leg work.[51] Conversely, some 50% of the bradycardiac training effect developed from regular leg exercise is clearly seen during arm testing.[52] Training also results in a reduction in effort-induced catecholamine levels, particularly noradrenaline, as well as a downregulation in the sensitivity of cardiac β adrenoreceptors.[53,54] This is the likely cause for the training bradycardia seen in the denervated hearts of trained cardiac transplantation patients.[55]

Resting and submaximal blood pressure is reduced by training, particularly in patients with mild to moderate hypertension.[56] The mechanisms are a drop in total peripheral resistance due to reduced vasomotor tone, redistribution of blood flow to active tissues, and increase in muscle vascularity. The reduction may be as much as 10 mm Hg for both systolic and diastolic levels.[56]

The product of the systolic blood pressure and the heart rate, commonly referred to as the double product, or rate pressure product, has been shown to correlate highly with directly measured myocardial oxygen consumption.[57] Thus the training-induced reduction in double product allows a greater external workload to be achieved at a lower myocardial oxygen cost.[58] For the patient with coronary heart disease, the implications are clear; a greater intensity of effort is possible before the anginal threshold is reached. Furthermore, the training bradycardia results in a marked prolongation of diastole, and since blood flow to the left ventricle wall occurs during the diastolic phase of the cardiac cycle, this tends to improve myocardial coronary perfusion.

Development of collaterals

Richard Lower first demonstrated the presence of coronary collateral vessels in a postmortem human heart in 1669. In 1873 Hyrtl, using a corrosion cast technique to outline the coronary tree, failed to demonstrate collaterals, and deduced that they did not exist. The pendulum swung between these two opposing views for the next 80 years. It was not until the 1960s that Fulton produced incontrovertible evidence that the normal human heart possesses a collateral circulation.[59]

Exercise-induced changes in the size and extent of collaterals have been demonstrated consistently in rats. These changes are maintained by a moderate level of training, but regress with deconditioning. Similar experiments have been carried out in dogs and in pigs.

In humans, we have seen that decreases in angina and the degree of ST segment depression occurring at any given level of effort can be explained by a reduction in double product, and therefore a lowering of myocardial oxygen demand. Conversely, if training is associated with the attainment of a higher double product before signs of ischaemia intervene, one can then speculate that myocardial oxygen supply has increased because of the development of collaterals.

Redwood et al[60] demonstrated that exercise training allowed patients to reach a higher double product before the onset of angina than they could prior to training. Sim and Neill[61] and Nolewajka et al[62] were unable to verify this. Raffo et al,[63] Laslett et al,[64] and Ehsani et al[65] used the degree of ST segment depression as an indicator of myocardial ischaemia; they observed higher double products at equivalent levels of ST segment depression in trained patients.

In individual cases, coronary angiography has revealed increased collateralisation after training. However, the same method used in group trials failed to detect any benefit from exercise. This may be due to the low intensity, short term training regimen used in all the angiography trials. Or, it may be due to the inadequacy of coronary angiography to identify small collaterals, or those lying in the subendocardium.

Verani et al used thallium-201 exercise scintigraphy to measure collateralisation, but could not demonstrate any benefit in a group of 16 patients who trained for 12 weeks.[66] This programme was considerably less intense than that used by Ehsani et al. More recently, Schuler et al showed a significant (54%) reduction in stress-induced myocardial ischaemia in a group of angina patients after one year of intensive exercise training and diet modification.[67] Finally, Todd and co-workers, from Glasgow, using scintigraphy, have been able to demonstrate an average 34% reduction in the exercise-induced area of ischaemia in 40 patients with angina who were exposed to a vigorous exercise programme.[68]

Thus, there is no direct evidence that exercise stimulates collateralisation in humans. Flaws in experimental design include the use of small groups and low intensity, short term exercise training programmes, and the inadequacy of coronary angiography for measuring collateral growth.

Further refinements in radionuclide exercise testing methods may provide the solution to this problem.

Regression of atherosclerotic plaques

Since the cause of the impaired myocardial blood supply in ischaemic heart disease is coronary stenosis due to atherosclerosis, it has long been the goal of various therapeutic strategies to reverse the atherosclerotic process. Indeed, since the 1930s, a number of animal studies have demonstrated consistently that the lesions induced experimentally by a high cholesterol diet could undergo a regression when low fat foodstuffs were susbstituted. In a relatively recent study, non-trained Macaque monkeys, fed an atherosclerotic diet, developed severe coronary atherosclerosis and fatal myocardial infarctions, whereas their treadmill-trained counterparts, who were fed the same diet, were found to have large-calibre coronary arteries free from atherosclerosis.[69]

The introduction of computerised techniques for serial angiogram analysis made it possible to carry out sophisticated trials to assess the effect of pharmacological and dietary interventions on plasma lipid levels and coronary lesions in humans. To date some eight randomised, controlled trials have demonstrated significant slowing of progression and stabilisation of atherosclerotic plaque in the treated groups, with six reporting significant regression.

Ornish et al[70] from California, have published the results of a lifestyle change trial in which patients were assigned either to a "usual care" control group, or to a non-pharmacological low fat vegetarian diet, combined with stress reduction techniques, and an exercise programme. Serial angiography showed an overall mean decrease in stenosis of 2·6% in the test group, and a 3·4% increase in the control group. Lipid lowering drugs were not used.

Schuler et al[71] in Heidelberg entered 18 patients into a rehabilitation programme consisting of a low fat Step II American Heart Association diet and a vigorous exercise programme. At the end of the year, in the intervention group significant regression was noted in seven subjects, with no change in six, and progression of disease in five. In the "usual care" group, regression occurred in only one, with no change in eleven, and progression in six.

The extent to which regular physical activity contributes to plaque regression has recently been examined by Hambrecht et al. In a group of 62 patients with stable angina, followed for 12 months, the greatest amount of disease progression was seen in the most sedentary. Those expending 1500 kcal (6270 kJ) of energy per week remained stable, whereas exercisers who spent an average of 2000 kcal (8360 kJ), or approximately five hours per week, had angiographic evidence of regression.[72]

While the full significance of these relatively small changes in atheroma size, and in particular, their relationship to symptomology and subsequent clinical events, is yet to be determined, it is of more than passing interest that the earlier epidemiological studies of Paffenbarger *et al* identified an energy expenditure of 2000 kcal (8360 kJ) per week with a 30% reduction in coronary mortality.[73]

Psychological effects of exercise training

There is virtual unanimity among health professionals working in the field of cardiac rehabilitation that exercise training is accompanied by an increase in self confidence, an improvement in mood, and an alleviation of depression.[74,75] Patients become more health conscious and are more successful in their attempts to stop smoking and follow a prudent low fat diet.[76] Some have attributed the elevation in mood to an exercise-induced increase in the secretion of β endorphins, the body's natural opiates.[77] The satisfaction obtained from mastering the discipline of the training regimen, or the distraction from daily worries afforded by the regular exercise workout, may be other important contributing factors. A recent meta-analysis of 80 studies into the antidepressant effect of exercise training concluded that it was as effective as psychotherapy, particularly in post-myocardial infarction patients, and that the greatest benefits came from programmes which last for at least six months and include three to four workouts a week.[78]

Risk factor modification

A number of the recognised coronary risk factors are favourably influenced by training. Body fat is lost, without the concomitant loss in lean body mass which inevitably accompanies dietary restriction alone. We have already seen that exercise is a valuable adjunct in the treatment of hypertension, and a recent meta-analysis has confirmed this.[79]

Although the reduction in total cholesterol and low density lipoprotein cholesterol is modest, training induces a significant increase in high density lipoprotein cholesterol, particularly when the exercise also results in weight loss.[80, 81] There is improvement in glucose metabolism, with an increased sensitivity to insulin, an important factor in the management of type II diabetes.[82] The reduction in circulating catecholamines[53,54] which accompanies regular training is plainly an advantage in helping one cope with stressful situations, since these substances are known to evoke the "fight or flight" response, with its attendant increase in heart rate, blood pressure, blood lipid and glucose levels, and enhanced clotting tendency. Excessive blood levels

---

The beneficial effects of aerobic training

- Improved efficiency of oxygen transport system, allowing an increase in maximal work capacity as well as greater tolerance for prolonged submaximal physical tasks

- Structural and functional changes in working muscles, with enhanced ability to store and utilise carbohydrate and fat, as well as extract more oxygen from circulating blood

- Increase in total blood volume and haemoglobin

- The rate pressure product (heart rate × systolic blood pressure) is decreased at the same submaximal levels of effort, thereby reducing the workload on the heart muscle. For the angina sufferer, this means that a higher level of effort is possible before the onset of symptoms

- The stroke volume is increased as a result of (a) augmentation in end-diastolic volume, and (b) enhanced myocardial contractility

- In the presence of coronary artery disease, possible stabilisation of atherosclerotic plaque, and/or improvement in blood supply to heart muscle by collateralisation and/or regression in plaque size

- Restoration of self confidence, improvement in mood, and alleviation of depression

- Reduction in CAD risk factors: decreased body fat, lowered serum triglycerides, increased HDL-cholesterol and decreased total cholesterol/HDL-cholesterol ratio, increased insulin sensitivity and glucose tolerance (important in Type II diabetes), enhanced fibrinolytic activity, decreased resting and exercise plasma catecholamine levels (with increased resistance to stress and increase in threshold for ventricular fibrillation)

---

of catecholamines are also a factor contributing to ventricular arrhythmias, and their reduction at any given work rate helps diminish the possibility of ventricular tachycardia or fibrillation. Finally, a number of studies have demonstrated that regular exercise increases fibrinolytic activity, with a reduction in platelet stickiness and an increase in the production of tissue plasminogen A.[83]

Patient selection

Following myocardial infarction

Historically, cardiac rehabilitation has its origin in the care of acute myocardial infarction survivors, and these still constitute a significant proportion of referrals to an exercise programme. However, the early selection of those suitable for revascularisation procedures has become more sophisticated in the past decade, and this has also resulted in a clearer separation of the various subsets referred for rehabilitation.

Judicious use of clinical observation and exercise testing 6–21 days after the event enables stratification of acute myocardial infarction patients into high, moderate, and low risk categories. Low risk patients are those who can perform more than 6 metabolic equivalents (METs) of exercise (oxygen intake of 21 ml/kg/min) without ischaemia. Those patients who can exercise to 8 or more METs (oxygen intake of 28 ml/kg/min) can perform most physical activities. For the latter subset of low risk patients, rehabilitation may be considered for psychological reasons, patient preferences, or because of inability to self regulate or understand recommended activity levels.

Moderate risk patients include those who develop angina or 1 to 2 mm of ST segment depression at less than 6 METs of exercise, experience non-sustained ventricular arrhythmias, or have a history of congestive heart failure.

Individuals considered to be at higher risk develop angina, ST segment depression greater than 2 mm, and/or inadequate heart rate or blood pressure response at exercise levels of 4·5 METs (15·75 ml/kg/min) or less. Other high risk patients include those with reduced ventricular function (ejection fraction < 30%), complex ventricular arrhythmias, and sudden death survivors. The high risk patients are generally referred for angiography and further intervention. Ideally, all high risk and many moderate risk patients will be identified before referral to rehabilitation programmes, although in practice some will be recognised only at the time of the admission exercise test or even later, during training sessions.

Typically, one half of post-myocardial infarction patients are in the low risk category. They will be referred to a rehabilitation programme on the basis of their needs, as perceived by themselves and their physicians. Some will require assistance to return to heavy labour or to vigorous recreational activity. For others, restoration of self confidence by demonstrating the ability to participate in a training programme will be necessary to attain full recovery. All low risk patients should be assessed for rehabilitation, as even those who consider themselves fit may be exercising at an inappropriately high intensity. This group will not require close monitoring or prolonged supervision, and can often continue on their own after attending classes for a few weeks to several months.

A significant proportion of the moderate to high risk patients will undergo revascularisation; the remainder will probably constitute less than 30% of myocardial infarction survivors, including the inoperable and those declining surgery. For some, exercise training will be absolutely contraindicated. Others will need varying degrees of close observation, including telemetry, ambulatory monitoring, and one to one supervision.

Contraindications to exercise

- Acute pericarditis, myocarditis
- Unstable angina
- Uncontrolled complex ventricular arrhythmias
- Severe aortic stenosis
- Uncontrolled resting hypertension (> 200/100 mm Hg)
- Symptomatic congestive heart failure
- Untreated third degree heart block
- Thrombophlebitis
- Recent pulmonary embolism
- Acute systemic illness or fever

Following coronary artery bypass grafting

A comparison of patients referred to the Toronto Rehabilitation Centre during 1968-75 and 1992, shows that the number of acute myocardial infarctions has reduced by 50%, whereas the number of coronary artery bypass graft (CABG) cases has increased threefold (table 3.1). This is hardly surprising, considering the dramatic worldwide increase of the procedure since it was first introduced in the 1960s. Although initially there was an expectation that the bypass patient had been "cured" of

Table 3.1 The patient referral pattern at the Toronto Rehabilitation Centre Cardiac Department

	1968-75 (n = 610, average age 48·6 years) (%)	1992 (n = 1500, average age 59·0 years) (%)
Male	100·0	83·0
Female	0	17·0
Acute myocardial infarction	85·0	40·5
Coronary artery bypass surgery	10·0	31·0
Chronic stable angina	5·0	11·0
Percutaneous transluminal coronary angioplasty	—	6·8
Other	—	10·7
(Cardiac transplantation valve, peripheral vascular disease, pacemaker, diabetes)		

coronary heart disease, subsequent experience proved this not to be so. In 1984 the Montreal Heart Institute published a 10 year follow up of 82 patients who had undergone saphenous vein bypass surgery.[84] Of all grafts that were patent one year after surgery, 62% were narrowed or occluded at the end of 10 years. Furthermore, of the native coronary vessels that were found to be healthy or minimally stenosed at the time of surgery, 50% showed evidence of advancing disease at long term follow up. These findings demonstrated dramatically the progressive nature of the atherosclerotic process and the need for prolonged risk factor modification following surgery.[85]

Post-CABG patients can be mobilised 24 h after surgery and progressed more rapidly than patients following myocardial infarction during the in-hospital phase. They can commence an endurance training regimen five to six weeks after surgery. The training programme requires little modification, apart from awareness that chest wall pain and, in the case of a venous graft, leg discomfort may slow the patient's progress. Upper limb exercises may be a valuable component in preventing adhesions, muscle weakness, and resultant poor posture, although obviously postsurgical sternal wound infection, or excessive sternal movement are contraindications.

With the increasing interest in cost effectiveness, CABG surgery should be evaluated for its ability to improve quality of life and facilitate return to work. Surgical patients are less likely to return to employment than medically treated post-myocardial infarction patients,[86,87] which may be because the CABG patient has more disease and thus is more disabled. Also, return to work may not be the primary goal, many patients being of the age group who may choose "early retirement" in order to pursue avocational interests. For instance, one study noted that 12 months after bypass surgery, patients participating in exercise rehabilitation reported significant increases in time spent on such activities as golf, bowling, walking, hiking, and bicycling.[88]

Once candidates have been chosen for exercise rehabilitation, the question of how soon to start after the acute event must be addressed. Although mobilisation with low level activities occurs just days after an uncomplicated myocardial infarction or CABG surgery, experience suggests that formal exercise training should not commence until eight weeks after the acute event.[27]

Following coronary angioplasty

Many patients who undergo percutaneous transluminal coronary angioplasty (PTCA) underestimate the chronic nature of their coronary artery disease and perceive the procedure as a "quick fix", not recognising the necessity for rehabilitation. Patients can start training two to four weeks after the procedure. The incidence of postoperative stenosis within the first 12 months has been estimated at between 25 and 30%. Whether a vigorously pursued rehabilitation regimen can favourably affect this outcome remains a subject for further research. However, the close observation, serial exercise testing, and telemetry associated with exercise training affords an excellent opportunity for early detection of restenosis.

Following valve surgery

Patients recovering from cardiac valve surgery, despite an excellent haemodynamic result, may be disabled by years of presurgical restricted activity and deconditioning; they are also candidates for exercise rehabilitation.[89] Patients with mechanical prosthetic valves, however, receive anticoagulant therapy and may not tolerate vigorous weightbearing activities. Also, mechanical prostheses have fixed orifices, which place some limitation, at least theoretically, on cardiac performance during maximal effort.

Following cardiac transplantation

With the introduction in the early '80s of effective immunosuppressant drugs and improved surgical techniques, cardiac transplantation has become a viable clinical procedure, with 5 and 10 year survival rates of 68 and 56%, respectively.[90] The typical heart transplant recipient is a 45 year old male who, as a result of severe ischaemic heart disease or cardiomyopathy, has developed New York Heart Association Class IV cardiac failure. He has experienced varying periods of preoperative invalidism, suffers from generalised muscle weakness, has not worked steadily for some time, and is depressed and fearful. It is hard to imagine a more appropriate candidate for exercise rehabilitation.

Barring complications, cardiac transplant patients are usually discharged from the hospital ward after approximately three weeks. On the second postsurgical day rehabilitation commences and takes the form of the customary physical therapy regimen. By the third to fifth day patients are walking in the room, and may also be using the cycle ergometer, pedalling at zero resistance for three to five minutes. By the time of discharge a low level incremental exercise test may be carried out either on the cycle ergometer or on the treamill, with power output increments of 1 MET. This allows the prescription of a walking or stationary cycling programme, which can be followed during the early outpatient phase of four to eight weeks.

As might be expected, there are relatively few reports in the literature on the effects of training after heart transplantation. To date, the most comprehensive report described the results of a pilot study between the Toronto Rehabilitation Centre and the Cardiac Transplantation Unit of Harefield Hospital, England.[55] Over a two year period, 36 orthotopic transplantation patients were trained for an average duration of 16 months using a walking/jogging programme. Compliance was very good, all patients progressing to an average distance of 24 km each week. Eight of the patients were highly motivated, and achieved 32 km or more a week. It was one of these eight who entered and finished the 42 km Boston Marathon 12 months after joining the programme and 15 months after undergoing the transplantation procedure.[91]

In terms of training effect, the peak work output increased by 49% (65% in the eight highly compliant), and peak oxygen intake by 27% (54% in the highly compliant). The resting heart rate for all patients was slightly reduced, but the greatest reduction occurred in those who were highly compliant. The group as a whole experienced only a few episodes of rejection or infection, and these were of such a minor nature that they had little effect on the training regimen.[55]

Chronic heart failure

It had been believed that patients with severe left ventricular dysfunction (that is, ejection fraction less than 30%) should avoid exercise, but in recent years our view has changed. Despite potential adverse effects, exercising training has been found to benefit patients with impaired ventricular function.[92] There have been reports of symptom relief, increased feeling of wellbeing, improvement in exercise capacity and $\dot{V}O_2$max, but no evidence of improved cardiac function.[93,94]

The first controlled, randomised cross-over trial into the effects of physical training in chronic heart failure (CHF) patients was reported in 1990.[94] Eight weeks of home-based cycle ergometer training resulted in an 18% increase in maximal oxygen intake, an 18% decrease in submaximal rate-pressure product, and an 8% reduction in resting heart rate. Recently the present author evaluated the effects of a one year supervised progressive walking programme on patients with documented clinical heart failure.[96] Over the year, the average weekly walking distance increased from 10·8 km to 23·6 km. Peak work rate improved by 16%, peak oxygen intake 14%, oxygen pulse 10%, and ventilatory threshold 15%. Compliance with the walking regimen was excellent, with no adverse incidents.

Thus, although it might be premature to advocate widespread admission of CHF patients to exercise programmes, there is increasing evidence that physical training will benefit a number of these patients.

Exercise training protocols

A training session should include a warm up and a cool down, with flexibility routines to reduce injuries. Patients should be instructed in pulse taking, recognition and interpretation of symptoms, the effect of various medications, the ability to cope with climatic conditions, and the choice of suitable footwear and clothing. Guidelines for a supervised cardiac rehabilitation programme have been published by the American Heart Association[97] and the American College of Sports Medicine,[98] which recommend that exercise sessions be attended by a physician or nurse with resuscitation equipment.

Prescribing exercise

The prescription of exercise requires that we define the type of activity, or *mode*, the *intensity* of effort to be expended, the *duration* of the training session, and the number of times it should be carried out each week, or *frequency*. Of these four factors, the intensity is the most critical in terms of eliciting a training effect. In the case of the cardiac patient there is the additional need to avoid precipitating adverse signs or symptoms.

Intensity

The most effective training intensity for attaining aerobic fitness is in the range of 50 to 70% of the subject's maximal capacity for effort. The latter is usually expressed in terms of maximum heart rate (HRmax) or maximal oxygen intake ($\dot{V}O_2$max). Both values can be determined most accurately from a maximal exercise test. In the absence of any form of exercise test, HRmax and $\dot{V}O_2$max can be estimated from an age-related equation (see box) or from age-gender population tables, although these values are subject to considerable individual variation and should not be used when prescribing exercise for cardiac patients.

A maximum exercise test is one in which the subject exercises to exhaustion, either on a treadmill or a cycle ergometer. Where the test has to be stopped before that point is reached because of the appearance of adverse signs or symptoms, it is referred to as a symptom-limited maximum test. If expired air is collected and analysed during the test, then objective evidence of peak effort is deduced from the failure of the oxygen intake to increase despite an increment in the work rate, the so-called "oxygen plateau".

Oxygen intake may be expressed in absolute units, litres per minute (l/min) or, to allow for body weight, in millilitres of oxygen per kilogram per minute (ml/kg/min). A popular and convenient concept is the use of metabolic equivalents (METs). One MET is the energy requirement for basal metabolism and is equal to 3·5 ml/kg/min. Thus multiples of resting levels are used to express levels of energy expenditure—for example, $\dot{V}O_2 = 21$ ml/kg/min = 6 METs.

Apart from direct measurement of $\dot{V}O_2$max, respiratory gas analysis has the added advantage of permitting identification of the oxygen intake level above which aerobic energy production is supplemented by anaerobic mechanisms. Termed the anaerobic, or ventilatory threshold (VT), this usually occurs at 50 to 60% of $\dot{V}O_2$max. In cases where maximal effort cannot be achieved on the test, the VT is useful to define a suitable aerobic training intensity level.

In many situations the equipment and expertise required for direct measurement of $\dot{V}O_2$max is not available, and clinicians generally rely on indirect methods. The commonest approach is to predict the $\dot{V}O_2$max from the maximal time of the treadmill, or the peak power output achieved on the cycle ergometer. Thus, for any given exercise test protocol, the energy requirements for a given work rate can be determined from tables, monograms, or formulas which take into account treadmill speed and grade, or power output on the cycle ergometer expressed in kilopond metres per minute (kpm/min^{-1}) (see box)

Once the $\dot{V}O_2$max (symptom-limited or otherwise) has been determined, it is a relatively simple matter to take a fixed percentage of this value and, using energy cost tables, convert it to the desired intensity of exercise or physical activity.[99]

There is a linear relationship between heart rate and oxygen intake during exercise, and since heart rate is the easier of the two to measure, it has become the preferred method for prescribing training intensity. As with $\dot{V}O_2$max, maximal heart rate can be determined from a maximum (or symptom-limited maximum) test or, in the absence of a test, from the age-related formula mentioned above.

There are two methods used to calculate the training heart rate. The first, and the simplest, utilises a percentage of HRmax. However, it should be noted that the heart rate reaches a maximum value before the oxygen intake, so that the 50–70% $\dot{V}O_2$max is equivalent to approximately 65 to 80% of HRmax (see box).[100]

The second method, initially described by Karvonen, introduces the resting heart rate into the equation. In Karvonen's formula the training heart rate is obtained by taking 65 to 80% of the difference between the maximum heart rate and the resting heart rate (referred to as the Heart Rate Reserve) and adding this to the resting heart rate (see box).[102] Resting heart rate is best obtained from the pulse rate taken in the morning before rising. Alternatively, it can be counted after five minutes resting in the sitting position. The Karvonen method gives a higher training heart rate than the percentage of HRmax, but has the advantage of taking into account the bradycardia produced by aerobic training, and has also been shown to relate more closely to the percentage $\dot{V}O_2$max.

Cardiac patients referred for exercise rehabilitation are often taking a β blocker. These drugs block cardiac adrenoceptors, resulting in reduced heart rate and blood pressure at rest and during exercise. Drug induced exercise bradycardia obviously invalidates the use of age-related heart rate tables for establishing maximal or target training rates, although the linear relationship of heart rate to oxygen intake remains unaltered. Therefore, exercise intensity can still be related to the usual percentage of the maximal heart rate achieved while the patient is taking a β blocker. It should also be noted that there is now considerable evidence that cardiac patients receiving β blockers can achieve a significant beneficial training effect.

The concept of perceived exertion is one in which the exercising subject interprets physiological cues from the working muscles and joints, as well

---

Formulas

(1) Estimating maximum heart rate from age
HR = 220 − (age in years).
Example. For a 60 year old HRmax = 220 − 60 = 160
(This estimation has a potential error of plus or minus 15 bts/min.)

(2) Predicting $\dot{V}O_2$max from maximal time achieved on treadmill (Bruce protocol)
$\dot{V}O_2$max (ml/kg/min) = 6·7−2·82 × (weighting factor for gender) + 0·056 × (treadmill time in seconds) where weighting factor for gender is one for men and two for women.[101]
Example. For a man who completes 6 minutes of treadmill (Stage II of Bruce).
$$\dot{V}O_2\text{max (ml/kg/min)} = (3\cdot8 \times 1) + (0\cdot056 \times 360)$$
$$= 23\cdot96 \text{ ml/kg/min}$$
$$= 6\cdot8 \text{ METs}$$

(3) Estimating $\dot{V}O_2$max from maximal power output (kilopond metres per minute) achieved on cycle ergometer test (300–1200 kpm/min)
$$\dot{V}O_2\text{max (ml/min)} = 2 \times \text{max kpm/min}$$
Example. For a subject who achieves 900 kpm/min.
$$\dot{V}O_2\text{max (ml/min)} = 2 \times 900$$
$$= 1800 \text{ ml/min or } 1\cdot8 \text{ l/min}$$
To correct to ml/kg/min^{-1}, for a 90 kg subject:

$$\frac{1800}{90} = 20\text{ml/kg/min} = 5\cdot7\text{METs}$$

(4) Training heart rate range (THR) by simple percentage of maximum heart rate
$$\text{THR} = 0\cdot65 \times \text{HRmax} - 0\cdot80 \times \text{HRmax}$$
Example. For a subject with HRmax of 160 bts/min^{-1}:
$$\text{THR} = 0\cdot65 \times 160 - 0\cdot80 \times 160$$
$$= 104 - 128 \text{ bts/min}^{-1}$$

(5) THR range by Karvonen method, using the heart rate reserve (HRmax − HRresting)
$$\text{THR} = 0\cdot65 - 0\cdot80 \times (\text{HRmax} - \text{HRresting}) + \text{HRresting}$$
Example. For a subject with a HRmax of 160 bts/min^{-1} and a HRrest of 60 bts/min^{-1}.
$$\text{THR range} = 0\cdot65 \,(160 - 60) + 60 - 0\cdot80\,(160 - 60) + 60$$
$$= 125 - 140 \text{ bts/min}$$

as the cardiorespiratory system, in order to identify a level of exertion. Rating scales have been devised which assign numerical values to various stages of effort. The most frequently used of these is the Borg 15 point Rating of Perceived Exertion scale which has values from 6 to 20, the lowest level being "very, very light" and the highest "very, very hard".[102] This scale has been shown to have a linear relationship with work rate and correlates highly with heart rate, oxygen intake, ventilation, and blood lactate levels. On this scale the training threshold lies between 12 and 14, or "somewhat hard". Borg later introduced a new "category-ratio" scale with numbers from zero to 10, and here the desired training range is 3-5 or "somewhat strong".

Mode

The aerobic training activity should involve repetitive movement of large muscle groups. Typical activities are brisk walking, slow jogging (the pace not to exceed a kilometre in 7·5 minutes), low intensity swimming, bicycling, cross-country skiing, and circuit training. Walking and jogging have been used in the programme at the Toronto Rehabilitation Centre for 25 years.[18,104]

The starting level is based on 50 to 70% of the patient's peak oxygen intake measurement, and progression takes place through a series of levels depending on the individual's training responses. As conditioning improves, patients can participate in other more vigorous forms of physical recreation.

Duration and frequency

If training intensity has been chosen appropriately, a workout at a constant pace for at least 20–30 minutes will not cause excessive fatigue or symptoms. As fitness improves, this can be extended to 45 minutes, provided that the intensity does not lead to disproportionate breathlessness or discomfort. A minimum of three training sessions a week is needed to gain a benefit. The Toronto Programme advocates five sessions weekly. One session is carried out at the centre under supervision; the remaining four are not supervised and are away from the centre.[105] Attendance is weekly for nine months, and then monthly for a further nine months, giving a total of 45 attendances.

For very high risk patients, supervision by suitably qualified medical personnel is advisable during all exercise sessions. Ideally, all staff should be trained in cardiopulmonary resuscitation techniques. Routine telemetry or Holter monitoring for all cardiac patients is prohibitively expensive and has not been shown to be a consistently effective safety measure, therefore it cannot be advocated. On the other hand, telemetry does provide a valuable safety net for high risk patients and those identified as having severe ST segment changes or frequent complex arrhythmias. It may also be helpful for those who, after starting the programme, report effort-induced bouts of pulse irregularity or symptoms consistent with cerebral ischaemia, such as lightheadedness or confusion.

Staffing cardiac exercise programmes

While the disciplinary background and professional qualifications of personnel involved in a cardiac rehabilitation programme will vary in accordance with local requirements, there is a basic staffing structure which is considered to be essential.[106] Core staff should include (a) a medical director or supervising physician, (b) a programme director, and (c) a registered nurse. The medical director could be a cardiologist, internist, or other physician with interest and experience in cardiac rehabilitation. Familiarity with exercise testing and prescription is also a further advantage. The programme director should have an advanced knowledge of exercise physiology and coronary risk factor modification strategies, and should preferably hold a masters degree or doctorate in a field related to cardiovascular rehabilitative services, usually applied physiology. The registered nurse should have experience or specialised training in cardiovascular rehabilitation and critical cardiac care.

Additional staff might include an exercise specialist or supervisor experienced in exercise programme planning and supervision, a nutritionist experienced in the areas of lipid disorders, obesity, and diabetes, a mental health professional experienced in psychological assessment, a vocational counsellor, a physical therapist, and an occupational therapist.

All staff members should be certified in basic life support and at least one senior staff member in advanced cardiac life support.

Safety of cardiac exercise training

Given that patients with ischaemic heart disease, latent or overt, are more likely to suffer a fatal myocardial infarction or cardiac arrest than their healthy counterparts, it is reassuring to know that medically supervised cardiac exercise programmes are safe. Haskell,[107] analysing 30 centres, found one fatal cardiovascular event for every 116 402 patient hours of exercise and one nonfatal event for every 34 673 patient hours. More recently, Van Camp and Peterson,[108] evaluating 157 cardiac programmes, reported one cardiac arrest in 112 000 patient hours of exercise, one nonfatal myocardial infarction in 294 000 patient hours, and one fatality in 783 972 patient hours of exercise. The Toronto Rehabilitation Centre's record for the years 1968-1991 is one fatal and one nonfatal cardiovascular event for every 347 579 and 405 509 patient hours of exercise, respectively.

A number of routine precautionary measures can minimise the risk of a

---

Exercise rules minimising risk

- Always warm up and warm down
- Avoid extremes of heat and cold
- Train regularly, avoiding excessive peaks of activity
- Avoid intensive competition
- Adhere to the prescribed limits
- Reduce the exercise load when either ischaemic symptoms or anxiety develops
- Report all symptoms, particularly lightheadedness, chest pain, or syncope, no matter how brief.

---

fatality. The training staff should caution patients to adhere to the exercise rules given in the box.

References

1 Dock W. The evil sequelae of complete bed rest. *JAMA* 1944; **125**: 1083–5.
2 Saltin B, Blomqvist G, Mitchell JH, Johnson RL, Wildenthal K, Chapman CB. Responses to exercise after bed rest and after training. *Circulation* 1968; 38 (5, suppl 7): 1–8.
3 Levine SA, Lown B. "Armchair" treatment of acute coronary thrombosis. *JAMA* 1952; **148**: 1365–9.
4 Chapman C, Fraser R. Studies on the effect of exercise on cardiovascular function: cardiovascular responses to exercise in patients with healed myocardial infarction. *Circulation* 1954; **9**: 347–51.
5 Newman L, Andrews M, Koblish M. Physical medicine and rehabilitation in acute myocardial infarction. *Arch Intern Med* 1952; **89**: 552–61.
6 Cain HD, Frasher WG, Stivelman R. Graded activity program for safe return to self-care after myocardial infarction. *JAMA* 1961; **177**: 111–15.
7 Wenger NK, Gilbert CA, Siegel W. Symposium: The use of physical activity in the rehabilitation of patients after myocardial infarction. *Southern Med J*, 1970; **63**: 891–7.
8 Zohman LR, Tobis JS. Cardiac Rehabilitation. New York: Grune & Stratton, 1970.
9 McNeer JF, Wallace AG, Wagner GS, Starmer CF, Rosati RA. The course of acute myocardial infarction. Feasibility of early discharge of uncomplicated patient. *Circulation* 1975; **51**: 410–3.
10 Gottheiner V. Long-range strenuous sports training for cardiac reconditioning and rehabilitation. *Am J Cardiol* 1968; **22**: 426–35.
11 Kellerman JJ, Modan B, Feldman S, Kariv I. Evaluation of physical work capacity in coronary patients after myocardial infarction who returned to work with and without a medically directed reconditioning program. In: Brunner D, Jokl E, editors. *Physical activity and aging*.Baltimore: University Park Press, 1970: 148–55.
12 Brunner D, Manelis G. Physical activity at work and ischaemic heart disease. In: Larsen OA, Malmborg RO, editors. *Coronary heart disease and physical fitness*. Baltimore: University Park Press, 1971: 424–37.
13 Hellerstein HK. Exercise therapy in coronary heart disease. *Bull N Y Acad Med* 1968; **44**: 1208–47.
14 Rechnitzer PA, Pickard HA, Paivio A, Huhasz MS, Cunningham DA. Long-term

follow-up study of survival and recurrence rates following myocardial infarction in exercising and control subjects. *Circulation* 1972; **45**: 853–7.

15 Kavanagh T, Shephard RJ, Chisholm AW, Qureshi S, Kennedy J. Prognostic indexes for patients with ischaemic heart disease enrolled in an exercise-centered rehabilitation program. *Am J Cardiol* 1979; **44**: 1230–40.

16 Kavanagh T, Shephard RJ, Pandit V. Marathon running after myocardial infarction. *JAMA* 1974; **229**: 1602–5.

17 Kavanagh T. Shephard RJ, Kennedy J. Characteristics of post-coronary marathon runners. In: Milvy P, editor. *The marathon: physiological, medical, epidemiological, and psychological studies.* Vol 1. New York: New York Academy of Sciences 1977: 455–65.

18 Kavanagh T. *The Healthy Heart Program.* 2nd ed. Toronto: Key Port Books Ltd, 1985.

19 Kentala E. Physical fitness and feasibility of physical rehabilitation after myocardial infarction in men of working age. *Ann Clin Res* 1972; 4 (suppl 9): 1–84.

20 Wilhelmsen L, Sanne H, Elmfeldt D, Grimby G, Tibblin G, Wedel H. A controlled trial of physical training after myocardial infarction: effects on risk factors, nonfatal reinfarction, and death. *Prev Med* 1975; **4**: 491–508.

21 Kallio V, Hamalainen H, Hakkila J, *et al.* Reduction in sudden deaths by a multifactorial intervention programme after acute myocardial infarction. *Lancet* 1979; **ii**: 1091–4.

22 Carson P, Phillips R, Lloyd M, *et al.* Exercise after myocardial infarction: a controlled trial. *J R Coll Physicians Lond* 1982; **16**: 147–51.

23 Vermuelen A, Liew KI, Durrer. Effects of cardiac rehabilitation after myocardial infarction: changes in coronary risk factors and long-term prognosis. *Am Heart J* 1983; **105**: 798–801.

24 Shaw LW. Effects of a prescribed supervised exercise program in mortality and cardiovascular morbidity in patients after myocardial infarction: the National Exercise and Heart Disease Project. *Am J Cardiol* 1981; **48**: 39–46.

25 Rechnitzer PA, Cunningham DA, Andrew GM, *et al.* Relation of exercise to recurrence rate of myocardial infarction in men: Ontario Exercise-Heart Collaborative Study. *Am J Cardiol* 1983; **51**: 65–9.

26 May GS, Eberlein KA, Furberg CD, Passamani ER, DeMets DL. Secondary prevention after myocardial infarction: a review of long-term trials. *Prog Cardiovasc Dis* 1982; **24**: 331–52.

27 O'Connor GT, Buring JE, Yusuf S, *et al.* An overview of randomized trials of rehabilitation with exercise after myocardial infarction. *Circulation* 1989; **80(2)**: 234–44.

28 Council on Scientific Affairs. Physician-supervised exercise program in rehabilitation of patients with coronary heart disease. *JAMA* 1981; **245**: 1463–6.

29 *Prevention of coronary heart disease. Report of a WHO Expert Committee.* Geneva: World Health Organization, 1982; Technical Report series 678.

30 Powell KE, Thompson PD, Caspersen CJ, Kendrick JS. Physical activity and the incidence of coronary heart disease. *Ann Rev Public Health* 1987; **8**: 253–87.

31 Leon AS, Connett J, Jacobs DR, Rauramaa R. Leisure-time physical activity levels and risk of coronary heart disease and death. The Multiple Risk Factor Intervention Trial. *JAMA* 1987; **258**: 2388–95.

32 Ekelund LG, Haskell WI, Johnson JL, Whaley FS, Criqui MH, Sheps DS. Physical fitness as a predictor of cardiovascular mortality in asymptomatic North American men. *N Engl J Med* 1988; **319**: 1379–84.

33 Blair SN, Kohl HW, Paffenbarger RS Jr, Clark DG, Cooper KH, Gibbons LW. Physical fitness and all-cause mortality. *JAMA* 1989; **262**: 2395–401.

34 American Heart Association. Benefits and recommendations for physical activity programs for all Americans. *Circulation* 1992; **86(1)**: 340–4.

35 Kavanagh T, Shephard RJ. Maximum exercise tests on post-coronary patients. *J Appl Physiol* 1976; **40**: 611–18.

36 Clausen JP. Circulatory adjustments to dynamic exercise and effect of physical training in normal subjects and in patients with coronary artery disease. In: Sonnenblick EH, Leseh M, editors. *Exercise and Heart Disease.* New York: Grune & Stratton, 1977: 39.

37 Kavanagh T, Shephard RJ, Doney H, Pandit V. Exercise versus hypnotherapy in coronary rehabilitation. *Can Family Phys* 1973; **Oct**: 68–72.

38 Kavanagh T, Shephard RJ. Importance of physical activity in post-coronary rehabilitation. *Am J Phys Med* 1973; **52**: 304–13.

39 Kavanagh T, Shephard RJ. The effects of continued training on the aging process. *Ann N Y Acad Sci* 1977; **301**: 656–70.

40 Kavanagh T, Shephard RJ. Conditioning of post-coronary patients. Comparison of continuous and interval training. *Arch Phys Med Rehabil* 1975; **56**: 72–6.

41 Wasserman K, Naimark A, McIlroy M. Continuous measurement of ventilatory exchange ratio during exercise. *J Appl Physiol* 1964; **19**: 644–52.

42 Detry JR, Rosseau M, Vandenbrouke G, *et al.* Increased arteriovenous oxygen difference after physical training in coronary heart disease. *Circulation* 1971; **64**: 109–18.

43 Paterson DH, Shephard RJ, Cunningham D, *et al.* Effects of physical training on cardiovascular function following myocardial infarction. *J Appl Physiol* 1979; **47**: 482–9.

44 Hindman MC, Wallace AG. Radionuclide exercise studies. In: Cohen LS, Mock MB, Ringqvist I, editors. *Physical conditioning and cardiovascular rehabilitation.* New York: John Wiley, 1981: 33–46.

45 Ehsani AA, Moslin WH, Heath GW, *et al.* Cardiac effects of prolonged and intense exercise training in patients with coronary artery disease. *Am J Cardiol* 1982; **50**: 246–53.

46 Ditchey RV, Watkins J, McKirnon MD, Froelicher V. Effects of exercise training on left ventricular mass in patients with ischaemic heart disease. *Am Heart J* 1981; **101**: 701–6.

47 DeBusk RF, Hung J. Exercise conditioning soon after myocardial infarction: effects on myocardial perfusion and ventricular function. *Ann N Y Acad Sci* 1982; **382**: 343–51.

48 Sklar J, Niccoli A, Leithner M. Changes in ventricular function after cardiac rehabilitation are not related to changes in myocardial perfusion. *Circulation* 1983; **64**: 187–93.

49 Jensen D, Atwood JE, Froelicher V, *et al.* Improvements in ventricular function during exercise studied with radionuclide ventriculography after cardiac rehabilitation. *Am, J Cardiol* 1980; **46**: 770–7.

50 Reading J, Goodman J, Pallandi D, *et al.* Central and peripheral cardiovascular adaptations to endurance training following coronary artery bypass surgery (CABS) [abstract]. *Med Sci Sports Exerc* 1993; **25** (suppl 4): S32.

51 Clausen JP, Trap-Jensen J, Lassen NA. The effects of training on the heart rate during arm and leg exercise. *Scand J Clin Lab Invest* 1970; **26**: 295–301.

52 Clausen JP, Klausen K, Rasmussen B, Trap-Jensen J. Central and peripheral circulatory changes after training of the arms or legs. *Am J Physiol* 1973; **225**: 675–82.

53 McCrimmon DR, Cunningham DA, Rechnitzer PA, Griffiths J. Effect of training on plasma catecholamines in postmyocardial infarction patients. *Med Sci Sports Exerc* 1976; **8**: 152–6.

54 Hartley LH, Mason JW, Hogan RP, *et al.* Multiple hormonal responses to graded exercise in relation to physical training. *J Appl Physiol* 1972; **33**: 602–6.

55 Kavanagh T, Yacoub MH, Mertens DJ, Kennedy J, Campbell RB, Sawyer P. Cardiorespiratory responses to exercise training after cardiac transplantation. *Circulation* 1988; **1**: 162–71.

56 Hagberg JM, Seals DR. Exercise training and hypertension. *Acta Med Scand* 1986; **711**: 131–6.

57 Kitamura K, Jorgensen CR, Gobel FL, Taylor HL, Yang Y. Hemodynamic correlates of myocardial oxygen consumption during upright exercise. *J Appl Physiol* 1972; **32**: 516–22.

58 Frick MH, Katila M. Hemodynamic consequences of physical training after myocardial infarction. *Circulation* 1968; **37**: 192–202.

59 Fulton WFM. *The coronary arteries: arteriography, microanatomy, and pathogenesis of obliterative coronary artery disease.* Springfield, IL: Charles C Thomas, 1965.

60 Redwood DR, Rosing DR, Epstein SE. Circulatory and symptomatic effects of physical training in patients with coronary artery disease and angina pectoris. *N Engl J Med* 1972; **286**: 959–65.

61 Sim DN, Neill WA. Investigation of the physiological basis for increased exercise threshold for angina pectoris after physical conditioning. *J Clin Invest* 1974; **54**: 763–70.

62 Nolewajka AJ, Kostuk WJ, Rechnitzer PA, *et al.* Exercise and human collateralization: an angiographic and scintigraphic assessment. *Circulation* 1979; **60**: 114–21.
63 Raffo JA, Luksix IY, Kappagoda CT, *et al.* Effects of physical training on myocardial ischaemia in patients with coronary artery disease. *Br Heart J* 1980; **43**: 262–9.
64 Laslett LJ, Paumer L, Amsterdam EA. Increase in myocardial oxygen consumption indexes by exercise training at onset of ischaemia in patients with coronary artery disease. *Circulation* 1984; **71**: 958–62.
65 Ehsani AA, Heath GW, Hagberg JM, *et al.* The effect of 7 years of intense exercise training on ischaemic ST segment depression in patients with coronary artery disease. *Circulation* 1981; **64**: 1116–24.
66 Verani MS, Hartung GH, Hoepful-Harris J, *et al.* Effects of exercise training on left ventricular performance and myocardial perfusion in patients with coronary artery disease. *Am J Cardiol* 1981; **47**: 797–803.
67 Schuler G, Schlierf G, Wirth A, *et al.* Low-fat diet and regular supervised physical exercise in patients with symptomatic coronary artery disease: reduction of stress-induced myocardial ischaemia. *Circulation* 1988; **77**: 172–81.
68 Todd IC, Bradnam MS, Cooke MBD, Ballantyne D. Effects of daily high-intensity exercise on myocardial perfusion in angina pectoris. *Am J Cardiol* 1991; **68**: 1593–9.
69 Kramsch DM, Aspen AJ, Abramowitz BM, *et al.* Reduction of coronary atherosclerosis by moderate conditioning exercise in monkeys on an atherogenic diet. *N Engl J Med* 1981; **305**: 1483–9.
70 Ornish D, Brown SE, Scherwitz LW, *et al.* Can lifestyle changes reverse coronary heart disease? The Lifestyle Heart Trial. *Lancet* 1990; **336**: 129–33.
71 Schuler G, Hambrecht R, Schlierf G, *et al.* Myocardial perfusion and regression of coronary artery disease in patients on a regimen of intensive physical exercise and low fat diet. *J Am Coll Cardiol* 1992; **19**: 34–42.
72 Hambrecht R, Niebauer J, Marburger C, *et al.* Various intensities of leisure time physical activities with coronary artery disease: effects on cardiorespiratory fitness and progression of coronary atherosclerotic lesions. *J Am Coll Cardiol* 1993; **22**: 468–77.
73 Paffenbarger RS Jr, Hyde RT, Wing AL, *et al.* Physical activity, all-cause mortality and longevity of college alumni. *N Engl J Med* 1986; **314**: 605–13.
74 Kavanagh T, Shephard RJ, Tuck JA. Depression after myocardial infarction. *Can Med Assoc J* 1975; **113**: 23–7.
75 Kavanagh T, Shephard RJ, Tuck JA, Qureshi S. Depression following myocardial infarction: the effects of distance running. *Ann N Y Acad Sci* 1977; **301**: 1029–38.
76 Fox SM, Naughton JP, Gorman PA. Physical activity and cardiovascular health. *Mod Concepts Cardiovasc Dis* 1972; **41**: 17–30.
77 Carr DB, Bullen BA, Skirnar GS, *et al.* Physical conditioning facilitates the exercise-induced secretion of beta-endorphine and beta-lipoprotein in women. *New Engl J Med* 1981; **305**: 560–2.
78 North TC, McCullagh P, Vu Tran Z. Effects of exercise on depression. *Exerc Sport Sci Rev* 1990; **18**: 379–415.
79 Fagard RH, Tipton CM. Physical activity, fitness, and hypertension. In: Bouchard C, Shephard RJ, Stephens T, eds. *Physical activity, fitness, and health. International proceedings and consensus statement.* Champaign, IL: Human Kinetics, 1994: 633–55.
80 Wood PD, Klein H, Lewis S, *et al.* The distribution of plasma lipoproteins in middle-aged male runners. *Metabolism* 1976; **25**: 1249–57.
81 Kavanagh T, Shephard RJ, Lindley LJ, Pieper M. Influence of exercise and lifestyle variables upon high density lipoprotein cholesterol after myocardial infarction. *Arteriosclerosis* 1983; **3**: 249–59.
82 Frisch RE, Wyshak G, Albright TE, Albright NL, Schiff I. Lower prevalence of diabetes in female former college athletes compared with nonathletes. *Diabetes* 1986; **35**: 1101–5.
83 Stratton JR, Chandler WL, Schwartz RS, *et al.* Effects of physical conditioning on fibrinolytic variables and fibrinogen in young and old healthy adults. *Circulation* 1991; **83**: 1692–7.
84 Campeau L, Enjalbert M, Lesperance J, *et al.* The relation of risk factors to the

development of atherosclerosis in saphenous-vein bypass grafts and the progression of disease in the native circulation. *N Engl J Med* 1984; **21:** 1329–32.

85 Leaman DM, Brower RW, Meester GT. Coronary artery bypass surgery—a stimulus to modify existing risk factors. *Chest* 1982; **81:** 16–19.

86 Oberman A, Wayne JB, Kouchouka NT, *et al.* Employment status after coronary artery bypass surgery. *Circulation* 1982; **65** (suppl II): 115–19.

87 Varnauskas E, and the European Coronary Surgery Group. Survival, myocardial infarction, and employment status in a prospective randomized study of coronary bypass surgery. *Circulation* 1985; **72** (suppl V): 90–101.

88 Barboriak JJ, Anderson AJ, Rimm AA. Changes in avocational activities following coronary artery bypass surgery. *J Cardiac Rehabil* 1983; **3:** 214–16.

89 Newell J, Kappagoda C, Stoker J. Physical training after heart valve replacement. *Br Heart J* 1980; **44:** 638–49.

90 Kaye P. The Registry of the International Society for Heart and Lung Transplantation: Tenth Official Report—1993. *J Heart Lung Transplant* 1993; **12:** 541–8.

91 Kavanagh T, Yacoub M, Campbell R, Mertens D. Marathon running after cardiac transplantation: a case report. *J Cardiopulmonary Rehabil* 1986; **6:** 16–20.

92 Letac B, Cribier A, Desplanches JF. A study of left ventricular function in coronary patients before and after physical training. *Circulation* 1977; **56:** 375–8.

93 Cobb FR, Williams RS, McEwan P, *et al.* Effects of exercise training on ventricular function in patients with recent myocardial infarction. *Circulation* 1982; **66:** 100–8.

94 Sullivan MJ, Higginbotham MB, Cobb FR. Exercise training in patients with chronic heart failure delays ventilatory anaerobic threshold and improves submaximal exercise performance. *Circulation* 1989; **79:** 324–9.

95 Coats AJS, Adamopoulos S, Meyer TE, Conway J, Sleight P. Effects of physical training in chronic heart failure. *Lancet* 1990; **335:** 63–6.

96 Kavanagh T, Myers MG, Baigrie RS, Mertens DJ, Sawyer P. Cardiorespiratory training responses to a one-year walking programme in patients with congestive heart failure [abstract]. *Eur Heart J* 1993; **14** (suppl): 415.

97 American Heart Association. *Exercise standards: a statement for health professionals.* Dallas: American Heart Association, 1991.

98 American College of Sports Medicine. *Guidelines for Exercise Testing and Prescription.* 4th ed. Philadelphia: Lea & Febiger, 1991; 121–58.

99 Fletcher GF, Froelicher VF, Hartley LH, Haskell WL, Pollock ML. Exercise standards: a statement for health professionals from the American Heart Association. *Circulation* 1990; **82:** 2286–322.

100 Mertens DJ, Kavanagh T, Shephard RJ. A simple formula for the estimation of maximal oxygen intake during cycle ergometry. *Eur Heart J* 1994; **15:** 1247–51.

101 Bruce RA, Kusumi F, Hosmer D. Maximal oxygen intake and nomographic assessment of functional aerobic impairment in cardiovascular disease. *Am Heart J* 1973; **85:** 546–62.

102 Karvonen M, Kentala K, Mustala O. The effects of training on heart rate: a longitudinal study. *Ann Med Exp Biol Fenn* 1957; **35:** 307–15.

103 Borg G. *Physical performance and perceived exertion.* Lund, Sweden: Gleerup, 1962: 1–63.

104 Kavanagh T, The Toronto Rehabilitation Centre's cardiac exercise program. *J Cardiac Rehabil* 1982; **6:** 496–502.

105 Kavanagh T. Take Heart! Key Porter Books, Toronto: 1992.

106 American Association of Cardiovascular and Pulmonary Rehabilitation. Guidelines for Cardiac Rehabilitation Programs. 2nd ed. Human Kinetics, Champaign, IL: 1994.

107 Haskell WL. Safety of out-patient cardiac exercise programs: issues regarding medical supervision. In: Franklin BA, Rubenfire M, editors. *Cardiac rehabilitation (Clinics in sports medicine).* Philadelphia: WB Saunders, 1984: 471.

108 Van Camp SP, Peterson RA. Cardiovascular complications of outpatient cardiac rehabilitation programs. *JAMA* 1986; **256:** 1160–3.

4 Psychological factors in cardiac rehabilitation

BOB LEWIN

Introduction

Early cardiac rehabilitation programmes for myocardial infarction patients were simple exercise programmes. It was hoped that, by increasing myocardial efficiency, patients could compensate for any residual impairment and thus minimise their disability. By the mid 1970s it had become clear that many patients could indeed become significantly fitter than they had been prior to the myocardial infarction but that, despite this, a sizeable proportion of these patients remained significantly disabled in some aspects of their lives. It was observed that this disability bore little relationship to the severity of the infarction and that psychosocial recovery was often more difficult to achieve than physical restitution. Psychiatrists and psychologists then became interested in rehabilitation. Twenty years on a good deal is known about the psychology of recovery from myocardial infarction, although this knowledge has yet to be incorporated into routine clinical practice. Surgery patients and those with angina and heart failure have yet to receive the same degree of attention, and what follows is almost exclusively restricted to myocardial infarction.

This chapter begins by describing the psychological process from the initial symptom appraisal and seeking of medical help to the problems of long term adjustment. The first section provides some practical recommendations on the psychological management of the most common problems.

It is not widely appreciated that, even without rehabilitation, sustaining a myocardial infarction can lead to an improved quality of life. This at least is the belief of 33% of patients looking back a year later.[1] This beneficial outcome is not the normal experience, however, and it should be the goal of rehabilitation to help as many patients as possible to achieve and maintain an optimum quality of life. In achieving this, it is helpful to understand why it is that suffering a myocardial infarction improves the perceived quality of life for some patients but significantly damages it for others. The second part of the chapter examines what is known about the predictors of good psychosocial outcome. Some evidence is provided that outcome would be significantly improved if psychological factors were taken into account in the routine medical management of acute myocardial infarction, and some guidelines are suggested.

The third and final part of the chapter briefly reviews a selection of psychological interventions that have been the subject of controlled trials and concludes by offering an opinion on the role of psychologists in cardiac rehabilitation.

Psychological processes in myocardial infarction and recovery

Onset of symptoms

The majority of myocardial infarction patients are poorly prepared for the acute event and fail to identify the true meaning of the symptoms. Valuable time is often wasted in inappropriate self treatment, in particular for angina and "indigestion".[2,3] Despite a reluctance to summon medical aid, many patients harbour a fear that the degree of pain, in many cases greater than any they have previously experienced, is not commensurate with their own diagnosis. This causes considerable anxiety, particularly if they are alone.[4] As the average time to mortality in those who die during acute myocardial infarction is 2·5 hours and a number of studies have reported average delays in hospital arrival time of 3–5 hours (with about half of the patients arriving within 3 hours), this delay can be lethal. Part of this time is occupied in travelling to the hospital but approximately 60% is "decision time", and it has been estimated that as many as 50% of deaths might have been avoided if prompt action had been taken.[5]

It is not clear which patients are most at risk in this way and in reviewing this area Doehrman[3] noted that patients experiencing re-infarction were just as likely to defer seeking help as those with a first myocardial infarction. Clinical experience suggests some of the reasons for the delay. There is often an unwillingness to "bother the doctor" and a fear of embarrassment should it prove to be a false alarm. Some patients are uncertain about a layman's authority to call an ambulance and some patients use "denial" as their preferred way of coping with anxiety. The delay is often greater when there is another person present, and it is important to discuss these issues with post-myocardial infarction patients and their families and to inform them of the correct procedure should they suspect re-infarction. Ideally, clear written advice should be given to patients, telling them how to act in the event of chest pain that does not remit following a 20 minute rest. An additional strategy, and one which is usually welcomed by patients and partners alike, is to provide cardiopulmonary resuscitation training for the patients and their families.

Admission and acute myocardial infarction

Anxiety is the predominant emotion during the first 24 hours. Even in the second and third days, when the acute crisis has passed, around 60% of patients experience clinically significant levels of anxiety.[6] In view of the widespread nature of this reaction and of patients' urgent need to seek help, heightened anxiety is often seen as an appropriate response and therefore not a feature requiring any intervention. Of course medical and nursing staff are usually extremely busy at the time of admission, and a definite diagnosis may not be established for hours or even days. Nevertheless, patients have pressing psychological needs at this time; firstly, for dealing with the pain and the accompanying somatic symptoms of anxiety; and secondly, for information about what is happening to them and why.

Rehabilitation should begin as soon as possible and it is unfortunate that, in most cases, the formal rehabilitation process does not begin for four to six weeks after discharge. At least two studies have examined the value of giving patients a relaxation tape to listen to whilst in the coronary care unit. Hase and Douglas[7] demonstrated a significant reduction in anxiety and a number of longer term benefits. For example, at four month follow up their experimental group claimed to be walking further (6·7 km each week v 2·7 km), reported significantly fewer episodes of chest pain (0·40 v 2·13), and there was a 50% reduction in the number of patients who reported "psychological problems" (10 patients v 25). Although this study was weakened by pseudo-randomisation (on a monthly basis) and a failure to control for the severity of infarction, there is no doubt that patients are enthusiastic about this simple and inexpensive intervention. Guzzetta[8] found that administering a relaxation tape in the coronary care unit led to significantly lower mean heart rates and higher peripheral temperature than a control group. When patients were asked "How helpful were the sessions in helping you to relax?", 29% said "extremely helpful" and 77% said that they would continue to practise these techniques following discharge from the coronary care unit.

The psychological reaction to the coronary care unit

In the early days of coronary care units the fear was often expressed that the high tech environment and witnessing cardiac deaths might increase the incidence of psychological distress. Reviews of the literature have revealed mutually contradictory data. What is clear is that discharge from the coronary care unit to a general ward often causes an increase in anxiety[9] and patients welcome the security of a "step down" ward that is sited close to the coronary care unit.

Psychological recovery whilst in hospital

Numerous surveys have established the temporal pattern of psychological adjustment during the days following the acute event. Anxiety is generally at its highest during the first few hours. As the clinical condition is stabilised and patients begin to believe that they are going to survive there is a rapid reduction in anxiety. In some patients there may even be a brief period of euphoria. Within a couple of days patients will begin to consider what the event means and its likely long term effect on their lives. In reviewing a series of 441 postmyocardial infarction patients referred for psychiatric consultation, Hackett and Cassem[10] found anxiety to be the most common problem in the first two days, with depression emerging as the dominant reason for psychiatric referral between the third and fifth days.

It is important to realise that the full extent of the patients' anxiety and depression are often deliberately hidden from medical staff and other patients. Although 40–60% of patients experience clinically significant levels of anxiety, the majority appear cheerful from the second or third day after admission until discharge. Dellipiani et al[11] found that, just prior to discharge, mean anxiety levels rose to be similar to those on admission.

The predominant fear is of sustaining another myocardial infarction. For some patients there are additional concerns about loss of employment and poverty. Younger patients and those with manual jobs are often more distressed than those with sedentary jobs, the elderly, or the retired.[6] During this period patients' families are usually more anxious than patients themselves. Their needs for reassurance and information and advice on how to manage patients after discharge are often not dealt with. Most of the fears they have will be unfounded and will reflect a poor understanding of myocardial infarction and coronary artery disease. It is at this time that patients and their families are most in need of education and most receptive to new ideas. Such counselling should not be confused with "hand-holding" or providing emotional support. In the past encouraging a "stiff upper lip" was generally regarded as the best response to encourage in patients. This often led to ignoring patients' valid concerns, thus perpetuating the distress. There are signs that this belief has now been reversed so that the equally unhelpful opposite idea—that "ventilating" emotions is always healthy and "keeping them in" is unhealthy—is becoming popular. Patients may be deliberately encouraged to disclose and display their emotional distress. There is no evidence to support this strategy or to suggest that cardiac patients either want or benefit from such "help".

What do patients want? Orzeck[12] devised a questionnaire to determine patients' perception of the support they required. Of the 50 "needs" presented in the questionnaire, patients rated the items concerning emotional support as *least* important. The ten most highly endorsed items (in descending order) were:

1 It is important for questions to be answered honestly
2 It is important for me to know specific facts about my heart condition
3 It is important to know what exercises are helpful or harmful
4 It is important for explanations to be understandable
5 I need to know what to do in case of an emergency situation
6 I need to know what can be done to prevent another heart attack
7 I need to know if I will ever be back to my previous lifestyle
8 I need to know my prognosis
9 I need to know when I can resume my normal activities
10 I need to know if returning to work is good or bad for my heart.

Denial

The tendency to put a good face on things has been discussed above but some patients appear to take this further and exhibit a particularly cavalier attitude. Hackett and Cassem[13] reported that approximately 23% of their patients claimed that they were *not at all worried*. In other studies,[14,15] 20–80% have repudiated feelings of anxiety or worry whilst in hospital. Some patients (12–20%) are sceptical about having had a heart attack or express doubt about the need for further treatment. A few baldly contradict the physician's diagnosis. In a small number even more extreme reactions have been reported: immediately following discharge, patients "test fate" by undertaking strenuous activity or indulging in "saturnalian excess".[16] Whether this behaviour actually produces an increase in mortality is not recorded, but there is evidence that the spouses of patients who behave in this way suffer particularly high levels of psychologcal distress.[17]

The idea of denial was popularised by Freud who described it as a primitive and pathological defence mechanism. Janis[18] attempted to de-pathologise the concept calling it "intellectual denial" or "minimisation". He also suggested that it may often be more simply understood as the result of misleading reassurance from health professionals or as a faulty understanding of the disease. Denial has also been viewed as being a healthy psychological strategy that aids patients in coping with their problems. It has been claimed to reduce mortality and speed recovery[19,20] and to be a predictor of better long term psychosocial adjustment to ischaemic heart disease, but at present these findings remain contentious and it has been suggested that the empirical evidence is either conflicting or absent.[21-23] At present the balance of evidence suggests that moderate levels of denial, in a well informed patient, may be a helpful short term coping strategy. Denial does present a problem if it interferes with medical compliance and the adoption of secondary prevention measures. When faced with high levels of denial it is worth remembering that frightening patients with dire warnings about what will happen if they do not alter their health behaviour has repeatedly been shown to be a very poor way of motivating them to make lifestyle changes. A more productive strategy is to emphasise the positive benefits of change.

Psychological adjustment following discharge

In the first weeks of home convalescence the prevalence of anxiety and depression remains high relative to the general population. It is only once they get home that most patients feel able to exhibit this distress. It may take the form of increased irritability, withdrawal from the family, and/or increased emotional lability. "Home-coming depression" is almost universal and the partners and families must be prepared for the sudden dip in patient's mood and be advised how best to react if this becomes a problem.[24] Many patients find that they feel tearful at the slightest provocation, some cry frequently. For the majority this emotional lability is distressing and patients often attribute it to their "mind being damaged during the heart attack".[25] In warning patients to expect this it is best to explain it as a part of the normal recovery process following survival of any kind of life threatening emergency and not specific to myocardial infarction. Patients must also be warned that after a week spent mostly in bed, they are likely to feel weak, especially when tackling stairs or household chores. Lay people often believe rest to be restorative and fail to comprehend the speed with which deconditioning occurs. If patients are not informed about this, they often interpret any breathlessness or increase in their pulse rate as an indication of further problems or of having taken insufficient "rest". This often raises their anxiety levels and sends them back to bed. In some cases it can lead to the development of a phobic avoidance of any but the lightest activity.

Relationship problems

For the family a common problem is the increased irritability of the patient. It is common for them to report that living with patients is like "walking on eggshells", "living with a volcano", or "sitting on a keg of dynamite". Partners commonly blame themselves for patients' newly presenting misery or bad temper or, having seen patients apparently happy whilst on the ward, regard it is a negative reflection on the quality of their relationship. Patients may actively encourage these beliefs and blame partners for their unhappiness or even for the infarct itself.[17] Many partners fear that confronting patients about their unreasonable demands or anger might lead to a row that could precipitate another myocardial infarction or death. These problems are often even more acute in homes where there are teenagers or young adults. In most cases the children quickly and quite appropriately resume their normal lifestyle. If this involves behaviour disapproved of by patients, such as playing loud music or staying out late, it may be interpreted by the parents as selfishly imposing stress on patients. Again the underlying fear is that this stress will lead to re-infarction. Both patients and their partners should be reassured that this is extremely unlikely to happen. In these situations the partner is often forced to become a mediator between the children and patients. Partners should be advised that it is better for patients' long term recovery to conduct family life as normal, even if this initially causes unpleasantness.

Partners are often terrified of the possibility of sudden death. A common fear is that patients have died whilst asleep. It is not uncommon for partners to repeatedly wake patients to check that they are still alive. Overprotectiveness may extend to never allowing patients out of their or other family members' sight or preventing them being physically active. This can lead to increased irritability, to patients accepting the restrictions and adopting the invalid role, or to patients exploiting their control over the family. Care givers should be strongly advised to try to avoid "wrapping patients in cotton wool" and warned of the dangers of imposing unnecessary rest. There is one exception to this: occasionally, female patients are expected to resume all of the household chores immediately following discharge, the husbands' attitude being "they wouldn't have let you out if you weren't OK again". This often leads to exhaustion and increased anxiety; patients and partners should be advised that all activities should be resumed on a systematic and gradual basis.

Long term psychological sequelae

One year after the acute event approximately 20-35% of the survivors of a heart attack have a formally diagnosable psychiatric illness.[6,26] Of course in some cases this psychiatric morbidity predates the infarction: in a retrospective study of 100 patients, one week after the acute myocardial infarction, Lloyd and Cawley[27] described three groups of patients. Firstly, there were those whose psychiatric problems appeared to predate the infarction (17%). Secondly, there was the group whose psychiatric distress appeared to result from the myocardial infarction (20%). Thirdly, there were those without a diagnosable psychiatric illness (63%). At 12 months 75% of the first group and 25% of the second were disturbed. It was the non-distressed group (the third group) that showed the greatest change: 19% developed a psychiatric illness by four months which fell to 11% at one year.

It seems clear that a myocardial infarction may precipitate clinical anxiety or depression in a significant number of patients and it is important that patients are formally assessed to detect this. When should this be done? It is hard to predict problems in adjustment from the psychological status at one week, and sampling at this point would include many cases that are in the process of rapid remission. A study by Mayou[28] demonstrated that 6–12 weeks post-infarction is the best time to assess the likely long term outcome in terms of psychiatric morbidity. Similarly, Stern et al[29] reported that 67% of patients who were anxious at three months were still depressed or anxious at one year follow up. In many hospitals patients attend a clinic at 4–12 weeks after discharge; this would be an ideal time to administer a simple questionnaire, such as the hospital anxiety and depression scale[30] or the general health questionnaire[31] to identify those patients who are likely to have long term problems.

It is sometimes suggested that using such questionnaires can interfere with the doctor-patient relationship. These fears have been demonstrated to be groundless, indeed many patients welcome the fact that care is being taken to assess their emotional state. A questionnaire can often allow a patient to express distress without feeling that they are moaning or taking up valuable time. Both of these questionnaires can be scored in a few minutes by any member of staff. A raised score can provide the opportunity for an enquiry such as, "I see that you are feeling a bit worried/fed up: is there anything in particular that is bothering you?" In some cases the problem may be a simple misunderstanding about the disease or the likely prognosis and can be resolved by a few minutes discussion. It is important to avoid being overguarded in expressing an opinion about prognosis. Those patients whose questionnaire scores demonstrate high levels of distress or who, in conversation, reveal complex psychosocial or psychiatric problems should be offered further assessment, preferably by a clinical psychologist, psychiatrist, social worker or nurse counsellor experienced in working with medical patients. A useful strategy is to compile a local resources file of agencies the patient or family can approach for help: Relate, the Citizens Advice Bureau, addiction clinics, support groups, social services, volunteer agencies, national charities, etc. If this can be given to patients to take home, so much the better.

Psychological health is an important objective in its own right and there is little point in striving to limit impairment and improve prognosis if patients are left disabled by anxiety or depression. For these reasons alone it should be attended to, but in addition there is an increasing amount of evidence that psychological status is independently related to survival. Anxiety and depression have been significantly associated with early mortality in several studies.[32-34] Data from the β blocker heart attack trial[35] showed that, in a cohort of 2320 male postmyocardial infarction patients, after controlling for other risk markers, patients who perceived themselves as being socially isolated and experiencing a high level of "life stress" were four times as likely to die over the following three years. Analysis of data generated by a four and a half year prospective psychological treatment trial involving 1012 postmyocardial infarction patients (the recurrent coronary prevention project) found that sudden cardiac death had predominantly psychosocial predictors, while non-sudden cardiac death and non-fatal recurrence were predominantly predicted by biological factors. The authors[36] claim that: "These results are the first demonstration of a direct relation between stress and sudden cardiac death in a large prospective clinical study."

Carney et al[37] followed up 52 patients who had angiography for suspected coronary artery disease. At 12 months 78% of the depressed patients had sustained at least one major cardiac event compared with 35% of the non-depressed. Multiple regression showed that depression was an independent predictor of events when all other demographic and physiological variables were entered. A significant weakness of the study is that one of the "major cardiac events" included was coronary artery bypass surgery: nearly twice the number of depressed patients went for surgery. This may have been as the result of a selection bias, the more depressed patients being more likely to report uncontrolled pain or to continue to demand further treatment.[38] This suggests a further reason for attending to psychological factors; poor psychological adjustment often leads to patients seeking further, perhaps unnecessary, investigations and treatments.

Reduced quality of life following myocardial infarction

Quality of life is harder to define and assess than psychiatric illness. One indicator is a subclinical, but still abnormal, score on questionnaires measuring anxiety or depression. A typical finding reported from a study of 400 postmyocardial infarction males, using the Zung self rating scale, found that, 6 months after myocardial infarction 50% of patients were more anxious than an age matched sample from the general population.[39]

Of course an unnecessarily poor quality of life may exist in the absence of raised levels of anxiety or depression; it may take the form of deleterious changes in discrete areas of patients' lives, such as poverty or loss of status due to a failure to return to work, a curtailment of previously enjoyed activities, and sexual or marital problems.

Return to work

In numerous studies the return to work rate has been reported as being between 62 and 92%.[40,41] One reason for this wide range is variation in the temporal sampling point. Although relatively large numbers return to work, many soon retire or are made redundant. For example, Mayou et *al*[42] described a cohort in which 90% initially returned to work but in which, 1 year later, only 70% were still employed.

An obvious predictor of failure to return to work is occupational disbarment: for example, a pilot or heavy goods vehicle driver usually loses his licence. Those whose jobs have a heavy manual element are also less likely to return to work. In many of these cases this caution may be unjustified, and such patients would benefit from rehabilitation programmes especially designed to assess the needs of their work and then restore them to the required level of strength and fitness.[40,41] However, this "work hardening" is unlikely to succeed without also taking the patient's own perceptions into account. It is known that there is a strong social class difference in the degree to which patients believe physical activity to be a risk factor following a myocardial infarction. Those in the lower socioeconomic classes tend to rate physical work as more dangerous.[42,43]

At a work assessment centre established by the Australian government to investigate why postmyocardial infarction patients so often failed to return to work, a psychiatrist, Wynn,[44] examined 400 male patients with coronary artery disease. He came to a number of instructive conclusions. He found that unwarranted emotional distress and invalidism were present in some 50% of the patients referred to the centre. One of his conclusions was that psychological distress contributed more to the patient's level of disability than did physical impairment, and he rated this as "moderate to severe" in 27, "severe" in 14, and "gross" in 9%. Other studies have concluded that for 40–50% of patients psychological causes were the primary reason for failure to return to work.[45,46] For most, it appeared to be fear of further damage that prevented the return. There is also evidence that, not surprisingly, patients who dislike their jobs are also less likely to return to work.[47] It has often been reported that there is a significant relationship between failure to return to work and anxiety and depression.[23,30,48-50] It is impossible to deduce the direction of causality in this relationship, although it is worth noting that a number of patients mention the "loss of ability to earn" or "fear of unemployment" as one of their major anxieties only a few days after the myocardial infarction.[48]

The average time before returning to work has reduced over the last 20 years and is now 60–70 days after myocardial infarction.[47] A number of factors are thought to influence the length of time off work. Physical complications during recovery have an unequivocal effect on return to work time, but the severity of coronary artery disease has only a modest association[46] and psychosocial factors are often a stronger determinant.[43,48,50]

Once back at work a substantial number of patients reduce their output or actively avoid responsibility or overtime. Thirty per cent of patients believe that reduced health status has harmed their work. Postmyocardial infarction patients often have reduced earnings and report greater work-related stress.[51]

It has become increasingly common to regard return to work as an unsuitable outcome measure for auditing rehabilitation programmes. In part this reluctance is justifiable because rates of return to work are influenced by factors that rehabilitation programmes cannot influence, such as high levels of unemployment and potential employers' pessimistic expectations. It has been suggested that cutting back on work, taking early retirement, or living on sickness benefit may be something to actively encourage in rehabilitation.[52] Obviously, work should be discussed with the patients: for those with secure and guaranteed retirement pensions who dislike their work, retirement may be a superior option, but it should be emphasised that this is to improve the quality of life rather than for prognostic reasons. Giving advice to retire early to patients who will have to depend on state entitlements is fraught with danger, especially in countries where unemployment benefits are low and the criteria for eligibility are liable to change unpredictably; it should be remembered that poverty is a strong predictor of early mortality.[53] As we have seen, as many as 50% of patients failing to return to work do so for psychological reasons, and the inability of rehabilitation programmes to influence return to work may reflect the almost universal lack of attention paid to psychological factors. It is important to establish whether a patient who is seeking to leave employment is motivated by unwarranted fears or undue illness behaviour. Where this appears to be the case it is important to try to correct the patient's misconceptions rather than exempt the patient on medical grounds; lengthy periods of work avoidance are likely to make the anxiety worse. Occasionally, personnel departments are prepared to negotiate a phased return to work for such patients. Work is often an important source of self validation and a major provider of social support. Depressed or anxious patients should be dissuaded from making any drastic changes in their employment before these problems have been treated. A patient who has lost his job may benefit from taking up voluntary work.

Relationships

The physical sequelae of a myocardial infarction are contained within patients but the psychological impact usually extends well beyond the individual. Often the patient's partner manifests the greatest distress, and their emotional and practical response may have a major influence on the eventual outcome.[54,55] The pre-existing quality of the marital and familial relationships has been seen as an important determinant of psychological recovery.[27,56] A substantial multicentre study in Germany showed that marriages "high in intimacy" appear to have a "buffering effect", protecting patients from anxiety and depression.[39] Ideally, the patients' families should be involved in the rehabilitation process. Members of a family often share lifestyles and the acute event for one member of the family may provide a useful opportunity for health promotion for the whole family.

Some disruption of the marital relationship is common in the first weeks after the acute event and, unless these problems are causing severe distress, it is probably better to explain them to the couple as part of the normal recovery process. If there are still problems several months later, the couple should be offered marital therapy from a suitably trained counsellor or psychologist. Where the problem is an unwillingness to leave the patient unattended, a simple strategy is to draw up a contract between patient and spouse whereby the patient is allowed to be alone, or to engage in an activity that the partner is fearful about, for a negotiated and *mutually* agreed period of time. An example might be going for an unaccompanied walk by himself. The initial period may need to be quite short, say a 10 minute walk once a day. It is essential that the patient sticks to the contract and does not take the opportunity to slip away for a longer period. After a week of such walks a new and longer period can be negotiated. Treated in this way the period of separation can usually be extended systematically over the ensuing weeks and the partner's anxiety will gradually subside. A similar method can be used to help patients who have become excessively fearful of exercise, work, or being alone.

Sexual adjustment

Several authors have reported that the myocardial infarction can improve the quality of the patient's sex life through bringing a couple closer and producing a general improvement in the marital relationship.[1,57] Such patients are in the minority, however; numerous surveys attest to the fact that 10-58% of patients complain of sexual difficulties or a reduction in the frequency of, or satisfaction with, sexual intercourse.[58-61]

It is not safe to assume that a patient's sexual difficulties are the result of the myocardial infarction. A sample of 131 postmyocardial infarction men with such difficulties were asked if they had sexual problems prior to myocardial infarction; 14% had been impotent, 28% reported a "substantial decrease of sexual interest and activity", and 8% reported premature ejaculation.[62] Sjörgen[61] avoided this difficulty by recruiting males who reported being sexually active before the myocardial infarction. These men exhibited a number of problems; 45% reported a reduction in "satisfaction with sex". Of those reporting particular problems, fatigue was mentioned by 45%, fear by 39%, a reduced libido by 8%, chest pain by 39%, and "erectile or orgasmic incompetence" by 22%. The majority of surveys of postmyocardial infarction patients have only recruited men; an exception was a study by Papadopoulos et al[63] who reported that 50% of women admitted to being afraid to recommence intercourse following myocardial infarction. In an interview study of 100 postmyocardial infarction,[64] women aged between 40 and 60, "sexual dissatisfaction" was reported by 65%; in an age matched sample on non-cardiac medical patients only 24% reported such problems. Interestingly, in both groups of women, the dissatisfaction was related mainly to sexual dysfunction in their partners.

It is likely that some of these problems are the result of drug therapy. It has been estimated that antihypertensive agents and diuretics may be responsible for impotence and ejaculatory problems in 30% of male patients.[65] β blockers can cause a number of problems, including impotence (in 15%), a decreased potency (inability to maintain erection to ejaculation; in 28%), and reduced libido (in 4%).[66] Even without the added complications of compromised arteries and medication it can be difficult to separate physiological from psychological causes of sexual difficulties. Removing the drug may not establish the original cause because, after a period of drug induced difficulties, the problem may be maintained by psychological factors alone. In males the continuation of morning erections and the ability to masturbate to ejaculation *may* indicate that psychological factors are predominant. If explicit reassurance about the safety of intercourse, given to both partners, does not help then referral to a clinical psychologist or psychiatrist experienced in assessing and treating sexual problems may be indicated.

The evidence reviewed here demonstrates that a number of patients and their partners feel scared about sex following a myocardial infarction. It has been noted that "there are many myths about sudden death from heart attack during sexual intercourse."[67] A common myth, quoted by Cooper,[68] is that "sexual exertion is somehow much more lethal than equally strenuous non-sexual exercise". Hackett and Cassem[69] claimed that the beliefs that "sexual intercourse should never again be attempted and that repeat infarctions tend to occur at orgasm" represent the most common misconception amongst cardiac patients. These misconceptions probably account for much of the fear reported above and should be explicitly countered before the patient leaves hospital.

Many patients find it difficult to volunteer information about sexual problems. A survey (admittedly conducted over 20 years ago) revealed that both patients and doctors assumed that only "psychiatrically disturbed patients spontaneously talk about sex".[70] Medical staff should take the risk of being thought psychiatrically disturbed and help patients by initiating the discussion. Both patients and their partners should be given information about the resumption of sexual activity and also given an invitation, separately and/or together, to discuss any fears that they have. Unfortunately, there is evidence that medical staff often neglect to do this. Freeman and King[67] established that 65% of physicians did not talk to patients about the resumption of sexual activity. Even worse, most junior doctors said that they would advise patients *not* to resume sex if they had experienced "a severe myocardial infarction" or had "many risk factors"!

Undue illness behaviour

Undue illness behaviour relating to the heart has been recognised under many names over the years; "neurocirculatory asthenia", "effort syndrome", and "soldier's heart" are a few of the euphemisms it has generated. Such patients usually manifest high levels of anxiety and a phobic avoidance of activity or effort, along with a hopeless and dependent attitude.

After a myocardial infarction most patients are cautious about physical exertion and reduce it. This often involves abandoning previously enjoyed activities. The self enforced lack of activity usually leads to increasing deconditioning and tiredness, boredom, and more time to look for new symptoms. The decline in fitness is often interpreted by patients and their families as evidence of a further deterioration of the heart. This leads to increased anxiety and an increase in resting time, leading to steadily increasing disability.

After a myocardial infarction most patients divert a great deal more attention to how they feel. Some continually scan their bodies for any minor symptoms or unusual somatic sensations, especially those emanating from the chest. This shift of attention to the chest can produce a quite startling degree of sensitisation to normally inaccessible somatic information. Many of these patients can report an accurate pulse rate by simply "feeling" each heart beat. For most patients these preoccupations slowly extinguish over time. For some they do not, and such patients are at high risk of commencing a life of unnecessary illness behaviour. It is particularly unfortunate for cardiac patients that many of the symptoms of high arousal and panic (palpitations, nausea, a sudden feeling of weakness, perspiration, etc) closely mimic the symptoms of myocardial infarction. A vicious circle often develops whereby any symptom noticed by patients, for example palpitations or a sudden feeling of faintness, produces more anxiety, leading to an increase in symptoms. The end result may either be a panic attack and/or a false alarm admission, or a constant anxiety state and feeling of being unwell. Such patients cause a number of problems for their doctors. Although it is now generally accepted that as many as 50% of medical consultations are primarily driven by psychological factors, it is often extremely difficult to determine which 50%. There is an understandable reluctance to assess psychological contributions to the presentation before all medical causes or treatments have been excluded. This is especially true when chest pain, breathlessness, and extreme fatigue are being reported. Repeated false alarm admissions to hospital and atypical chest pain in the absence of evidence of an accompanying ischaemic episode should alert medical staff to the need for a psychological assessment.

A longitudinal study by Mæland[71] of 383 postmyocardial infarction patients showed that the major predictors of readmission to the hospital were raised levels of anxiety and depression at discharge, poor cardiac lifestyle knowledge, and the number of previous admissions. The use of the hospital services did not correlate with peak enzymes in the initial myocardial infarction, and in 20% of cases no clear diagnosis could be attached to the readmission. In these patients, being female and the patient's own estimate (prior to discharge) of the amount of "emotional control" they would have once they got home were the major predictors of readmission. Having examined the use of health resources following myocardial infarction Mæland concluded that "psychological factors influence health service utilisation to a comparable extent as medical factors."

Psychological management and outcome

One third of patients claim that their lives have been improved by the myocardial infarction. What is it that differentiates them from those who fail to achieve a good quality of life? It would seem reasonable to expect that the more ill a patient is the more anxious or depressed he will be but, in general, this is not the case. It has repeatedly been demonstrated that there is no significant association between the psychological reaction to myocardial infarction or the rehabilitative outcomes and the severity of the infarct or the underlying illness.[1,6,11,24,26–29]

Why do patients who have reasonably good prognosis and little in the way of residual impairment continue to behave as if they are dangerously ill? One suggestion is that such behaviour is a rational response to mistaken beliefs about the seriousness of an illness and its long term prognosis. Garrity and Klien[72] showed that, in male myocardial infarction patients, differences in many rehabilitative outcomes are influenced by the way patients perceive their health status. Psychological adjustment, return to work, and community involvement covaried with perceived health status. Once again there was only a weak relationship between clinical measures of health and patients' perception of their health status.

There is no doubt that sustaining a myocardial infarction has a powerful effect on how patients view their health. In the cohort of Mæland and Havik[73] 67% rated their pre-infarction health as high. Following discharge from hospital the number who regarded themselves as healthy had sunk to 21%, and even at three to five years only 42% regarded themselves as having recovered their health. Patients' perceived health shifted little after the first six weeks, another reason why rehabilitation should begin as early as possible. There was no relationship between perceived health and the severity of the myocardial infarction but there was a strong association between perceived health and a number of measures of recovery, including psychological adjustment, "involvement with symptoms", anxiety, and depression. Interestingly, when asked for a subjective estimate of their exercise capacity patients were generally accurate (as measured by treadmill performance), showing that they made a clear distinction between their functional ability and how healthy they were. This may help to explain why exercise programmes alone do not improve long term psychological outcome[74-78] or rates of return to work.[79] Given that most patients had a normal functional capacity prior to the myocardial infarction, it is not surprising that they do not regard the return of this ability as indicating a good health status.

Wynn[44] believed that a certain type of personality was at particular risk of distress, a type of man who had previously dealt with anxiety by "compulsive hard work". For such patients the main cause of the emotional problem was being told to "take it easy" or being given a certificate that only allowed them to do "light work". In the largely working class group he was seeing, Wynn identified this as the major precipitator of distress in 25% of cases. He considered that in 22% of his patients anxiety was caused by the advice given by medical attendants: "Often it was the symbolic significance of the doctor's remarks, rather than his words, which did so much harm. Thus 'lie still and you will be all right' often signifies 'move and you will die' to the patient."

In the convalescent phase, comments such as "you will be all right if you are careful" were interpreted by some patients as "if I am not careful I will die." Few doctors issuing this type of caution explicitly defined "careful" and, not unreasonably, for many frightened patients this injunction resulted in a severe restriction of activity. Other commonly used and frightening phrases were "you were lucky this time", the patient's interpretation being "I won't be lucky next time"; or "it is only a warning", the patient's interpretation being "something terrible is yet to come."

Wynn found that 11% "were suffering the dire psychological distress of anticipating early death" and stated that "This was usually because the patient had been given an overly cautious or guarded prognosis by their doctor." Sometimes the opinion had been given to wives or family members in confidence but had been passed on to the patient. Thirty eight per cent were primarily upset due to an inadequate understanding of what had happened: "patients not infrequently made comments like 'the main artery to my heart is blocking up' or 'half my heart is dead and the other half is dying'." Patients with angina often believed that each episode was another small heart attack.

Havik and Mæland also found that such "cardiac misconceptions were an important predictor of poor adjustment, for example in predicting "false alarm" readmissions due to patients "believing that the infarction had left a weak area in the heart wall that easily could rupture; or that the risk for recurrence would remain high indefinitely seemed to be of special importance".

Patient attributions for myocardial infarction

It seems that what the patient believes about the cause of myocardial infarction has an important bearing on eventual rehabilitation status. In a survey[80] 102 postmyocardial infarction patients were asked to list the factors that they believed had "caused their heart attacks" in order of perceived pathogenicity and were then asked to rate how controllable each of those causes would be. Eighty per cent of patients gave stress, worry, overwork, or smoking as the primary cause. This was a particularly startling finding as these patients had all been counselled about the "official" risk factors, of smoking, hypertension, high cholesterol levels, diet, sedentary lifestyle, etc, in "educational" sessions that were part of their rehabilitation programme. Although these "official" risk factors were mentioned by many patients, they were all (except smoking) perceived to be less important and much more controllable than the psychological or behavioural factors. A similar study by Murray[81] confirmed these findings.

In work carried out at the British Heart Foundation Rehabilitation Research Unit in Edinburgh, involving more than 180 patients, the same beliefs emerged. Many patients appeared to view the heart as a kind of battery or fuel tank, and "energy" it "contains" as used up by work, worry, stress, and emotional arousal. They often saw the heart attack as "a warning" that they had experienced too much of these in their own lives and that very little energy was left. Given these two beliefs, the most logical thing for a patient to do if he or she wishes to live as long as possible is to conserve the remaining energy by avoiding any further work, worry, stress, or excitement. Rest, or "taking things easy", is often seen as recuperative, and it is easy to understand how such beliefs may lead to restricted lifestyle. As we have seen, prolonged rest carries medical and psychological dangers.

The patients' beliefs do not match those of most medical staff and Fielding[80] has criticised rehabilitation programmes and suggested that they fail the patient because "the focus on biological factors in rehabilitation . . . fails to address those specific areas of concern held by myocardial infarction patients."

These cardiac misconceptions and patients' beliefs about the causes of myocardial infarction are socially normative and in many cases they are reinforced by the patient's family and friends and the media. As rehabilitation programmes become more psychologically oriented, these problems may be compounded if staff present patients with a naive understanding of the dangers of "stress" or of "type A behaviour". Sometimes the actions of therapists, just as much as what is actually said, may reinforce these mistaken beliefs. For example, some patients remarked to us that they believed that the relaxation training they received after their exercise classes was intended to "rest the heart" to "make up for" the exercise.

Recommendations for psychological management

The evidence reviewed above carries a number of practical implications for the psychological management of myocardial infarction, and a number of recommendations can be made (see box).

There is some evidence that by following these guidelines patients can be helped to a significantly improved psychological outcome. A controlled trial conducted by Thompson[82] showed the profound impact that relatively brief, in-hospital, nurse-led counselling can produce. The intervention was aimed at reducing the misconceptions about the illness and was designed to include the following features:

- Early initiation of psychological intervention (within 24 hours of admission to the hospital)
- Inclusion of the patient's spouse
- Examination of specific sources of anxiety
- A structured plan for the systematic and early resumption of activity following discharge.

The intervention brought about highly significant and clinically worthwhile reductions in anxiety in both patient and spouse, and these were maintained to six months (the extent of the follow up). It also produced a significant improvement in sexual adjustment, resumption of leisure activities, and a number of other important areas affecting the patients' quality of life. This intervention was carried out by a highly experienced nurse who also holds a PhD in psychology. Such staff are rare: in the United Kingdom few rehabilitation programmes have a psychology input of any type.

As a response to this problem a self help six week rehabilitation programme, *The Heart Manual*, based on a work book and two audio tapes, has been developed (see Lewin *et al*[83]). It is administered by a facilitator, who can be any member of the medical staff who has attended the two day training course. The facilitator introduces and explains the programme and also provides brief contacts to encourage compliance and detect and solve problems of adjustment. The programme is designed to

---

Recommendations for psychological management after myocardial infarction

- Rehabilitation should start as soon as possible following the acute event

- Early rehabilitation should be aimed at reversing the cardiac misconceptions that cause anxiety and underpin much of the failure to regain a good quality of life

- Medical staff must be careful not to unintentionally reinforce these misconceptions and should attempt to elicit them from patients and then help the patients to achieve a more accurate and helpful understanding of their disease

- A fear that stress, worry, overwork or emotional or physical arousal will lead to reinfarction is central to much of the poor adjustment manifested by post-myocardial infarction patients; these misconceptions must be addressed in a believable and sympathetic manner if undue illness behaviour and disability are to be avoided

- Advice and education must take account of the lay understanding of the disease rather than regarding patients as blank slates on which to write the current medical explanation

- Patients and their families should be prepared for the likely psychological sequelae and be given honest practical advice about the management of these difficulties

- The physiological and psychological symptoms of anxiety should be explained to patients and their families, and they should be warned to expect them and given advice on how to distinguish them from cardiac symptoms and how to deal with them

- Prior to discharge the patients and their families should be given a clear, understandable, and practical strategy for systematically returning to as many as possible of their previous activities

- A simple home based exercise programme, or a programme of daily walking, increasing in a controlled manner, can be commenced from discharge

- Many patients appreciate being given a hospital telephone number to call if they have problems following discharge; in practice this facility is rarely abused

- To achieve the best outcome following myocardial infarction it is important to assess formally and, where necessary, provide treatment for clinically significant psychological problems following myocardial infarction; this assessment is probably best done 6-12 weeks after discharge

- Equal attention should be paid to the spouse's and family members' problems of adjustment

undermine the most common unhelpful attributions and cardiac misconceptions. There is a separate tape for the spouse, who is encouraged to take part and to encourage the patient to comply. This tape also helps the family with some of the common difficulties they are likely to face. If the self help advice and time do not significantly reduce the psychosocial problems, patients are encouraged to make appropriate self referral for further help. The programme includes a simple home-based exercise programme aimed at leading the patient into regular exercise and provides advice on secondary prevention. It also includes a relaxation and stress management programme, the intention of which is to increase the patient's feeling of control over work, stress, and worry, and thereby reduce anxiety about returning to a "normal" life. In a placebo controlled trial[83] the package produced marked improvements in both anxiety and depression. It also significantly reduced both the number of contacts with patients' general practitioners and readmissions to hospital over the following 12 months.

Psychological interventions and their role in rehabilitation

The use of psychological therapies in rehabilitation

A "psychological" technique that has been widely adopted in rehabilitation is relaxation training. This is often popular with patients and staff, as it accords with their own views about the pathogenic nature of stress. A study that compared the efficacy of exercise training with and without relaxation classes showed that adding relaxation training improved the training success by 50% as well as significantly reducing ST segment abnormalities.[84] Follow up at two to three years[85] revealed that patients who received both treatments had significantly fewer cardiac events (17 v 37%) than those who had undergone exercise training alone. A study of relaxation training in high risk (moderately hypertensive) patients has demonstrated useful reduction in blood pressure and fewer acute cardiac events over four years.[86]

An increasing number of centres are offering stress management training programmes. There is little standardisation of these, and the term is used to cover a multitude of procedures. Most have relaxation training at their core and include additional techniques for dealing with stress. A controlled comparison between stress management training and relaxation alone produced significant improvement in a number of rehabilitative end points in both treated groups. At six months the patients who had received stress management training had fewer cardiac complications (10 v 31%) than those who had been trained relaxation alone.[55] A controlled trial that did not *teach* stress management but simply monitored patients for a rise in emotional distress and then sent a nurse to solve the underlying problem halved the death rate in the year after myocardial infarction. However, following the withdrawal of this service, mortality rates in this group became similar to those in the control group.[87]

Another obvious role for psychological input is risk factor reduction and lifestyle change. Many rehabilitation programmes now include some form of education classes and these have been shown to encourage short term changes in health behaviours but do not appear to lead to long term (one to five years) changes in smoking,[88] diet,[89] or compliance with exercise advice,[90,91] or reduce clinical levels of psychological disturbance.[92] A more promising approach seems to be the development of cognitive-behavioural treatments for producing changes in lifestyle. Cognitive-behaviour therapy differs from education and advice in that the beliefs, motivations, and environmental factors that are maintaining the patient's unwanted behaviours are examined and the patient is involved in systematically practising alternative behaviours. Exercise programmes that have incorporated cognitive-behaviour therapy methods have shown worthwhile gains in long term compliance with exercise, which is otherwise generally poor.[91] A controlled trial of a cognitive-behaviour therapy programme designed to reduce cardiac risk factors in a high risk but well group produced a 41% reduction in coronary heart disease risk one year later.[93]

Psychotherapy is sometimes advocated for myocardial infarction patients. Unfortunately most research in this area is of very poor quality. There are problems of definition, there are many schools of psychotherapy, and these may vary widely in their theoretical basis and application. The success of Thompson's study, in which the counselling was directly aimed at removing cardiac misconceptions, has already been mentioned. Another study that met scientific standards compared education and relaxation training (both delivered on audio tapes in the hospital) with the same package plus six one-hour sessions of individual counselling. The addition of counselling did not improve outcome; both groups made significant and nearly identical psychological and lifestyle gains when compared with a control group.[94]

Who should deliver psychological treatment?

This chapter has presented evidence indicating the importance of attending to psychological factors in the rehabilitation process. In response to such evidence the question is often posed, should a rehabilitation team include a psychologist? In some countries a psychologist is almost always a member of the multidisciplinary rehabilitation team; in others, such as the United Kingdom, psychologists are scarce and are rarely found in cardiac rehabilitation settings.[95] Certainly it is well established that a small proportion of patients will manifest clinical levels of anxiety, depression, and other psychological problems that require formal psychological or psychiatric help. At present most of the patients who might benefit are not treated; as a result there is probably a large hidden cost to the health service in the subsequent unnecessary use of medical resources. Such patients should be identified through routine screening at follow up clinics and be referred for appropriate treatment. The choice of whether to employ a psychologist specifically for such work must depend on the numbers requiring treatment and on the availability of skilled help elsewhere in the locality. As with any other worker a psychologist's results are likely to improve with increasing experience of a particular area, and therefore the more a psychologist is able to specialise in "cardiac psychology" the greater their success rate is liable to be. Where a full time worker can not be justified, "psychology time" can often be bought in on a sessional basis.

The source of many of the common problems of adjustment and of the widely experienced reduction in quality of life are the "cardiac misconceptions" held by patients and their families. Medical and nursing staff are best placed to identify and reverse such faulty beliefs, and research[82,83] suggests that a good deal of psychological distress could be mitigated without the need for specialist psychological input *if* the routine management of myocardial infarction was designed in such a way as to optimise psychological as well as physical recovery.

An important goal of comprehensive rehabilitation is to change health behaviours such as smoking, diet, and compliance with exercise. The evidence suggests that in many cases, such goals are unlikely to be met without invoking psychological knowledge about behaviour change and the maintenance of new behaviours. Psychologists do not have any claim to being indispensible in such services but their expertise may be valuable in developing and evaluating more successful behaviour change programmes.

References

1 Laerum E, Johnsen N, Smith P, Larsen S. Myocardial infarction may include positive changes in lifestyle and in the quality of life. *Scand J Prim Health Care* 1988; 6: 67–71.
2 Greene WA, Moss AJ, Goldstein S. Delay, denial and death in coronary heart disease. In: Eliot RS, editor. *Stress and the heart*. Mount Kisco, NY: Futura, 1974: 123–42.
3 Doehrman SR. Psycho-social aspects of recovery from coronary heart disease: a review. *Soc Sci Med* 1977; 11: 199–218.
4 Finlayson A, McEwan J. *Coronary heart disease and patterns of living*. London: Croom Helm, 1977.
5 Hackett TP, Rosenbaum JF. Emotion, psychiatric disorders and the heart. In: Braunwald E, editor. *Heart Disease: A textbook of cardiovascular medicine*, 1923–1943. Philadelphia: WB Saunders, 1980.
6 Cay EL, Vetter N, Philip A, Dugard P. Psychological status during recovery from an acute heart attack. *J Psychosom Res* 1972; 16: 425–35.
7 Hase S, Douglas A. Effects of relaxation training on recovery from myocardial infarction. *Aust J Adv Nurse* 1987; 5: 18–26.

8 Guzzetta CE. Effects of relaxation and music therapy on patients in a coronary care unit with presumptive acute myocardial infarction. *Heart Lung* 1989; **18**: 609–16.

9 Byrne DG, Byrne AE. Anxiety and coronary heart disease. In: Byrne DG, Rosenman RH, editors. *Anxiety and the heart*. New York: Hemisphere, 1990: 213–29.

10 Hackett TP, Cassem NH. Psychiatric consultation in a coronary care unit. *Ann Intern Med* 1971; **75**: 9–14.

11 Dellipiani AW, Cay EL, Philip AE, *et al*. Anxiety after a heart attack. *Br Heart J* 1976; **38**: 752–7.

12 Orzeck SA. Comparison of patients and spouses: needs during the post hospital convalescence phase of myocardial infarction. *J Cardiopulmonary Rehabil* 1987; 7: 59–65.

13 Hackett TP, Cassem NH. Factors contributing to delay in responding to the signs and symptoms of acute myocardial infarction. *Am J Cardiol* 1969; **24**: 651–9.

14 Almeida D, Wenger NK. Emotional responses of patients with acute myocardial infarction to their disease. *Cardiology* 1982; **69**: 303–9.

15 Baile WF, Bigelow GE, Gottlieb SH, Stitzer ML, Sactor JD. Rapid resumption of cigarette smoking following myocardial infarction. *Addict Behav* 1982; 7: 373–80.

16 Gulledge AD. Psychological aftermaths of myocardial infarction. In: Gentry WD, Williams RB, editors. *Psychological aspects of myocardial infarction and coronary care*. St. Louis: CV Mosby, 1979: 113–30.

17 Stern MJ, Pascal L. Psychosocial adaptation to post-myocardial infarction: the spouse's dilemma. *J Psychosom Res* 1979: **23**: 83–7.

18 Janis IL. *Psychological stress: psychoanalytic and behavioural studies of surgical patients*. New York: Academic Press, 1958.

19 Tesar GT, Hackett TP. Psychiatric management of the hospitalised cardiac patient. *J Cardiopulmonary Rehabil* 1985; **5**: 219–25.

20 Krantz DS, Schulz R. A model of crisis, control and health outcomes: cardiac rehabilitation and relocation of the elderly. In: Baum A, Singer I, editors. *Advances in environmental psychology*. Hillsdale, New Jersey: Lawrence Earlbaum, 1980: 23–57.

21 Croog SH, Shapiro DS, Levine S. Denial among heart patients. *Psychosom Med* 1971; **33**: 385–97.

22 Stern MJ, Pascal L, Ackerman A. Life adjustment postmyocardial infarction. Determining predictive variables. *Arch Intern Med* 1977; **137**: 1680–5.

23 Croog SH. Recovery and rehabilitation of heart patients: psychosocial aspects. In: Krantz DS, Baum A, Singer JS, editors. *Handbook of psychology and health*. Vol. 3: *Cardiovascular disorders and behaviour*. Hillsdale: Lawrence Erlbaum, 1983: 295–334.

24 Wiklund I, Sanne H, Vedin A, Wilhelmsson C. Determinants of return to work one year after a first myocardial infarction. *J Cardiopulmonary Rehabil* 1985; **5**: 62–72.

25 Wishnie HA, Hackett TP, Cassem NH. Psychological hazards of convalescence following myocardial infarction. *J Am Med* 1971; **215**: 1296–9.

26 Lloyd GG, Crawley RH. Psychiatric morbidity after myocardial infarction. *QJ Med* 1982; **51**: 33–42.

27 Lloyd GG, Cawley RH. Distress or illness? A study of psychological symptoms after myocardial infarction. *Br J Psychiatry* 1983; **142**: 120–5.

28 Mayou R. Prediction of emotional and social outcome after a heart attack. *J Psychosom Res* 1984; **28**: 17–25.

29 Stern MJ, Pascal L, McLoone JB. Psychosocial adaption following an acute myocardial infarction. *J Chron Dis* 1976; **29**: 513–26.

30 Zigmond AS, Snaith RP. The hospital anxiety and depression scale. *Acta Psychiatr Scand* 1983; **67**: 361–70.

31 Vieweg BW, Hedlund JL. The general health questionnaire (GHQ): a comprehensive review. *J Oper Psychiatry* 1983; **14**: 74–81.

32 Obier KM, MacPherson M, Haywood JL. Predictive value of psychosocial profiles following acute myocardial infarction. *JAMA* 1977; **69**: 59–63.

33 Kennedy GJ, Hofer MA, Cohen D. Significance of depression and cognitive impairment in patients undergoing programmed stimulation of cardiac arrhythmias. *Psychosom Med* 1987; **49**: 410–14.

34 Crisp AH, Queenan M. Myocardial infarction and the emotional climate. *Lancet* 1984; **i**: 616–19.

35 Ruberman W, Weinblatt E, Goldberg JD, Chaudhary BS. Psychosocial influences on mortality after myocardial infarction. *N Engl J Med* 1984; **311**: 552–9.
36 Brackett CD, Powell LH. Psychosocial and physiological predictors of sudden cardiac death after healing of acute myocardial infarction. *Am J Cardiol* 1988; **61**: 979–83.
37 Carney RM, Rich MW, Freedland KE, *et al*. Major depressive disorder predicts cardiac events in patients with coronary artery disease. *J Psychosom Med* 1988; **50**: 627–33.
38 Channer KS, O'Connor S, Britton S. Psychological factors influence the success of coronary artery surgery. *J R Soc Med* 1988; **11**: 629–32.
39 Waltz M, Badura B, Pfaff H, Schott T. Marriage and the psychological consequences of a heart attack: a longitudinal study of adaption to chronic illness after 3 years. *Soc Sci Med* 1988; **27**: 149–58.
40 Wicklund I, Sanne H, Vedin A, Wilhelmsson C. Coping with myocardial infarction: a model with clinical applications, a literature review. *Int Rehabil Med* 1985; **7**: 167–75.
41 Smith GR, O'Rourke DF. Return to work after myocardial infarction: a test of multiple hypotheses. *JAMA* 1988; **259**: 1673–7.
42 Mayou R, Foster A, Williamson B. Psychosocial adjustment in patients one year after myocardial infarction. *J Psychosom Res* 1978; **22**: 447–53.
43 Shanfield SB. Return to work after an acute myocardial infarction: a review. *Heart Lung* 1990; **19**: 109–17.
44 Wynn A. Unwarranted emotional distress in men with ischaemic heart disease. *Med J Aust* 1967; **2**: 847–51.
45 Goble AJ. Rehabilitation of the cardiac patient. *Med J Aust* 1963; **2**: 975–82.
46 Nagel R. Factors influencing return to work after myocardial infarction. *Lancet* 1971; **2**: 454–6.
47 Vuopla V. Resumption of work after myocardial infarction in northern Finland. *Acta Med Scand* 1986; **530** (suppl): 3–53.
48 Cay EL, Vetter N, Philip A, Dugard P. Return to work after a heart attack. *J Psychosom Res* 1973; **17**: 231–43.
49 Mayou R. The course and determinants of reactions to myocardial infarction. *Br J Psychiatry* 1979; **134**: 588–94.
50 Maeland JG, Havik OE. Return to work after a myocardial infarction: the influence of background factors, work characteristics and illness severity. *Scand J Soc Med* 1986; **14**: 183–95.
51 Hinohara S. Psychological aspects in rehabilitation of coronary heart disease. *Scand J Rehabil Med* 1970; **2**: 53–9.
52 Wenger N. Research related to rehabilitation. *Circulation* 1979; **60**: 1636–9.
53 Davey Smith G, Bartley M, Blane D. The Black report on socioeconomic inequalities in health 10 years on. *BMJ* 1990; **301**: 373–7.
54 Cay EL. Psychological problems in patients after a myocardial infarction. *Adv Cardiol* 1982; **22**: 108–12.
55 Langosch W, Seer P, Brodner G, Kallinke D, Kulick B, Heim P. Behaviour therapy with coronary heart patients: results of a comparative study. *J Psychosom Res* 1982; **26**: 475–84.
56 Taylor CB, Bandura A, Ewart CK. Exercise testing to enhance wives, confidence in their husband's cardiac capability soon after clinically uncomplicated acute myocardial infarction. *Am J Cardiol* 1985; **55**: 635–8.
57 Hellerstein HK, Friedman EH. Sexual activity and the postcoronary patient. *Arch Intern Med* 1970; **125**: 987–97.
58 Horgan JH, Craig AJ. Resumption of sexual activity after myocardial infarction. *J Irish Med Assoc* 1978; **71**: 540–2.
59 Masur FT. Resumption of sexual activity following myocardial infarction. *Sex Disabil* 1979; **2**: 98–114.
60 Mehta J, Krop H. The effect of myocardial infarction on sexual functioning. *Sex Disabil* 1979; **2**: 115–21.
61 Sjörgen K, Fugl-Meyer A. Some factors influencing quality of sexual life after myocardial infarction. *Int Rehabil Med* 1983; **5**: 197–201.
62 Wabreck AJ, Burchell RC. Male sexual dysfunction associated with coronary heart disease. *Arch Sex Behav* 1980; **9**: 69–75.

63 Papadopoulos C, Beaumont C, Shelley SI, Larrimore P. Myocardial infarction and sexual activity of the female patient. *Arch Intern Med* 1983; **143**: 1528–33.

64 Abramov LA. Sexual life and sexual frigidity among women developing acute myocardial infarction. *Psychosom Med* 1976; **38**: 418–23.

65 Reichgott MJ. Problems of sexual function in patients with hypertension. *Cardiovasc Med* 1979; **4**: 149–52.

66 Burnet WC, Chahine RA. Sexual dysfunction as a complication of propranolol therapy in men. *Cardiovasc Med* 1979; **4**: 811–13.

67 Freeman LJ, King JC. Sex and the post-infarction patient. *Cardiol Pract* 1986; **Nov**: 6–8.

68 Cooper AJ. Myocardial infarction and advice on sexual activity. *Practitioner* 1985; **229**: 575–9.

69 Hackett TP, Cassem NH. Psychological adaption in myocardial infarction patients. In: Naughton JP, Hellerstein HK, editors. *Exercise testing and exercise training in coronary heart disease*. New York: Academic Press, 1973: 253.

70 Pinderhughes CA, Grace EB, Reyna LJ, Anderson RT. Interrelationships between sexual functioning and medical conditions. *Med Aspects Hum Sex* 1972; **6**: 52–84.

71 Mæland JG, Havik OE. Use of Health Services after a myocardial infarction. *Scand J Soc Med* 1989; **17**: 93–102.

72 Garrity TF, Klien RF. Emotional response and clinical severity as early determinants of six-months mortality after myocardial infarction. *Heart Lung* 1975; **4**: 730–7.

73 Mæland JG, Havik OE. Self-assessment of health before and after a myocardial infarction. *Soc Sci Med* 1988; **27**: 597–605.

74 Naughton J, Taylor J, Gorman P, Rios J. Editorial: National exercise and heart disease project. *Med Ann District Columbia* 1973; **43**: 5–6.

75 Plavsic C, Turkulin K, Perman Z, *et al.* The results of exercise therapy in coronary prone individuals and coronary patients. *J Ital Cardiol* 1976; **6**: 422–32.

76 Mayou R, MacMahon D, Sleight P, Florencio MJ. Early rehabilitation after myocardial infarction. *Lancet* 1981; **ii**: 1399–1401.

77 Stern MJ, Cleary P. The National Exercise and Heart Disease Project: long term psychosocial outcome. *Arch Intern Med* 1982; **142**: 1093–7.

78 O'Rourke A, Lewin B, Whitecross S, Pacey W. The effects of physical exercise training and cardiac education on levels of anxiety and depression in the rehabilitation of coronary artery bypass graft patients. *Int Disabil Stud* 1990; **12**: 104–6.

79 Danchin N, Goepfert PC. Exercise training, cardiac rehabilitation and return to work in patients with coronary artery disease. *Eur Heart J* 1988; **9**: 43–6.

80 Fielding R. Patients' beliefs regarding the causes of myocardial infarction: implications for information-giving and compliance. *Patient Educ Counselling* 1987; **9**: 121–34.

81 Murray PJ. Rehabilitation information and health beliefs in the post-coronary patient: do we meet their information needs? *J Adv Nurs* 1989; **14**: 689–93.

82 Thompson DR. A randomized and controlled trial of in-hospital nursing support for first time myocardial infarction patients and their partners: effects on anxiety and depression. *J Adv Nurs* 1989; **14**: 291–7.

83 Lewin B, Robertson IH, Cay EL, Irving JB, Campbell M. A self help post-MI rehabilitation package - The Heart manual: effects of self-help post-myocardial-infarction rehabilitation on psychological adjustment and use of health services. *Lancet* 1992; **339**: 1036–40.

84 Van Dixhoorn J, Duivenvoorden HJ, Staal HA, Pool J. Physical training and relaxation therapy in cardiac rehabilitation assessed through a composite criterion for training outcome. *Am Heart J* 1989; **118**: 545–52.

85 Van Dixhoorn J, Duivenvoorden HJ, Staal HA, Pool J, Verhage F. Cardiac events after myocardial infarction: possible effect of relaxation therapy. *Eur Heart J* 1987; **8**: 1210–14.

86 Patel C, Marmot MG, Terry DJ, Carruthers M, Hunt B, Patel M. Trial of relaxation in reducing coronary risk: four year follow-up. *BMJ* 1985; **290**: 1103–6.

87 Frasure-Smith N, Price R. Long-term follow-up of the ischaemic heart disease life stress monitoring program. *Psychosom Med* 1989; **51**: 485–513.

88 Sivarajan ES, Newton KM, Almes MJ. Limited effects of outpatients teaching and counselling after myocardial infarction: a controlled study. *Heart Lung* 1983; **12**: 65–73.

89 Barbarowicz P, Nelson M, DeBusk RF, Haskell WL. A comparison of in-hospital education approaches for coronary bypass patients. *Heart Lung* 1980; **9**: 127–33.
90 Oldridge NB. Cardiac Rehabilitation Exercise Programme compliance and compliance enhancing strategies. *Sports Med* 1988; **6**: 42–55.
91 Martin JE, Dubbert PM. Behavioural management strategies for improving health and fitness. *J Cardiac Rehabil* 1984; **4**: 200–8.
92 Horlick L, Cameron R, Firor W, Baltzan J. The effects of education and group discussion in the post myocardial infarction patient. *J Psychosom Res* 1984; **28**: 485–92.
93 Lovibond SH, Birrell P, Langeluddecke P. Changing coronary heart disease risk-factor status: the effects of three behavioural programs. *J Behav Med* 1986; **9**: 415–37.
94 Oldenburg B, Perkins RJ. Controlled trial of psychological intervention in myocardial infarction. *J Consult Clinical Psychol* 1985; **53**: 852–9.
95 Maes S. Psychosocial aspects of cardiac rehabilitation in Europe. *Br J Clin Psychol* 1992; **31**: 473–83.

5 Selecting patients for rehabilitation and rehabilitation for patients

VEIKKO KALLIO

Introduction

The beginning of a new era

Rehabilitation of patients with coronary heart disease has undergone many changes over the last 40 years. In the early 1950s, it was common practice to confine the patient to bed for several weeks after an acute myocardial infarction. This resulted in severe physical and psychological problems, described by the American cardiologists Levine and Lown[1] as follows:

> The abruptness of the onset of coronary thrombosis, with its grave prognostic connotations, afflicting as it frequently does the highly active and previously healthy person, when coupled with long continued bed-rest, saps morale, provokes desperation, unleashes anxiety and ushers in hopelessness with respect to resumption of normal living.

"Armchair" treatment—a new method for rehabilitation

In the "armchair" treatment method proposed by Levine and Lown, the majority of patients were allowed to sit in an armchair for one to two hours during the first day, then for longer periods, so that by the end of the first week they spent most of the day in a chair. The contraindications to this approach were a continuing state of shock, marked debility, and concomitant cerebrovascular accident. No complications attributable to the "armchair" treatment were seen. Besides resulting in less deconditioning, this method of treatment also appeared to have beneficial effects on the psychological state of the patients and facilitated the rehabilitation process. Hospital treatment was still maintained for about four weeks.

It took some time to change the policy of long lasting bed rest into "armchair" treatment and early ambulation. Several controlled studies on early ambulation were published in the '70s and reviewed by Swan et al.[2] They showed no increase in mortality or morbidity of patients randomised into the early ambulation group. The gains, in terms of a short stay in hospital and physical and psychosocial improvement, are considerable.

Cardiac rehabilitation—physical exercise or a comprehensive discipline?

In order to emphasise the multifactorial approach to cardiac rehabilitation, it is worth noting the European Society of Cardiology definition of cardiac rehabilitation,[3] which is:

> The rehabilitation of patients with coronary heart disease is defined as the sum of interventions required to ensure the best possible physical, psychological and social conditions so that patients with chronic post-acute cardiac disease may, by their own efforts, preserve or reserve the proper place in society.

Cardiac rehabilitation has often been used as a synonym for physical exercise and training. Although physical exercise is the core of cardiac rehabilitation, there are many other important activities that must be included in the programme. A comprehensive rehabilitation programme thus consists of elements such as physical exercise training, advice on psychological and social problems, and health education. It should be available to cardiac patients recovering from myocardial infarction or after invasive interventions, such as coronary artery bypass graft surgery and percutaneous transluminal coronary angioplasty. However, it is not necessary that all patients with coronary heart disease undergo the whole programme.[4] It is important to emphasise that the rehabilitation strategies used must depend on a careful assessment of each individual's needs and requirements. This type of patient selection gives optimal results in terms of psychosocial adaptation, physical conditioning, and the safety of the exercise training.

Physical exercise testing is a prerequisite for patients to be considered as participants in exercise programmes after acute myocardial infarction, stable angina pectoris, coronary artery bypass graft surgery, and percutaneous transluminal coronary angioplasty. In the case of acute myocardial infarction, the test is usually performed three to six weeks after the event, provided that there are no contraindications to testing. Exercise testing is usually considered to be contraindicated in the acute stage of myocardial infarction, unstable angina pectoris, serious arrhythmias, severe left ventricular dysfunction and uncontrolled left heart failure, and

110

tight aortic stenosis. In addition to these absolute contraindications, there are relative contraindications such as high blood pressure, asthma, and other serious diseases. The need for and timing of the exercise test have to be carefully considered and related to the severity of the patient's disease. The contraindications are not always absolute if the importance of the information that can be obtained outweighs the risk.

Selection of patients for formal physical exercise programmes has undergone changes during the last 30 years. In the '60s and '70s these programmes were provided for almost all patients after an acute myocardial infarction. However, due to early ambulation, reduced hospital stay, and thrombolytic therapy, patients become less deconditioned, and consequently the need for and interest in instituting strictly formal supervised physical rehabilitation programmes for all patients after acute myocardial infarction has recently been on the wane. This does not mean that exercise rehabilitation has lost its importance in the comprehensive treatment of patients with coronary heart disease. On the contrary, the beneficial effects of long term physical training are well known. Formal supervised training courses should, however, be considered like any medication: they should be prescribed only when there are indications for them.

The amount and intensity of exercise training is determined, in accordance with the aims of treatment, using data recorded during a treadmill or bicycle exercise test. This allows the physician to plan the treatment according to the patient's individual needs, tailoring a programme for them. Risk stratification, discussed later in more detail, helps the physician to organize the training with a view to what equipment and supervision are required for maximal benefit and safety.

Several studies have indicated that subsequent cardiac mortality is high in myocardial infarction patients who have contraindications to the exercise test.[5,6] On the other hand, patients whose tests showed no ischaemia, no complicated arrhythmias, and good functional capacity $\geqslant$6-8 metabolic equivalents (METs) or >100 W had very low mortality during follow up of several years. Such patients belong to the low risk group and they do not need a formal exercise rehabilitation programme. They should, however, be advised and encouraged to take regular exercise by themselves, as part of risk factor modification and generally keeping fit.

The variables often used to define patients with intermediate risk for cardiac events include ischaemia at high threshold (>6–8 METs or >100 W), left ventricular dysfunction and complex arrhythmias. Those most likely to benefit from a supervised exercise programme are patients in intermediate risk group.

Acute myocardial infarction patients belonging to a high risk group are characterised by severe myocardial ischaemia at low threshold (<6 METs or < 100 W), enlarged heart, and complex and sustained arrhythmias. They need further evaluation of their physical condition including non-invasive and invasive examinations, and, if indicated, angioplasty or operative treatment. However, it has been shown that even a high risk patient may benefit from a physical exercise programme under close supervision and electrocardiogram monitoring.[7,8]

During the last few decades cardiac rehabilitation has been targeted at secondary prevention after acute myocardial infarction, coronary artery bypass graft surgery, and percutaneous transluminal coronary angioplasty.[9] There have also been major developments in pharmaceutical therapy, including anticoagulants, thrombolytic agents, and β blocking agents. However, there are still many reasons in favour of comprehensive rehabilitation of myocardial infarction patients as well as patients who have had coronary artery bypass graft surgery and percutaneous transluminal coronary angioplasty.

Risk stratification of acute myocardial infarction patients in rehabilitation planning

There are quite a number of factors that influence the outcome of patients after myocardial infarction in terms of morbidity and mortality. The first group of factors is related to the degree of damage to the heart muscle. The second group includes variables related to the status of the coronary arteries and risk of an advancing atherosclerotic process in the coronary arteries. The third group of variables is related to the thrombotic component and the fourth to electrical instability of the heart. Any of these mechanisms can be responsible for a new cardiac event, be it a fatal or non-fatal myocardial infarction or a sudden or non-sudden cardiac death.

In the following review the prognostic significance of various historical and clinical factors registered during the hospital stay is examined in order to stratify patients into risk categories by the end of hospitalisation. Stratification is into low risk, intermediate risk, and high risk of a recurrent cardiac event. The stratification is useful from the point of view of planning the individual's rehabilitation programme, and in considering requirements for non-invasive and invasive examinations and further measures such as coronary artery bypass graft surgery and percutaneous transluminal coronary angioplasty. The aim is to provide patients with the type of rehabilitation that can be expected to improve physical working capacity, raise the angina threshold, and prevent recurrences of cardiac events or other complications. The importance of psychosocial variables will be briefly reviewed in order to highlight various approaches to risk stratification. Finally, some factors related to risk of not returning to work[10] will be reviewed.

Severity of infarction

The available information regarding morbidity and mortality in patients with ischaemic heart disease has been reviewed by Pryor *et al* [11] Important prognostic characteristics from the initial assessment include the patient's gender, age, coronary artery disease risk factors, symptoms, evidence of myocardial damage, and associated vascular disease. The presence of significant myocardial damage is often associated with symptoms of congestive heart failure, which has been found in almost all studies to be an important predictor of outcome. Non-invasive testing, such as treadmill exercise test, nuclear studies, and ambulatory electrocardiography, are able to identify high and low risk subgroups among patients with chronic coronary artery disease.

Peel and Norris and their coworkers were among the first to construct prognostic indices for acute myocardial infarction patients. [12,13] The Peel index includes clinical factors, present on admission to hospital, which were associated with mortality in a group of 757 patients. The main factors predicting survival in hospital and for three years after discharge from hospital included age and severity of the infarction.

Grande *et al* compared 218 acute myocardial infarction patients below 70 years of age with 102 patients admitted to hospital because of anginal pain but with no signs of prior myocardial infarction. [14] The two groups were similar with regard to distribution of age, sex, and coronary risk factors. There was a highly significant difference in the one year survival rate between those with ischaemic heart disease without acute myocardial infarction and those with acute infarction ($p = 0.001$). The infarction size was estimated using serum creatinine kinase measurements. The median infarction size of those who died during the first year was significantly greater than that of survivors. It was greater in patients with heart failure than in those without heart failure.

In another study of 364 men after myocardial infarction, the four year mortality was 13·5%. Only severity of the attack was significantly associated with poor four year survival. [15] This study was among the first to include cigarette consumption in the baseline characteristics, and it was found that cigarette consumption after infarction had been significantly less among those surviving the four year period than among the deceased. In this study no significant differences between survivors and deceased were noted in serum cholesterol levels and in mean body weight.

A number of enzyme variables reflecting infarction size have been studied in 727 patients and related to the five year mortality rate. [16] The results from lactate dehydrogenase and aspartate aminotransferase analysis clearly indicated that there was an association between infarction size and five year mortality. Another important message from this study was that after the first year of follow up, the mortality rate during the remaining four years appeared to be independent of the original infarction size. From a clinical standpoint, this means that a patient surviving the first year of first small infarction has a long term prognosis similar to that of a patient surviving the first year after the first large infarction.

History and clinical and exercise test characteristics

DeBusk et al studied the relative value of the history and clinical and exercise test characteristics in distinguishing patients with a high risk of subsequent cardiac events from those with a low risk.[5] The patient population consisted of 702 consecutive men aged less than 70 years who were alive 21 days after infarction. Characteristics in the history, such as previous angina pectoris or myocardial infarction, identified 10% of the patients with the highest rate of reinfarction and death within six months (18%). Clinical contraindications to exercise testing identified another 40% of the patients as having a cardiac event rate of 6·4%. In patients who underwent a treadmill testing three weeks after myocardial infarction, the rates of cardiac events within six months were 3·9% in those with a negative test and 9·7% in those with a positive test.

The stepwise classification procedure correctly classified 72% of the patients who experienced significant medical events within six months of infarction. The authors indicated that most patients who had experienced a subsequent cardiac event had been correctly classified on the basis of history and clinical risk characteristics (for example, previous angina or myocardial infarction). In patients without these risk characteristics, early treadmill testing is useful for further discrimination of high risk and very low risk patients.

In patients classified on historical and clinical grounds as having a relatively high risk of cardiac events, it seems appropriate to consider additional diagnostic evaluation in order to identify very high risk subsets which may benefit from aggressive medical and surgical intervention. The risk stratification proposed in the study by DeBusk et al appears to facilitate and to direct diagnostic, therapeutic, and rehabilitation resources toward patients most likely to benefit from these interventions.

The prognostic value of an exercise test within three months after the acute myocardial infarction was studied by De Backer et al.[17] Among 112 men, ST segment depression of 2 mm or more at low work load and the maximal exercise parameters was indicative of future mortality and of non-fatal recurrent infarction.

Murray et al combined the results of clinical assessment, routine diagnostic investigations, and pre-discharge exercise testing in 350 consecutive patients who were followed up for one year.[6] Twenty six per cent of the 50 patients with contraindications to pre-discharge exercise testing (mainly heart failure) died or had reinfarctions, compared with 9%

of the patients who were given an exercise test. In the 300 exercise tested patients, extensive myocardial damage, reciprocal change on the electrocardiogram (ECG), and ST depression were the major risk markers which identified at least 75% of the patients who had cardiac events during the follow up. Patients with exercise-induced angina pectoris or clinical contraindications to β blockade were particularly at risk; 43% of them died or had reinfarction.

In a study by Tibbits et al, 866 patients after myocardial infarction were enrolled to determine optimal predictors of long term prognosis.[18] Twenty nine variables (historical, physical examination, various blood samples, ambulatory monitoring, radionuclide ventriculogram, and exercise test variables) revealed that the only exercise test variable that contributed independently to prediction was whether the patients took the test. The improvement in sensitivity and specificity by addition of information from the radionuclide scan and exercise test was insignificant. The results imply that costly tests after myocardial infarction should be reserved for specific indications and should not be universally applied in assessing prognosis.

The low risk group was characterised by a non-ischaemic response to treadmill exercise test, such as absence of chest pain, ST segment changes, and reversible perfusion defects. Patients with an ischaemic response need further diagnostic examinations.

Electrocardiographic site of infarction

Hands et al studied the prognostic significance of the ECG site of infarction among 398 patients with anterior and 391 patients with inferior infarction.[19] The one year mortality was higher in patients with anterior myocardial infarction than in those with inferior infarction (18·4% v 10·5%, p = 0·002). Further multivariate analysis confirmed the prognostic significance of infarct location independent of peak creatinine kinase level. The authors concluded that the location of myocardial infarction, independent of size, is an important prognostic indicator and warrants risk stratification in the clinical management and rehabilitation of patients suffering from their first myocardial infarction.

Persistent ST depression

The prognostic significance of persistent ST depression on ECG after an acute myocardial infarction has been studied in connection with the β-Blocker Heart Attack Trial.[20] The patients were divided into three groups on the basis of the presence or absence of ≥ 1 mm ST segment depression in ECGs taken during the first few days after admission and at the time of randomisation, which was done at $9·7 \pm 3·3$ days after the index infarction. Group one included patients with no ST segment depression, group two comprised patients with transient ST segment depression in the first few days after admission or at the time of randomisation.[8] Group three included patients with persistent ST segment depression in the first few days after admission, and at the time of randomisation. At a median follow up time of 26 months, the mortality rates were 4·9% in group one, 7·6% in group two, and 13·6% in group three. The differences between the three groups were highly significant. The authors concluded that persistent and transient ST segment depression in patients after the first myocardial infarction were strong predictors of increased long term mortality, in contrast to patients without ST segment depression.

Congestive heart failure and ventricular dysfunction

In a series of 202 patients a two month follow up revealed the following independent prognostic factors: early clinical signs of heart failure, peak creatinine kinase level, and increased cardiothoracic ratio on chest x ray.[21] Ventricular dysfunction and simple clinical data predicted early death after acute myocardial infarction, cardiac mortality being 5·4% during the first two months. The results suggest that, before discharge from hospital, patients at high risk of early death can be easily separated from a very low risk group, and so could be subjected to appropriate non-invasive and invasive examinations and active intervention, including coronary risk factor modification.

In a non-selected group of 1256 myocardial infarction patients, 37% died during the five year follow up.[22] A high risk group consisted of patients with signs of left heart failure and a history of two or more myocardial infarctions. Rehabilitation programmes including physical exercise have been shown to be feasible in these patients.[7,8]

Anterior infarction, ventricular dysfunction, ventricular premature beats and Q wave infarction

A five year follow up of 940 patients was carried out by Davis et al[23] in order to identify subsets of patients with different survival patterns. A combination of anterior infarction with left ventricular dysfunction and ventricular premature depolarisation identified a high risk subset, which made up 15% of the myocardial infarction populations. This group had six month and three year survival rates of 85 and 70%, respectively. A low risk subset that made up 24% of the population was identified by the absence of three of the above factors; three year survival in these patients was 94%. The authors concluded that the intermediate and high risk groups seemed to have the greatest potential for mortality reduction by appropriate interventions, including rehabilitation.

Comparison of Q wave and non-Q wave myocardial infarction has indicated that patients with a non-Q wave infarction have a significantly higher rate of re-infarction than patients with a Q wave.[24] In this study, there were no differences, basis of Q wave status, in coronary heart disease death rates. Subjects with an initial Q wave infarction had a higher rate of subsequent congestive heart failure, while those with non-Q wave infarctions had a significantly higher rate of coronary insufficiency. Subjects with a history of hypertension prior to an initial myocardial infarction were at particularly high risk of re-infarction. Because of the greater morbidity and mortality, subjects with initial non-Q wave myocardial infarction need non-invasive and invasive examinations and, later on, close follow up. The study indicated that they could apparently benefit from a supervised exercise rehabilitation programme, including risk factor intervention.

Serum cholesterol, smoking, and other risk factors

The coronary drug project included 2789 men who had sustained at least one myocardial infarction. The mortality from all causes was 21·2%[25] during a five year follow up period. Serum cholesterol was among the 10 baseline variables that were most strongly related to death from all causes. Baseline cholesterol and smoking were positively related to the risk of four major end points: death from all causes, sudden cardiovascular death, coronary death, and coronary death or definite non-fatal myocardial infarction. There was a possible weak association between moderate or vigorous physical activity and decreased mortality during the next five years. These findings suggested a potential benefit of lowering serum cholesterol, taking physical exercise, and stopping cigarette smoking after recovery from one or more myocardial infarctions. These data are important from the point of view of secondary prevention, suggesting that these patients should be included in a health education and exercise programme.

Low ejection fraction, ventricular ectopy, low functional class, and rales in the lungs

The study by the multicenter postinfarction research group, consisting of 866 patients after acute myocardial infarction, found four independent risk factors predicting mortality: an ejection fraction below 0·40, ventricular ectopy of 10 or more per hour, advanced New York Heart Association functional class, and rales heard in the upper two thirds of the lung fields.[26] Various combinations of these four factors identified five risk subgroups with two year mortality rates ranging from 3% (no factors) to 60% (all four factors).

Hypertension

Blood pressure after myocardial infarction was investigated in the Framingham study.[27] Hypertensive patients had almost three times the mortality of normotensive patients. Blood pressure after myocardial infarction was unrelated to survival over the next five years. A decrease in blood pressure suggested a severely damaged myocardium. Confusion about the prognostic role of blood pressure after myocardial infarction derives from failure to separate subjects whose blood pressure is low due to severe myocardial damage from those who have always had low blood pressure.

Three-vessel disease and ejection fraction

Patients with three-vessel disease were followed up for a mean of 43 months in a study by Castaner et al.[28] The ejection fraction was identified as the only predictor of survival (p < 0·001). Patients were stratified in risk categories according to the ejection fraction. The four-year relative probability of survival was 1·0 in participants with an ejection fraction of ⩾50%, 0·77 in those with an ejection fraction of 21–49%, and 0·22 in patients with more severe left ventricular dysfunction and an ejection fraction of <20%. A normal ejection fraction was found in about 25% of infarct survivors with three-vessel disease. This subset of patients had a low incidence of early and intermediate range coronary events.

Influence of thrombolytic therapy

A study by Volpi et al aimed to determine whether and to what extent the available information and proposed prognostic criteria are applicable in the thrombolytic era.[29] The patient population consisted of 10 219 survivors of myocardial infarction. In the group originally allocated to streptokinase therapy, a 24% reduction in post-discharge six month mortality was seen. Ineligibility for exercise testing, early left ventricular failure, and recovery-phase left ventricular dysfunction were the most powerful predictors of mortality among these patients. The lack of an independent adverse influence of early postmyocardial infarction angina on six month survival represents a major difference between this study and those of the pre-thrombolytic era.

Psychological and social indicators of new cardiac events

Several studies have examined the relation between psychosocial factors and recurrent cardiac events. An extensive analysis of social and psychological predictors of sudden cardiac death has been made using data from the recurrent coronary prevention project, a prospective trial of 1012 postinfarction patients.[30] The "no recurrence" group was compared with the sudden cardiac death, non-sudden cardiac death, and non-fatal recurrence groups. Type A behaviour score was an independent predictor of sudden, but not of non-sudden, cardiac death. The authors of this study considered that the likely pathophysiological mechanism of this association is that patients with type A behaviour have a greater sympathetic response to a given environmental stressor, and this sympathetic response makes the heart more vulnerable to ventricular

118

fibrillation. This conclusion is in accordance with a recent finding that a long term comprehensive rehabilitation programme decreases the neuroadrenergic activity, the arrhythmogenic effect of catecholamines and, consequently, the incidence of ventricular arrhythmias.[31]

The prognostic importance of somatic and psychosocial variables in patients who had had their first infarction was studied by Wiklund et al in 201 consecutive infarction patients.[32] Age, marital status, previous emotional complaints, and educational level were recorded at the time of myocardial infarction. Two to three months after the infarction emotional instability, preoccupation with health, pessimism, subjective cardiac complaints, subjective emotional complaints, neuroticism, frequency of self assessed chest pain, life dissatisfaction, and use of sedatives were recorded. Three types of indices were studied: the severity of the infarction, a myocardial infarction recurrence index including history of angina pectoris and hypertension, maximum serum aspartate aminotransferase level during the hospital phase, and smoking status after the infarction. Being single increased risk of death and all events, whereas an index reflecting infarction size was correlated to risk of death only. Early identification of patients who have both phychosocial and medical risk factors is important. Special attention should be directed toward single patients, who lack social support, for example by means of offering more frequent appointments and referral to groups for physical exercise and counselling.

Type A behaviour and baseline anxiety were analysed by comparing the three end point groups—(a) no complications, (b) hospitalised due to angina pectoris, angioplasty, or bypass surgery, and (c) recurrent myocardial infarction or cardiac death. It was found that the level of anxiety was significantly higher in patients who had suffered a fatal or non-fatal cardiac event during the year after the initial infarction.[33] Anxiety may be an indicator of a poor coping style, which should be given due attention as part of a rehabilitation programme.

High stress has been associated with an almost threefold increase in risk of cardiac mortality over five years and an approximately 1·5–fold increase in risk of non-fatal infarction over the same period.[34] The results of Frasure-Smith's study[34] suggested that the patients who benefit most from interventions to alter this risk factor could and should be identified before hospital discharge.

The outcome of group psychotherapy has been reviewed by Kolman.[35] Positive findings included modification of type A behaviour, increased employment, fewer re-infarctions, and less social isolation. Negative findings were increased anxiety and raised serum cholesterol.

Friedman et al studied 862 post-myocardial infarction patients selected randomly from a group that received cardiologic counselling on the commonly accepted risk factors and a group that received both the above and type A behaviour counselling.[36] Reduction of type A behaviour at the end of three years was observed in 44% of the participants. The three year cumulative cardiac recurrence rate was 7·2% in participants who initially were enrolled to receive cardiologic and type A behavioural counselling. This was significantly less than that (13%) observed in participants who initially were enrolled to receive only cardiologic counselling.

Coping with myocardial infarction has been reviewed by Wiklund et al.[37] They pointed out that the high incidence of emotional disturbance, pessimism, self reported symptoms, avoidance behaviour, and sexual decline indicate that a majority of the patients unjustifiably consider themselves severely impaired both during convalescence and one year after myocardial infarction. The authors emphasised the importance of comprehensive rehabilitation. Selection criteria for rehabilitation should include emotional instability before and after the myocardial infarction, concern about health, resisting angina pectoris, and a pessimistic and displeased attitude. Post-myocardial infarction adjustment can benefit from psychological measures, which should be especially included since psychological reactions are of greater significance and may be easier to prevent than cardiac dysfunction.

Conroy et al studied 299 consecutive male patients aged under 60 years in order to examine the relationship between social class and initial risk factors, change in risk factors at one year follow up, return to work, and three year mortality.[38] A significant positive correlation was found between smoking on admission and social class. Lower class patients also had a significantly higher weekly alcohol intake. Mean in-hospital blood pressure was higher in lower class patients. No relationship was found as to the amount of leisure exercise, serum cholesterol, or degree of overweight. There were highly significant associations between social class and successful smoking cessation, increase in leisure exercise, and weight reduction over the first year after discharge. There was no significant association between social class and three year mortality, a correlation which has been found by others—for example, Ruberman et al.[39]

The support provided by a person's social network may be related to the incidence of coronary artery disease.[40] Enhanced support may improve adherence to more healthy nutritional and exercise habits. It has been recommended by Davidson[40] that future research should aim to develop a behavioural risk profile analogous to the physiological risk profile concept that has been helpful in managing patients' risk for cardiac events and the recurrence of such events. In order to identify these high risk patients a type of screening method would also have to be developed to enable us to identify patients who need to strengthen their social network.

With the present state of knowledge it is difficult to reach agreement on the prognostic role of psychosocial variables due to insufficient numbers of patients in controlled studies. No doubt, risk stratification based on the relevant psychosocial variables would be of help in planning psychosocial rehabilitation in cardiac patients.

Indicators used in risk stratification of patients with acute myocardial infarction

HISTORY AND CLINICAL FINDINGS

- Severity of infarction - assessed from enzyme levels, congestive heart failure symptoms, physical working capacity, and ischaemia signs during exercise testing - is one of the most important risk indicators

- A history of angina pectoris or previous myocardial infarction is an important risk indicator

- The presence of contraindications to exercise testing (mainly heart failure) indicates high risk, and exercise testing can distinguish high and very low risk patients (however, its low sensitivity and specificity are such that it should be reserved for specific indications)

ELECTROCARDIOGRAPHIC CHARACTERISTICS

- The ECG site of the infarction has prognostic significance: one-year mortality is higher in anterior than in inferior myocardial infarction

- Persistent ST segment depression ($\geqslant 1$mm) in the first few days increases mortality threefold

- Combined anterior infarction, ventricular premature beats, and signs of left ventricular dysfunction identifies a high risk subset of patients

- In non-Q wave infarction the re-infarction rate is significantly higher than in Q wave infarction; Q wave infarction predicts a higher rate of subsequent congestive heart failure, and non-Q wave a higher rate of coronary insufficiency

CONVENTIONAL RISK FACTORS

- High serum cholesterol and smoking increase death from all causes, sudden cardiovascular death, coronary death, and non-fatal myocardial infarction

- An ejection fraction below 40%, ventricular ectopy of $\geqslant 10$/hour, advanced New York Heart Association functional class, and rales in the upper two-thirds of the lung fields are independent risk factors for mortality

- A history of hypertension is linked with a threefold rise in mortality

- Low physical activity is weekly associated with mortality

- Type A behaviour is an independent predictor of sudden cardiac death, and high stress has been associated with an almost threefold increase in cardiac deaths

Summary

Risk stratification is useful in planning an individual rehabilitation programme and assessing the need for non-invasive and invasive examinations. The somatic and psychosocial variables are briefly reviewed and discussed here, paying special attention to factors indicating a high, intermediate, or low risk after hospitalisation.

In the recommendations by the working group on rehabilitation of the European Society of Cardiology it has been pointed out that we are unable to predict the progression of coronary artery disease.[41] Consequently, the risk stratification should be based on the severity of myocardial damage assuming stable or slowly progressive coronary artery disease. The measurable determinants of the outcome of patients with established ischaemic heart disease, mentioned in the report of the European working group, are the degree of left ventricular dysfunction, the severity of myocardial ischaemia, the presence of threatening arrhythmias, and associated conditions that may aggravate the ischaemic disease or favour its expression. Prognostic resting variables of left ventricular dysfunction include, above all, left ventricular ejection fraction of $\leqslant 40\%$, wall motion abnormalities of $\geqslant 45\%$, and increased left ventricular end systolic and diastolic volumes. Many prognostic parameters, such as ST depression after an acute myocardial infarction determined by resting ECG, are easily available. Exercise testing reveals the extent and severity of inducible myocardial ischaemia.

Risk stratification and return to work

Return to work after acute myocardial infarction, coronary artery bypass graft surgery, and percutaneous transluminal coronary angioplasty is considered to be a major objective of cardiac rehabilitation. While about two thirds of patients have a clinically mild infarction,[42] there is always a risk of recurrent coronary events, which causes anxiety for patients and their families. DeBusk et al[42] suggested that exercise testing be performed soon after myocardial infarction because it has considerable prognostic significance, especially in patients with clinically mild myocardial infarction. A normal test may relieve the anxiety and thus motivate return to work.

After an acute myocardial infarction, patients who were over 50 years of age, who had experienced cardiac complications, and who had a physical working capacity less than 100 W have been reported to be less likely to return to work than younger patients. In this study the rehabilitation programme improved the rate of return to work in patients belonging to a low social class and in those who had a strenuous job.[43]

The determinants of return to work after cardiac events include medical, psychological, sociodemographic, economic, and cultural factors.[44] Patients' perception of present health and medical risk may be the strongest predictor of return to work. The medical community can thus have a strong impact on return to work. A need for better physician education exists, particularly in avoiding placing unnecessary physical restrictions on patients whose hospital course and early evaluations suggest that they are at a low risk for recurrence of a cardiac event. Individualisation of cardiac rehabilitation services by an interdisciplinary team is essential.

Sheldahl *et al* emphasised a prescription for exercise conditioning, which may result in physiological and psychological benefits that enhance the patient's ability to resume work.[45] They pointed out that potential occupational problem areas may be improved through medical treatment, surgical treatment, or rehabilitation procedures such as exercise training courses. As pointed out earlier, exercise testing has proved to be of considerable value in helping health professionals to develop realistic occupational and non-occupational activity recommendations for cardiac patients. Sheldahl *et al* emphasised that an exercise training course may restore patient's work tolerance so that they will be able to resume occupational work within 4–12 weeks of hospital discharge.

Psychological predictors for return to work after a myocardial infarction have been studied by Mæland and Havik.[46] Patients' in-hospital expectations of their future work capacity proved to be a strong predictor of return to work. Findings support the view that the patient's role in the coping and readaptation after the acute event is important. Early return to physical activity could lead to less pessimistic expectations of future physical ability and more rapid resumption of previous physical activities.

Education, physical activity associated with employment, severity of myocardial infarction, and perception of health status have been found to be important independent variables in predicting return to work.[47]

A randomised trial on early return to work after uncomplicated myocardial infarction was designed by Dennis *et al*[48] to study whether the interval between uncomplicated myocardial infarction and return to work could be shortened by the following: (a) identifying patients at low risk for cardiac events, (b) demonstrating a well preserved physical capacity, and (c) providing explicit advice regarding prognosis, physical capacity, and return to work to patients and to their primary physicians. The intervention included pre-discharge risk stratification, early treadmill testing, and explicit medical advice. The study confirmed the results of previous studies, demonstrating that the majority of patients eligible for exercise testing after myocardial infarction have no prognostically significant abnormalities during treadmill testing and accordingly have low rates of cardiac events during follow up.

Early discharge followed by early rehabilitation and return to work after acute myocardial infarction was studied by Saeterhaug and Nygaard.[49] They concluded that a successful rehabilitation can be achieved by a thorough explanation to the patient and his family of his illness and the problems he will meet among friends, relatives, and employers. Early mobilisation and discharge from the hospital and individualised treatment with early rehabilitation after acute myocardial infarction have made it possible to get a large number of the patients to return to work quickly.

A report on guidelines for assessing occupational working capacity in patients with ischaemic heart disease has been published by Haskell et al.[50] They proposed that evaluation for return to work can be performed within five weeks after medically uncomplicated myocardial infarction, seven weeks after coronary artery bypass graft surgery, and one week after successful coronary angioplasty. The recommendations of this group stressed the importance of early evaluation of occupational working capacity, including an exercise test and, in the case of uninterpretable exercise test, further non-invasive testing to establish the safe working capacity.

Patients' expectations, during hospitalisation, of their future work capacity have been indicated to be strong predictors for return to work.[51] Based on results of a randomised trial, it was suggested that the clinically uncomplicated cases who underwent an occupational work evaluation three weeks after myocardial infarction returned to work earlier than patients who received usual care. The majority of patients eligible for exercise testing after myocardial infarction were shown to have low rates of cardiac events during follow up.

In summary, it has been proposed that return-to-work evaluation can be performed within five weeks after medically uncomplicated myocardial infarction. Participating in an exercise test is considered to give the most useful information in assessing occupational working capacity.

Summary

Since the American cardiologists Levine and Lown published their experiences on early mobilisation and "armchair" treatment in 1952, cardiac rehabilitation has made immense progress. The selection criteria for participation in a formal exercise rehabilitation programme have favoured patients with low risk for new cardiac events. According to present practice, this group of patients can exercise unsupervised in health education programmes, which are less costly. Supervised exercise rehabilitation can thus be reserved for patients with intermediate or moderately high risk of a new cardiac event.

Risk stratification is a helpful tool for planning exercise rehabilitation or further invasive or non-invasive examinations. Supervised formal exercise rehabilitation can be compared with medication, prescribed when needed.

Secondary prevention, including risk factor modification and drug treatment, is an important part of comprehensive rehabilitation. As high total cholesterol and low high density lipoprotein cholesterol values are risk factors for recurrent coronary events, they should be attacked vigorously, together with antismoking campaign and treatment of high blood pressure.

Cardiac rehabilitation has often been used as a synonym for exercise training. However, it is important to emphasise that the development of atherosclerosis, thrombosis, and the damage to the heart muscle are multifactorial processes that have to be approached in a comprehensive way and according to the needs of the individual patient.

Psychological and social factors play an important role in everyday life. It is no wonder that they play a role in the development of coronary artery disease both before and after a coronary event. There have been attempts to develop risk stratification based on various psychological and social variables, such as stress, anxiety, living alone, and lack of a good social network. Attempts to develop risk stratification to help rehabilitation planning may encounter difficulties due to the cultural and other national differences. In principle it seems possible, however.

Return to work has often been considered the main goal and outcome measure of cardiac rehabilitation. It is well known that return to work has medical, psychological, and social determinants. Risk stratification, based on medical variables recorded before discharge from hospital, is recommended as it would help in planning return to work when the medical background including an exercise test result is clear. Patients in the low risk group can usually return to work without any formal rehabilitation programme, while those at intermediate or high risk would receive benefit from formal exercise rehabilitation.

References

1 Levine SA, Lown B. Armchair treatment of acute coronary thrombosis. *JAMA* 1952; **148**: 1365–9.
2 Swan HJC, Blackburn HW, DeSanetis R, *et al.* Duration of hospitalization in "uncomplicated completed acute myocardial infarction". *Am J Cardiol* 1976; **37**: 413–19.
3 Task Force of the Working Group on Cardiac Rehabilitation of the European Society of Cardiology. Cardiac rehabilitation: definition and goals. *Eur Heat J* 1992; **13** (suppl C): 1–2.
4 Lipkin DP. Is cardiac rehabilitation necessary [editorial]? *Br Heart J* 1991; **65**: 237–8.
5 DeBusk RF, Kraemer HC, Nash E, Berger WE, Lew H. Stepwise risk stratification soon after acute myocardial infarction. *Am J Cardiol* 1983; **52**: 1161–6.
6 Murray DP, Salih M, Tan LB, Murray RG, Littler WA. Prognostic stratification of patients after myocardial infarction. *Br Heart J* 1987; **57**: 313–18.
7 Conn EH, Williams RS, Wallace AG. Exercise responses before and after physical

conditioning in patients with severely depressed left ventricular dysfunction. *Am J Cardiol* 1982; **49**: 296–300.

8 Coats AJS, Adamopoulos S, Meyer TE, Conway J, Sleight P. Effects of physical training in chronic heart failure. *Lancet* 1990; **335**: 63–6.

9 Kallio V, Hämäläinen H, Hakkila J, Luurila O. Reduction in sudden deaths by a multifactorial intervention programme after acute myocardial infarction, *Lancet* 1979; **2**: 1091–4.

10 Cintron GB. After the infarct: what? *Cardiovasc Rev Rep* 1984; **5**: 665–77.

11 Pryor DB, Bruce RA, Chaitman BR, *et al.* Task Force I: determination of prognosis in patients with ischaemic heart disease. *J Am Coll Cardiol* 1989; **14**: 1016–25.

12 Peel AAF, Semple T, Wang I, Lancaster WM, Dall JLG. A coronary prognostic index for grading the severity of infarction. *Br Heart J* 1962; **24**: 745–60.

13 Norris RM, Caughey DE, Mercer C-C, Scott PJ. Prognosis after myocardial infarction. Six-year follow-up. *Br Heart J* 1974; **36**: 786–90.

14 Grande P, Christiansen C, Pedersen A. Influence of acute myocardial infarct size on acute and one-year mortality. *Eur Heart J* 1983; **4**: 20–5.

15 Mulcahy R, Hickey N, Graham I, McKenzie G. Factors influencing long-term prognosis in male patients surviving a first coronary attack. *Br Heart J* 1975; **37**: 156–65.

16 Herlitz J, Hjalmarson Å, Waldenström J. Five-year mortality rate in relation to enzyme-estimated infarct size in acute myocardial infarction. *Am Heart J* 1987; **114**: 731–7.

17 De Backer GG, Weyne T, Derese A. Prognostic value of exercise testing: a 6-year follow-up in postmyocardial infarction patients. *Cardiology* 1981; **68** (suppl 2): 71–7.

18 Tibbits PA, Evaul JE, Goldstein RE, *et al.* Serial acquisition of data to predict one-year mortality rate after acute myocardial infarction. *Am J Cardiol* 1987; **60**: 451–5.

19 Hands ME, Lloyd BL, Robinson JS, De Klerk N, Thompson PL. Prognostic significance of electrocardiographic site of infarction after correction for enzymatic size of infarction. *Circulation* 1986; **73**: 885–91.

20 Gheorghiade M, Shivkumar K, Schultz L, Jafri S, Tilley B, Goldstein S. Prognostic significance of electrocardiographic persistent ST depression in patients with their first myocardial infarction in the placebo arm of the Beta-Blocker Heart Attack Trial. *Am Heart J* 1993; **126**: 271–8.

21 Cleempoel H, Vainsel H, Bernard R, *et al.* Predictors of early death after acute myocardial infarction: two months follow-up. *Eur Heart J* 1986; **7**: 305–11.

22 Henning R, Wedel H. The long-term prognosis after myocardial infarction: a five year follow-up study. *Eur Heart J* 1981; **2**: 65–74.

23 Davis HT, DeCamilla J, Bayer LW, Moss AJ. Survivorship patterns in the posthospital phase of myocardial infarction. *Circulation* 1979; **60**: 1252–8.

24 Berger CJ, Murabito JM, Evans JC, Anderson KM, Levy D. Prognosis after first myocardial infarction. Comparison of Q-wave and non-Q-wave myocardial infarction in the Framingham Heart study. *'JAMA* 1992; **268**: 1545–51.

25 Schlant RC, Forman S, Stamler J, Canner PL. The natural history of coronary heart disease: prognostic factors after recovery from myocardial infarction in 2789 men. The 5-year findings of the Coronary Drug Project. *Circulation* 1982; **66**: 401–14.

26 The Multicenter Postinfarction Research Group. Risk stratification and survival after myocardial infarction. *N Engl J Med* 1983; **309**: 331–6.

27 Kannel WB, Sorlie P, Castelli WP, McGee D. Blood pressure and survival after myocardial infarction: the Framingham Study. *Am J Cardiol* 1980; **45**: 326–30.

28 Castaner A, Betriu A, Roig E, *et al.* Clinical course and risk stratification of myocardial infarct survivors with three-vessel disease. *Am Heart J* 1986; **112**: 1201–9.

29 Volpi A, De Vita C, Franzosi MG, *et al.* Determinants of 6–month mortality in survivors of myocardial infarction after thrombolysis. Results of the GISSI-2 data base. *Circulation* 1993; **88**: 416–29.

30 Thoresen CE, Friedman M, Gill JK, Ulmer DK. The recurrent coronary prevention project. Some preliminary findings. *Acta Med Scand* 1982; **660** (suppl): 172–92.

31 Hertzeanu HL, Shemesh J, Aron LA, *et al.* Ventricular arrhythmias in rehabilitated and nonrehabilitated postmyocardial infarction patients with left ventricular dysfunction. *Am J Cardiol* 1993; **71**: 24–7.

32 Wiklund I, Oden A, Sanne H, Ulvenstam G, Wilhelmsson C, Wilhelmsen L. Prognostic

importance of somatic and psychosocial variables after a first myocardial infarction. *Am J Epidemiol* 1988; **128**: 786–95.

33 Julkunen J, Idänpään-Heikkilä U, Saarinen T. Type A behaviour, anxiety and the first-year prognosis of a myocardial infarction. In: Schmidt LR, Schwenkmezger P, Weinman J, Maes S, editors. *Theoretical and applied aspects of health psychology.* New York: Harwood Academic Publishers, 1990.

34 Frasure-Smith N. In-hospital symptoms of psychological stress as predictors of long-term outcome after acute myocardial infarction in men. *Am J Cardiol* 1991; **67**: 121–7.

35 Kolman PBR. The value of group psychotherapy after myocardial infarction: a critical review. *J Cardiol Rehabil* 1983; **3**: 360–6.

36 Friedman M, Thoresen CE, Gill JJ, *et al.* Alteration of type A behavior and reduction in cardiac recurrences in postmyocardial infarction patients. *Am Heart J* 1984; **108**: 237–48.

37 Wiklund I, Sanne H, Vedin A, Wilhelmsson C. Coping with myocardial infarction: a model with clinical applications, a literature review. *Int Rehabil Med* 1985; **7**: 167–75.

38 Conroy RM, Cahill S, Mulcahy R, Johnson H, Graham IM, Hickey N. The relation of social class to risk factors, rehabilitation, compliance and mortality in survivors of acute coronary heart disease. *Scand J Soc Med* 1986; **14**: 51–6.

39 Ruberman W, Weinblatt E, Goldberg JD, Chaudhary BS. Psychosocial influences on mortality after myocardial infarction. *N Engl J Med* 1984; **311**: 552–9.

40 Davidson DM. Social support and cardiac rehabilitation: a review. *J Cardiopulmonary Rehabil* 1987; **7**: 196–200.

41 Task Force of the Working Group on Cardiac Rehabilitation of the European Society of Cardiology. Risk of cardiac events (in patients with established ischaemic heart disease). *Eur Heart J* 1992; **13** (suppl C): 14–19.

42 DeBusk RF, Domanico L, Luft HS, Harrison DC. Return to work following myocardial infarction: a medical and economic critique of the work evaluation unit [editorial]. *J Chron Dis* 1977; **30**: 325–30.

43 Velasco JA, Tormo V, Ridocci F, Grima A. From Spain: return to work after a comprehensive cardiac rehabilitation program. *J Cardiac Rehabil* 1983; **3**: 725–8.

44 Davidson DM. Return to work after cardiac events: a review. *J Cardiac Rehabil* 1983; **3**: 60–9.

45 Sheldahl LM, Wilke NA, Tristani FE. Exercise prescription for return to work. *J Cardiopulmonary Rehabil* 1985; **5**: 567–75.

46 Mæland JG, Havik OE. Psychological predictors for return to work after a myocardial infarction. *J Psychosom Res* 1987; **31**: 471–81.

47 Smith GR, O'Rourke DF. Return to work after a first myocardial infarction. A test of multiple hypotheses. *JAMA* 1988; **259**: 1673–7.

48 Dennis C, Houston-Miller N, Schwatz RG, *et al.* Early return to work after uncomplicated myocardial infarction. Results of a randomized trial. *JAMA* 1988; **260**: 214–20.

49 Saeterhaug A, Nygaard P. Early discharge and early rehabilitation and return to work after acute myocardial infarction. *J Cardiopulmonary Rehabil* 1989; **7**: 268–72.

50 Haskell WL, Brachfeld N, Bruce RA, *et al.* Task Force II: Determination of occupational working capacity in patients with ischaemic heart disease. *J Am Coll Cardiol* 1989; **14**: 1025–34.

51 Engblom E, Hämäläinen H, Rönnemaa T, Vänttinen E, Kallio V, Knuts L-R. Cardiac rehabilitation and return to work after coronary artery bypass surgery. *Quality of Life Research* 1994; **3**: 207–13.

6 Rehabilitation after cardiac surgery

JEAN-PAUL BROUSTET AND HERVÉ DOUARD

Introduction

The methods and results of rehabilitation following coronary artery bypass graft (CABG), percutaneous transluminal coronary angioplasty (PTCA), and other forms of cardiac surgery vary from country to country and depend on the availability of facilities for cardiac rehabilitation, which in turn depends on the strength (or weakness) of the local economy and medical services in general. Outcome also depends on the preoperative status of the patient. In countries where interventional cardiology and cardiac surgery are performed on a large scale, such as in Western Europe and the United States, cardiac patients usually undergo PTCA, CABG, or valve replacement early on in the course of their disease and before the occurrence of severe impairment or cardiac failure. Postoperative recovery of these patients is therefore more straightforward than for a patient who has had a long wait before surgery. Patients in the latter category often suffer from advanced cardiac failure.

In economically developed countries, the age of those undergoing CABG or valve replacement is steadily increasing and it is not always possible for elderly people to undertake physical training (simply because of their age): in any case, their need for a high level of physical activity is obviously reduced. They are nevertheless faced with a need to maintain their physical autonomy, and therefore their independence, as long as possible, in order to put off admission to a nursing home or complete dependency on the family. In addition, in elderly patients, psychological and neurological disorders are much more common after cardiac surgery. Assessment of these factors and corrective treatment are the main features of rehabilitation for this category of patient.

For younger patients who have not retired, the ultimate aim of cardiac surgery is obviously to return to work. The rate of return depends on a number of factors, and an accurate knowledge of these is necessary in order to understand why, after successful operation and a satisfactory exercise test, patients may be reluctant to resume their previous occupations.

To maintain the results obtained either by surgery or by PTCA, and to control long term risk factors, secondary prevention is fundamental, and this involves educating the patient.

In this chapter, we will discuss these different points in the light of our 20 years' experience in cardiac rehabilitation. We do not intend to present flow charts or rigid steps to be followed: rehabilitation depends more on social aspects and availability of resources than on pure science. Nor do we intend to present an exhaustive overview of the literature on rehabilitation, as the finding of evaluations are inconsistent and because to do so would be repetitive.

After surgery there are three phases, the first of which is the patient's admission to rehabilitation, or the assessment phase. The second phase concerns the rehabilitation process proper—that is, training and teaching. The third phase is the return to daily life. For patients who are still active, this means return to work. For all patients, it means secondary prevention and as active a life as possible.

Let us first of all look at phase I, the assessment phase, and when it should be scheduled. Depending on local facilities, and after a stay of 5–10 days in postoperative care, patients are discharged either to their homes or to a recovery clinic (what is called a sanatorium in Eastern Europe) for a stay of two to six weeks. The optimum time for preliminary assessment, before physical training begins, is around the 10th day after the operation (the 15th in cases in which complications have arisen). Earlier than this, many patients are still suffering from anaemia, haematoma, and pleural and/or pericardial effusion, all of which impair their ability to train, and the electrocardiogram (ECG) may show signs of pericarditis.

Concerning ECG abnormalities, one of the main difficulties for the rehabilitation team is to separate out those which may follow on from the surgical procedure from those which existed prior to surgery. A common complaint to be heard among rehabilitation teams is the lack of accurate and detailed information about the pre- and postoperative status of patients who are discharged from surgical departments. The preoperative report and the data which led to the decision to undertake surgery are not always transmitted to them. For example, echocardiographic data, the preoperative ECG at rest, and the results of the exercise test (if any) are often missing. However, whether pre- or postoperative, abnormalities have to be identified and quantified.

Coronary artery bypass graft

Cardiac status

Some of the abnormalities of cardiac status that we shall be looking at are due to arrhythmia: sinus tachycardia, supraventricular arrhythmias, ventricular arrhythmia, heart failure, and myocardial ischaemia or are concerned with pericardial impairment.

Sinus tachycardia

Although not a real complication sinus tachycardia is a constant. It is the result of a deregulation of the autonomic nervous system due to the patient's excessive adrenergic status. The causes are many: for example, duration and amount of preoperative bed rest and period of physical inactivity, and postoperative insomnia (some patients appear to present hyperthyroidosis with a rhythm that is usually 100 to 110 beats/min. In most cases, β blocking agents are recommended but, when possible, the first exercise test should be carried out before these are administered.

Sinus tachycardia is sometimes brought on or aggravated by one of four factors: anxiety (which decreases in importance as the patient talks about it and is reassured), hypovolaemia (in elderly patients who have been given too many diuretics and who lose their sensation of thirst), unnecessary vasodilator drugs, and anaemia (which has become much more frequent since blood transfusions began to be avoided except where necessary for a better and more prompt recovery). Apart from these benign causes one should always be on the look out for cardiac failure, pulmonary embolism, pericardial effusions, and infectious diseases.

Supraventricular arrhythmias

Transitory atrial fibrillation is a common form of supraventricular arrhythmia, which is encountered in about 20% of coronary patients,[1-3] particularly among those who were deprived of β blocking drugs at time of surgery. It will be found in a higher percentage of valve replacement patients, especially those having undergone mitral valve surgery. It is triggered by the hyperadrenergic status already mentioned, by pericardial effusion, or by inflammation. The pre- and postoperative use of β blocking drugs is recommended here.[4] In cases in which sinus rhythm reappears, β blockers should be maintained for some weeks but not indefinitely. In cases of persistent atrial fibrillation (provided it is not long established or secondary to pre-existing left atrium enlargement), amiodarone in loading dosage is effective. However, a maintenance drug is not necessary, particularly in coronary patients. Anticoagulants should be maintained for at least six months, for as long as there is a possible risk of relapse.

After mitral valve repair or replacement, atrial fibrillation is common. In cases of longstanding preoperative atrial fibrillation, it is wise to wait three to six months before attempting a conversion to sinus rhythm and to check whether haemodynamic improvement and a decrease in left atrial dimension are obvious. Only then is a tentative reduction reasonable, even if the probability of success is low. Surprisingly, a large proportion of patients will remain is sinus rhythm for several years and the thrombotic risk will be substantially reduced. However, in such cases transoesophageal echocardiography is needed before any attempt at reduction. Such determination to restore and maintain a sinus rhythm is justified by haemodynamic data. During exercise, the loss of maximum cardiac output due to the absence of atrial contraction is in the range of 20–30% and this hampers the process and benefit of physical training.[5,6]

Ventricular arrhythmias

Monomorphic and isolated extrasystoles are common ventricular arrythmias occurring during the immediate postoperative period and will disappear in a few days, especially if the patient is given β blocking drugs. They do not constitute a contraindication to physical training.

If the extrasystoles increase in number, become closer to the previous R wave, or become polymorphic during the first exercise test or the first few training sessions, caution is needed, especially in patients with dyskinesia of a myocardial segment and/or poor pre- or postoperative left ventricular function.

Holter monitoring and/or telemetry may be necessary for such patients and their training sessions must be carefully monitored. If the symptoms persist after the patient has been prescribed β blocking drugs or amiodarone, a search for late potentials should be made. When such patients complain of dizziness or lipothymia, bouts of ventricular tachycardia should be suspected and a search for late potentials and/or Holter monitoring is necessary to identify the risk of ventricular tachycardia. Myocardial re-vascularisation should not be considered as appropriate preventive treatment for patients who have had an episode, or episodes, of ventricular tachycardia before surgery, especially when a postmyocardial infarction scar remains. In fact, ventricular arrhythmia is the main risk of controlled physical training.

Heart Failure

Preoperative congestive right heart failure has a poor prognosis. Physical training should be restricted to respiratory exercises and segmental musculation in an armchair.

Impairments of left ventricular function (contraction, active relaxation, or passive diastolic filling) are more common and are caused by many factors. One is the preoperative myocardial status (large myocardial infarction scar, well established hypertension, late intervention in valve replacement surgery). Others are to do with perioperative complications, such as a non-Q wave infarction camouflaged by the usual signs of pericarditis and a misinterpretation of the reduction in amplitude of R waves on precordial leads, or an anterior myocardial infarction after an emergency salvaging of an unsuccessful attempt at PTCA for unstable angina, or after a distal surgical endarteriectomy, needed because the distal bed is too small in diameter. Other possible causes are loss of contractility due to imperfect myocardial protection during extracorporeal circulation, arrhythmias such as atrial fibrillation, early closure of grafts, thrombosis, or early removal of prosthetic valves. Echocardiography and/ or exercise ventriculography with technetium-99m provide non-invasive measurements of heart failure and will help to define appropriate treatment. The exercise test will show two rather specific patterns of exercise-induced cardiac failure—that is firstly a poor exercise capacity compared to the elevation in blood pressure, and secondly a poor increase or even a decrease in systolic blood pressure in spite of the rapid increase in heart rate. In such cases β blockers might be proposed (with great caution); they can be continued only if a new exercise test demonstrates increasing exercise capacity without an increase in pulmonary congestion.

In the case of cardiac failure, angiotensin converting enzyme inhibitors, sometimes diuretics and often β blockers are necessary before launching a programme of moderate physical training. Very often, in spite of patient's heart failure at the outset of rehabilitation, there will be a big improvement in exercise capacity. A determination of peak VO_2 helps place the patient in the Weber classification, and this can be used as a benchmark for future tests. Surprisingly, many patients improve rapidly. They become asymptomatic and are able to follow a rehabilitation programme after a few weeks.

The occurrence of acute pulmonary oedema during exercise is very rare. There are three possible explanations: exercise-induced ischaemia, or arrhythmia, or both. In either case, training sessions must be stopped.

Myocardial ischaemia

The aim of a coronary bypass is usually to reduce or eradicate myocardial ischaemia and its consequences. In most cases, therefore, angina if not ischaemia should no longer be a handicap. But nobody is perfect, not even surgeons! Also the extent of coronary lesions is, more often than not such that grafting does not concern the totality of stenosed or occluded arteries. In many cases the anticipated programme of re-vascularisation is not completed. The diameter of the distal bed is found to be smaller than predicted, the prolongation of extracorporeal circulation is judged to be detrimental or, later on, an acute closure of the graft is not picked up because pre-established collateral circulation has preserved the area on which the occluded graft depends. Therefore, although angina is rarely present after surgery, silent ischaemia is frequent

Table 6.1 Symptoms, signs, and diagnostic comparisons before and after revascularisation†

Symptom	Before re-vascularisation	After re-vascularisation
Chest pain	Truly ischaemic?	Ischaemic? Parietal (painful and/or mobile thorax when coughing?) Worsening of pre-existing cervical arthrosis? Pleuropericardial pain?
Dyspnoea	Early shortness of breath (respiratory, muscular) or chest discomfort (cardiac failure and/or ischaemia)? Need for preoperative respiratory function test for reference (particularly for heavy smokers)	Excess weight? Prolonged (pre-operative) bed rest? Excess drugs (β blockers)?
Palpitations, extrasystoles	Many extrasystoles pre-date surgery (and even coronary heart disease)	If pre-operative abscence certain, consider perioperative myocardial infarction
Atrial fibrillation	Rare in heart disease patients; usually transitory	Frequent after surgery (20% of cases). Try at least one attempt at defibrillation
Dizziness, faintness	History of neurocirculatory asthenia or vagotonia or prolonged bed rest?	β Blockers?
Loss of memory	Rare before 65 years	Rare before 65 years but cases occur as a consequence of thrombotic microemboli during bypass
Fatigue	Not specific enough	Consider: Depression. Heart failure. Excess vasodilators or β blockers. Hepatitis?
Leg oedema	Excess vasodilators, heart failure or varicose veins	Same as preoperative? Loss of veins (grafts)? Pericardial constriction?
Pulmonary rales or gallop	Left heart failure	Left heart failure persistent? Aggravated (perioperative myocardial infarction)?
Hypertension	Unknown? Masked β blockers or calcium channel inhibitors?	Reappearance after withdrawal of antianginal medication
Leg arteries	Intermittent claudication masked by angina and bed rest	As preoperative
Complementary investigations		
ECG at rest	Were there Q waves and on what leads? Bundle branch block (L or R)? Reduction of R waves amplitude?	Identification of new Q waves? Subendocardial infarction?
Chest x ray	Heart enlargement? Emphysema? Other abnormalities	Comparative chest x ray: Pericardial effusion? Pleural effusion?
Echocardiography and Doppler	Left ventricular diastolic and systolic function? Valvular dysfunction?	As preoperative? Pericardial effusion?
Exercise stress test	Establish preoperative baseline, which may be: contraindication (what?) Masked by drugs. Not useful. Lost. Not done (why?—no reason not uncommon)	As preoperative. Perform test and compare maximum or critical values of: heart rate, systolic blood pressure, ST segment variations, exercise capacity, criteria for cessation (pain, fatigue, arrhythmia, claudication, lack of motivation)

†Comparisons should be made dispassionately, disregarding the surgeon's optimism.

at the time of the unmasked symptom-limited exercise test that is performed just before rehabilitation begins.

Table 6.1 summarises some of the questions that need to be asked. The answers should be as neutral and as objective as possible. The questions chosen are the result of considerable experience of the gap between surgeons' optimism and careful review of the patients using data from clinical examinations, echocardiography, and the unmasked exercise test.

Pericardial effusions

Among pericardial abnormalities, pericardial effusions are common. They disappear within a few weeks, leaving no haemodynamic or electrocardiographic trace. They are most frequently located around the inferior wall of the left ventricle and they can be identified by systematic echocardiography. In some cases they look like a cyst opposite the right cavities, especially the right atrium, and they are large enough to produce localised compression. Signs of right congestive failure may appear as well. In some rare cases, compression of the left atrium by a posterior haemorrhagic effusion may cause a pulmonary oedema.

Abundant, circumferential effusions are rare and might be aggravated by anticoagulants. The echocardiography and measurement of cutaneous pressure should be repeated. Physical training has to be postponed until after the effusion, which sometimes requires pericardial drainage, has disappeared.

Diagnosing tamponade is not easy since pallor is frequently attributed to anaemia, fatigue, and anorexia, which are all common in the postoperative period. Low blood pressure has many other possible explanations (for example bed rest, vasodilators, angiotensin converting enzyme inhibitors, and β blockers). One should always bear this possibility in mind. In such cases cessation of anticoagulants is recommended, unless the patient has had a valve replacement.

Pulmonary and pleural repercussions of surgery

Chest opening always has adverse consequences on respiratory function. There are three main types of event that can occur. Pleural extravasation is common but in most cases disappears spontaneously. It sometimes recurs with loculation and symphysis; breathing is painful. Paralysis of a hemidiaphragm is not uncommon. Although it is not painful, it will reduce the maximum tidal flow and would, in some cases, explain shortness of breath during training. Localised areas of atelectasis are also common. The final result of these events is a restrictive respiratory insufficiency.

Secondary prevention after surgery

After surgery, the progression of coronary lesions is obvious and the bypassed lesions are the first concerned. More than 70% of stenoses will progress to complete occlusion within six months of surgical procedure. Should an occlusion or stenosis of the graft occur, the patient's situation will be even more critical than prior to surgery. The main bypassed arteries may be either angiographically normal, or show mild, isolated, or diffused stenosis.

The control of risk factors has not proved to be effective in preventing graft occlusion. However, cessation of smoking is vital to the preservation of a good prognosis. The coronary artery surgery study[7] reported that the benefit of surgery was totally cancelled out in smokers and the same was observed in re-stenosis after PTCA.[8]

No rehabilitation programme is complete without teaching about one of the greatest risk factors—smoking. In our experience, cessation of smoking is common after CABG, when motivation is stronger than after PTCA. The stay in hospital and in recovery clinics (in France, at least), makes total withdrawal easier, and this is still the only successful way to stop smoking. A very real risk of relapse occurs after three to six months: memories of the operation have vanished and the patient is asymptomatic and active. The most common causes of relapse are psychological stress (occupational or social) and consumption of alcohol, especially during and/or after a good meal with good friends who smoke. Patients should be informed of the risk of being tempted to take up smoking again in this sort of situation.

The second risk, which sometimes occurs with the cessation of smoking, is putting on excess weight. Here too, motivation tends to decrease after six months: having to go out to a restaurant or eat in cafeterias and self service restaurants in the workplace favours excessive calorie intake. This risk is also common in women. If a second intervention should be necessary five to ten years later, the patient's condition will have worsened. Excess weight also probably increases the progression of coronary lesions. Patients must be made aware of these facts, which should be incorporated in the rehabilitation phase. The risk of diabetes becomes more frequent as age increases. It is also more frequent in patients who have a sedentary lifestyle and those who are overweight. We are accustomed to saying that coronary patients, especially those having undergone an operation, need to live like athletes, jockeys, or boxers: excess weight, lack of exercise, and smoking are all detrimental.

Return to work

It is well known that the rate of return to work depends on two factors: the length of time off work before surgery (if it is more than six months, the probability of returning to work after surgery is extremely low) and the duration of convalescence (those patients who have not returned to work six months after surgery are not likely to ever return to work).[9,10]

Surprisingly, there is no correlation between postoperative exercise capacity and the rate of return to work. The same has been observed after PTCA.[11-13]

Table 6.2 shows the main reasons that prevent return to work. Medical reasons play a modest part for most patients. Psychological and sociological factors carry much more weight. The level of social security

Table 6.2 Factors contributing to non-return to work.

Medical
   Extent of coronary lesions and left ventricular function
   Associated diseases
   Non-anginal thoracic pain
   Adverse effects of drugs
   Various and often contradictory advice of general practitioner, cardiologist, social services
      (and works doctor) about ability to work

Psychological
   Preoperative profile: anxiety, depression
   Effects of disease: anxiety, depression, poor coping
   Type A or B behaviour
   Dependency on alcohol or drugs

Perception of work before re-vascularisation
   Weariness, conflicts, lack of consderation, "syndrome of Peter"
   History of unemployment, dismissal or redundancy
   Previous reluctance to return to work after infarction (or surgery)
   Excess work considered responsible for the disease
   Spouse's opinion regarding past activity and return to work

Socioeconomic factors
   Age, sex, nearness to retirement age
   Level of education, training, and qualifications
   Balance between needs and sick pay availability
   nsurance in case of prolonged disease or infirmity
   Generous long duration (6 months) sick leave and pay
   Request for transfer refused by employers
   Re-education or re-training to more appropriate work not possible
   Level of unemployment and amount of unemployment compensation
   Impossibility of finding other suitable work, considering cardiovascular condition and
      professional qualifications (for example farmers)
   Employment regulations in special jobs (for example, pilots)
   Dismissal after long period of continuous absence (6 months)
   Inability of the service to re-employ handicapped persons

After coronary surgery
   Poor surgical outcome: early occlusion of graft(s)
   Perioperative myocardial infarction
   Long lasting and persistent chest pain secondary to thoracotomy; osteitis of sternum
   Depression regarding loss of health

After angioplasty
   Waiting for anticipated re-stenosis (30–50%)
   True re-stenosis, new percutaneous transluminal coronary angioplasty and second period
      of invalidity
   Bleeding secondary to anticoagulant therapy after stent implantation

coverage, the level of personal and/or complementary health insurance, the employment market, and how close the patient is to the legal retirement age are all factors that come into play.

In a study undertaken in our hospital, we found that out of 270 patients under 60 who were active before surgery, 70 went back to work within an average period of four months and 10 days.[10]

Follow up

When the preoperative, unmasked exercise test has been carried out and has shown strong ischaemia (that is low values of critical heart rate, exercise capacity, anginal pain, and important ST segment depression), the task is easy. The extent of correction of the abnormalities seen in the preoperative exercise test has to be checked at the beginning of follow up. All subsequent tests in the years to come will be compared with these figures.

A postoperative reference exercise test should be carried out at three months. Before this time, muscular weakness and pericardial effusions make an accurate assessment of the ECG and a true symptom-limited exercise test difficult.

The results of such an exercise test might be compared to those of a drug trial. Preoperative and future postoperative test criteria to be compared are: the critical maximum value of heart rate, blood pressure, double product, and ST segment depression; the relationship between the heart rate and the ST segment depression (if any); the duration of exercise and the heart rate at the same submaximum stage; the appearance of new Q waves on resting ECG and/or segment elevation on exercise ECG. Firm reference data are then available for future comparison. In cases where correction has been incomplete, considerable improvement can nevertheless be seen even when the exercise test remains abnormal. The task is much more delicate if the coronary bypass was performed without a preoperative exercise test (because of a justified or unjustified contra-indication such as recent infarction or unstable angina), or without cessation of powerful anti-ischaemic drugs, or when the preoperative ECG showed Q waves on multiple leads or left bundle branch block.

In all such cases, one has to ask if the poor exercise test result is due to the patient's preoperative status or early dysfunction of grafts. Thallium imaging may be helpful in these cases. In some instances a second exercise test after the prescription of antihypertensive, antiarrhythmic or antiischaemic drugs is useful for correct adjustment. Further exercise tests should be undertaken after six months, and annually thereafter. As far as possible, these tests should be performed after cessation of drugs so that comparison between pre- and postoperative exercise tests remains valid.

Such a programme will not predict or preclude an abrupt closure of the graft. Nevertheless, it is commonly observed that progression of lessions on native arteries, stenosis of the main graft, or closure of secondary grafts (right coronary, diagonal, or marginal) are very often detected after deterioration in the exercise test data of a patient who is still asymptomatic.

Physiotherapy and physical training after surgery

After the patient has been extubated and the suction drain and perfusion catheter have been removed, we recommend that the patient be encouraged to become mobile as early as possible in order to prevent thromboembolism. Strong bandages around the thorax and legs are also recommended if a saphenous graft was carried out. From the third to the fifth day, sitting upright on the edge of the bed and walking in the room is sufficient exercise for a start. But the physiotherapist should encourage breathing exercises and coughing to get bronchial secretions moving. All too often pleural and/or pericardial effusion and paralysis of the diaphragmatic cupola reduces the depth of respiration and delays the onset of active training.

After discharge, between days 6 and 10 after the operation, depending on local custom (and in cases without complications), the patient either goes home (in Britain and the United States for example) or moves to a recovery clinic (in France, Germany, and Italy). It is clearly a great advantage in terms of safety, clinical care, and efficiency of training if one can benefit from such clinics, where the staff are well-trained and specialised in the identification, prevention, and treatment of post-operative complications, rehabilitation, physical training, and teaching about secondary prevention.

Table 6.3 shows the aims and corresponding techniques of exercise training, with the appropriate time at which to schedule them in. First of all, disjunction of the sternum must be avoided, so wide open arm movements, even with light dumb-bells, must be done slowly and very carefully. Secondly, the rehabilitation team needs to assess the physical capacity of the patient as a whole and not restrict training to the respiratory system alone. The age of coronary bypass patients is increasing and they are reoperated more frequently. The preoperative rest period may be harmful for patients with severe disabling but stable angina, who have been on the waiting list for some time. Back pain, arthritis, intermittent claudication, and cervical arthrosis are common. Older smokers have restricted capacities: bronchial secretions cause repetitive coughing, which may jeopardise consolidation of the sternum.

Endurance training

Endurance training to improve aerobic capacity requires that the patient be able to sustain at least a daily session on a bicycle, treadmill, or walking uphill at a heart rate of at least 70% of predicted maximum. When

Table 6.3 Aims and techniques of exercise training.

Aims to improve	Technique	Postoperative period† Days 8-30	After day 30
Endurance capacity	Walk or slow jog for long periods	+	+ + +
Aerobic capacity	Endurance training at 70% of maximum predictive heart rate	+ +	+ + +
Muscular power	Sprint, dash, jump	Harmful and proscribed	Harmful and Proscribed
Muscular strength	Body building (successive segmental work recommended	+	+ + +
Respiratory capacity	Respiratory exercises	+ + +	+
Joint flexibility	Exercises light dumb-bells	+ + +	+ +
Neural coordination Sense of space and posture	Exercises and game	+	+ + +
Excess weight	Prolonged activity at low level (walking uphill or swimming)	0	+ + +
Stiffness of joints (back, knees)	Specific exercises	+ + (Learning)	+ + +

† Appropriateness of the exercise at this stage is shown by + signs.

β blocking agents are judged necessary, it is difficult to fix the proper heart rate figure. If the patient is in a recovery clinic, it is simple enough to compare the data from two exercise tests performed without β blocking drugs. Otherwise the mean decrease of pulse rate under β blocking agents ranges from 15 to 30 beats/min.

Variety in training is necessary to prevent the patient from becoming tired in his daily activities when he returns home. Long distance endurance training in order to resume cycling or low level hill walking will take place later, after the convalescence period.

Muscle power

Activities such as a sprint, dash, or jump, which produce an increase in "explosive" anaerobic power, are definitively over for the patient. Whatever the surgical results, the risk to joints and muscles increases in patients over 40.

Muscle strength

The need to reinforce muscle strength is obvious. Older people need more muscular strength than a high level of VO_2max to carry out daily activities: cleaning a bedroom, making a bed, hanging out the washing, putting a saucepan full of water on a stove, or loading and unloading the contents of a supermarket trolley are difficult, even painful, tasks for many patients who have undergone surgery, especially older women.

A training programme that deals consecutively with different muscular groups, relying on adapted bodybuilding technique has proved very effective[14,15] and not at all harmful. This kind of exercise is probably better suited to the fragility of joints in older patients. Those who are still weak can nevertheless exercise efficiently while sitting in an armchair.[16]

Flexibility of joints

The classical swedish gymnastics with or without light dumb-bells remains the most appropriate method. Everybody knows this type of exercise but few will practice on their own. It is tedious unless performed in groups.

Coordination, sense of space, and posture

In some instances patients need help to recover their sense of space and posture, especially if they have been obliged to stay in bed for a long time before and/or after surgery (in cases of complicated postoperative recovery). Among the many possibilities, exercises to recover coordination (dribbling a ball, for example), swimming, walking blindfold (to improve the sense of posture and the feeling of the ground underfoot), are the most useful.

Exercises for patients with excess weight

Although excess weight is common in patients who have undergone an operation, especially in non-smokers, diabetics, and women, it is illusory to trust in physical activity during convalescence to produce a weight loss. If one remembers that one hour of cycling at 16 km/h produces a loss of about 50 g of dry weight, it seems wise to postpone this approach until after the convalescent phase. Of primary importance, on the other hand, is teaching the patient about lifestyle and nutrition (how much and what to eat) with the help of a dietitian, and to "train" him by putting him on a low calorie diet. Obviously, the facilities provided in recovery clinics are a great advantage over home care, hasty explanations provided during hospital stay, or advice from the busy physician in his office. The time has unfortunately not yet come when a special body of health technicians is available to go out and teach patients about lifestyle and dietary techniques in the home after re-vascularisation or myocardial infarction. Nevertheless, as soon as the patient is back at home, he may resume low level but prolonged endurance training to increase the daily expenditure of calories as a part of a weight loss programme.

Special programmes

Among operated patients, many of them (such as former sportsmen and the obese) will be noted to have degenerative or traumatic impairments of the vertebrae, hips or knees. Mobilisation has to be undertaken with caution. However, provided the physiotherapist is aware of any problems this is a good opportunity to teach these patients about special precautions.

Drug regimen

Recovery clinics are an ideal facility in which to observe circulatory response, persistence of angina, reappearance of hypertension, persistence, or occurrence of arrhythmias. Appropriate drugs can be administered and results observed with ease. Corrections can be made when necessary. It is often observed that blood levels of lipids and cholesterol decrease for some weeks after surgery, but the patient must be made aware of the temporary nature of this decrease and these levels should be checked again after three months, especially if he has regained weight after having ceased smoking.

Percutaneous transluminal coronary angioplasty

After PTCA, patients do not need to be admitted to recovery clinics, which are costly. They can benefit from out-patient training,[11] but problems may arise over motivation and the expectation of re-stenosis. Motivation for rehabilitation depends mostly on the extent of anxiety and suffering provoked by pre- and postoperative symptoms. In PTCA patients, the situation is completely different. Many of them are dilated after hasty angiography showing a "dilatable" lesion, even though ischaemia is often mild, absent, or unproved.[12] The memory of symptoms is often therefore not sufficient to galvanise them into action, and the resumption of smoking is more frequent in PTCA patients than in those having undergone coronary surgery. Observance of dietary restrictions is also poor in such cases. Many lack confidence in their ability to return to work, even when physically capable of doing so.[13]

The spectre of re-stenosis

Many patients are aware of the frequency of re-stenosis. However the phenomenon is not simple for the patient to grasp, especially if his PTCA was not preceded by stable angina or a strongly positive exercise test. The patient is therefore cautious and anxious: cautious to avoid re-stenosis (but he cannot know if or when it will occur, any more than his cardiologist can), and anxious while waiting for the signs and symptoms of re-stenosis which may (or may not) appear in due course. A coronary angiograph is planned but is not carried out too early, in order to retain its predictive value. Many patients therefore wait cautiously for the results of the angiography before resuming a normal life. A normal exercise test can be predictive of the absence of ischaemia but not of the absence of re-stenosis; the reverse is also true. Many patients having undergone successful angiography still have a silent ST segment depression. Which is why (except in the case of spontaneous angina pectoris, registered at the time of an attack and showing significant ischaemia) it is absolutely necessary to have an unmasked symptom-limited exercise test before angioplasty is carried out, to quantify the ischaemia. Precise benchmarks are then available: critical values of heart rate, ST segment depression, exercise capacity, and criteria for limiting or stopping the exercise test. It will then be easy to compare these with the exercise test results after the angioplasty procedure. Such precautions limit the number of costly scans required and repeated coronarangiography.

However, when angioplasty is undertaken immediately after infarction there are no elements for comparison. In such cases, the results of the exercise test should be considered as if angioplasty had not taken place: if they are poor, a coronarography is essential and re-vascularisation will probably be necessary; if they are good, it does not much matter whether re-stenosis occurs or not.

Conclusions

Rehabilitation after myocardial re-vascularisation has four objectives: to improve physical capacity as much as possible, taking the patient's previous state into account; to restore the patient's confidence and hopes for the long term; to prevent recurrence and progression of heart disease by educating the patient and monitoring risk factors; and to encourage full and rapid return to work or normal activity wherever possible.

Postsurgical recovery clinics employing full-time cardiologists, physiotherapists, and dietitians, working together with the social services, are appropriate but unfortunately costly facilities. They should be used only for surgical patients, who should be transferred to them 8-10 days after their operation, for a period of two to four weeks. After angioplasty, return to a normal life with all its usual activities should take place a few days after the procedure. There is no scientific evidence to show that activity fosters re-stenosis or that rest prevents it.

For patients having undergone a bypass on the left anterior descending artery a coronary angiogram should automatically be obtained 10 years afterwards, even if functional status is good. The progression of lesions above the bypass means that the patients are totally dependent on the bypass and that they must constantly observe the preventive measures, reducing risk factors.

References

1 Forts L, Molgaard H, Christiansen EH, Hjortholm K, Paulsen PK, Thomsem PE. Atrial fibrillation and flutter after coronary artery bypass surgery: epidemiology, risk factors and preventive trials. *Int J Cardiol* 1992; **36**: 253–61

2 Yousif H, Davies G, Oakley CM. Peri-operative supraventricular arrhythmias in coronary bypass surgery. *Int J Cardiol* 1990; **26(3)**: 313–18.

3 Ormerod OJ, McGregor CG, Stone DL, Wisbey C, Petch MC. Arrhythmias after bypass coronary surgery. *Br Heart J* 1984; **51(6)**: 618–21.

4 Daudon P, Corcos T, Gandjbakhch I, Levasseur JP, Cabrol A, Cabrol C. Prevention of atrial fibrillation or flutter by acebutolol after coronary bypass grafting. *Am J Cardiol* 1981; **58(10)**: 933-6.

5 Kuo LC, Quinones MA, Rokey R, Sartori M, Abinader EG, Zoghbi WA. Quantification of atrial contribution to left ventricular filing by pulsed Doppler-echocardiography and the effect of age in normal and diseased hearts. *Am J Cardiol* 1987; **59(12)**: 1174–8.

6 Lundstrom T, Karlsson O. Improved ventilatory response to exercise after cardioversion of chronic atrial fibrillation to sinus rhythm. *Chest* 1992; **102(4)**: 1017-22.

7 Cavender JP, Rogers WJ, Fisher LD, Gersh BJ, Coggin CJ, Myers WO. Effects of smoking on survival and morbidity in patients randomized to medical or surgical therapy in the Coronary Artery Surgery Study (CASS) 10 year follow-up: CASS investigations. *J Am Coll Cardiol* 1992; **20**: 287–94.

8 Galan KM, Deligonul V, Kern MJ, Chaitman BR, Vandormael MG. Increased frequency of restenosis in patients continuing to smoke cigarettes after percutaneous transluminal coronary angioplasty. *Am J Cardiol* 1988; **61**: 260–3.

9 Gehrin J, Koenig W, Rana NW, Mathes P. The influence of the type of occupation on return to work after myocardial infarction, coronary angioplasty and coronary bypass surgery. *Eur Heart J* 1988; **9** (suppl L): 109–14.

10 Blaquière C, Mazaudier E, Douard H, Koch M, Broustet JP. Results of a regional work aptitude consultation. Proceedings of the Vth World Congress on Cardiac Rehabilitation. Intercept LTD-Andover, 1993 pp 467–71.

11 Danchin N, Juillère Y, Selton-Suty C, Vaillant G, Pernot C. Return to work after percutaneous transluminal coronary angioplasty: a continuing problem. *Eur Heart J* 1989; **10** (suppl G): 54–7.

12 Cay EL, Walker DD. Psychological factors and return to work. *Eur Heart J* 1988; **9**(suppl L): 74–81.

13 Fitzgerald ST, Becker DM, Celentano DD, Swank R, Brinker J. Return to work after percutaneous transluminal angioplasty. *Am J Cardiol* 1989; **64**: 1108–12.

14 McCartney N, McKelvie RS, Haslam DR, Jones NL. Usefulness of weight lifting training in improving strength and maximal power output in coronary artery disease. *Am J Cardiol* 1991; **67**: 939–45.

15 Frontera WR, Meredith CN, O'Reilly KP, Knuttgen HG, Evans WJ. Strength conditioning in older men: skeletal muscle hypertrophy and improved function. *J Appl Physiol* 1988; **64**: 1038–44.

16 Koch M, Douard H, Broustet JP. The benefit of graded exercise in chronic heart failure. *Chest* 1992; **101** (5 suppl): 231–5.

7 Cardiac rehabilitation in the district hospital

CHRISTOPHER DAVIDSON

Introduction

Despite the many changes occurring in the health service it seems likely that cardiac rehabilitation services in the United Kingdom will be based on the district hospital for the foreseeable future. The therapeutic breakthrough of thrombolysis has overtaken the debate about whether patients with myocardial infarction should be treated at home or in hospital; most patients with definite or suspected myocardial infarction, particularly in the big conurbations, are likely to be admitted to their local district hospital. Hospital statistics show that patients with cardiac disease comprise the largest group of patients occupying acute medical beds (22·5% in 1990-91), and the numbers with myocardial infarction remains relatively constant, with a slight upward trend in the numbers admitted with angina (fig 7.1). As a result, most district hospitals discharge 200-400 patients a year, more than enough to justify running a rehabilitation programme.

The management of myocardial infarction whilst in hospital is becoming relatively uniform, with a short period in a cardiac care unit followed by a period of 4–10 days in a general ward before discharge. However, there are wide variations in practice after discharge, when a period of recuperation at home may or may not be supplemented by a formal cardiac rehabilitation programme. The expected (but often unstated) goal is to return to normal activities and occupation within two to four months of the initial event. As we shall see, only a small minority of patients are formally investigated with exercise tests, and then mainly when symptoms develop during the convalescent period.

Given this pattern of care it is not surprising that cardiac rehabilitation

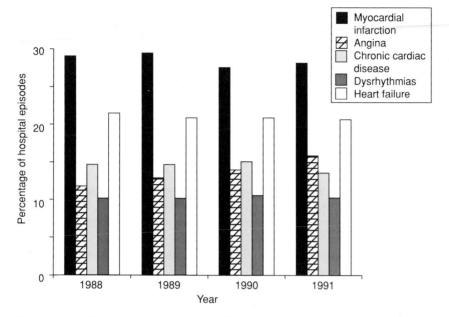

Figure 7.1 Diagnostic categories (% of hospital episodes) of patients with heart disease admitted to acute medical beds in the United Kingdom 1988–91. Source: Department of Health, hospital episode statistics

programmes have, in the main, been in district hospitals, particularly in those with an active cardiac care unit. Most of the necessary requirements in terms of personnel and facilities are already in place and it only needs some coordination to get a programme off the ground. In historical terms the United Kingdom has been a late starter, the first programmes not being established for a decade or more after pioneering work in Israel and North America.[1,2] The earliest programmes were set up in the late 1960s and early '70s by physicians and cardiologists and have formed the basis of practice in this country ever since. The focus has been on phase II, the period between leaving hospital and returning to work or full household duties, and has been structured with regular exercise sessions over a 4-12 week period, usually supplemented by educational sessions aimed at secondary prevention.

From these early beginnings there has been a steady increase in the number of rehabilitation programmes based in district hospitals, often instigated by nurses or physiotherapists rather than cardiologists or physicians. Although these programmes may have attracted only lukewarm support from the medical profession, they have become firmly established and cater for large numbers of patients. In 1989 the British Cardiac Society set up a working party to report on the status of cardiac

145

rehabilitation in the United Kingdom at that time and to assess future developments. The working party undertook a survey of all district hospitals,[3] in collaboration with the Coronary Prevention Group and funded by the British Heart Foundation; this survey will be referred to at various stages in this chapter, supplemented by newer information where it is available.[4] The recommendations from this report are shown in the box.

Recommendations of the British Cardiac Society Working Party on Cardiac Rehabilitation (1989)

- Every major district hospital caring for cardiac patients should provide a cardiac rehabilitation service; at present only a minority do

- The programme should be multidisciplinary and will usually be exercise based, depending on the resources available; a local coordinator is essential

- The expertise available for a comprehensive programme is available in most district and major cardiothoracic centres, but requires consultant leadership, most appropriately a cardiologist

- There is a continued need for research in the evaluation not only of the physiological response, but also of the social and psychological aspects of rehabilitation

- The role of vocational rehabilitation in recovery needs greater recognition

- The special problems of female patients and children together with certain ethnic groups need to be addressed

- Rehabilitation should be tailored to the individual needs of patients and special groups requirements; arrhythmia monitoring is necessary for high risk patients

- Individual programmes should evaluate their outcome, and a standard format of audit could be agreed nationally to allow comparison

---

As a result of this report, which showed that less than half the districts in the United Kingdom had established cardiac rehabilitation services, the British Heart Foundation and the Chest, Heart and Stroke Association offered a series of "pump-priming" grants, which have had a major impact on the number of active cardiac rehabilitation programmes in the United Kingdom (fig 7.2). This welcome initiative has been further expanded by the British Heart Foundation. By 1992 it was estimated that almost 25 000 patients had been treated by the 147 rehabilitation programmes in the United Kingdom for which the information was available.[4]

A major factor that has governed the rather slow development of cardiac rehabilitation services in the United Kingdom has been the lack of support

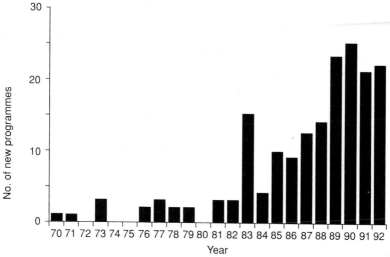

Figure 7.2   Number of new cardiac rehabilitation programmes established each year in the United Kingdom (source : British Cardiac Society survey, 1993), showing the rapid increase in the number of new programmes resulting from the Chest, Heart and Stroke Association and British Heart Foundation initiative.

by consultants as a whole and cardiologists in particular. In the 1989 British Cardiac Society survey only two thirds of the then 89 programmes were actively supported by a consultant and only half of these were cardiologists. The reason for this lack of support may not be immediately apparent, since at the outset a number of pioneering centres were run by cardiologists. Indeed one of the earliest, based in the cardiac centre at Stoke, provided one of the largest controlled trials of the effects of cardiac rehabilitation after myocardial infarction and was funded by the Department of Health.[5]

Even now the profession remains divided. Despite the publication of two meta-analyses[6,7] opponents to formal rehabilitation programmes remain unconvinced that the patient benefits in terms of reduced morbidity. There is also the feeling that a formal programme may make the patient more conscious of his condition rather than allowing it to become a thing of the past. Finally, many still feel concerned about the dangers of an active exercise programme so soon after cardiac injury, particularly after a major anterior infarction.[8] Perhaps this is one area in which the meta-analyses have provided a convincing answer, since, overall, treated groups have not had a higher morbidity than control groups. It seems clear that, at least with selection procedures in published trials, the safety record of rehabilitation programmes is very good both in North America and the United Kingdom. In North America the fatal event rates have been reported as one in 160 000[9] and one in 784 000[10]

Table 7.1 Exercise testing before and after cardiac rehabilitation programmes (data from British Cardiac Society survey of 89 rehabilitation programmes 1989).

	Exercise test before rehabilitation	Exercise test after rehabilitation
Always	28	17
Often	13	5
Sometimes	28	35
Never	12	24
Not stated	9	9

patient hours of exercise. In the British Cardiac Society working party survey in the United Kingdom only one myocardial infarction, five cardiac arrests, and two deaths were reported from an estimated 12 000 patients treated in the previous year, which, given an average of 15 hours of supervised exercise per patient, produces a very similar figure. The British experience is interesting in that, unlike North America, exercise tests have been carried out only in a minority of patients before entering the programmes (table 7.1).

The initiative by the British Heart Foundation and the Chest, Heart and Stroke Association has helped to change the inertia within the profession, and most of the new programmes have been set up in conjunction with the local cardiologist. Whatever doctors might feel about the theoretical benefit of rehabilitation in scientific terms, the organised rehabilitation programme remains a highly cost effective way of delivering quality care to the large numbers of patients with cardiac disease who pass through district hospitals, a fact not lost on the new purchasing authorities. In an ideal world, it might be possible to give each patient, after leaving hospital, individual advice and a high level of support through primary care teams; however, the numbers being dealt with by individual teams would be small and the level of support could become fragmented and inconsistent. Furthermore, such an approach fails to provide the very tangible benefits of group activity, which is such a central part of current programmes in the United Kingdom. The establishment of a *district based* service outside the hospital and supervised by a general practitioner is, however, both practicable and effective[11] and is dealt with in Chapter 8.

Setting up a district based programme

The resources needed to establish a cardiac rehabilitation programme are present in most district hospitals. Group based exercise is best carried out in a gym. Most district hospitals have their own gymnasium, but successful programmes have been established in sports centres outside hospitals and even in a large factory. The personnel required for exercise supervision—physiotherapists or remedial gymnasts—are also available in district hospitals, and the first step in establishing a programme is to agree a sessional allocation both for physiotherapists and for the gym. Sessional commitments from other health care professionals—for example, nurses, dietitians, occupational therapists, clinical psychologists, and vocational advisers—can be negotiated as the course becomes established and can be tailored to suit patients' requirements.

There are two further key factors in setting up and maintaining a satisfactory cardiac rehabilitation programme. The first is commitment and support from a consultant cardiologist or physician, and the second is a programme coordinator, usually a senior nurse with experience in treating cardiac patients.

The pivotal role of the consultant has recently been underlined in a review by Kellerman,[12] one of the pioneers of cardiac rehabilitation. Although he stresses that rehabilitation must be multidisciplinary in approach, "it is the full responsibility of the cardiologist to consolidate and conduct the effort of the team." Specific duties should include:

- *Allocation of resources*—to determine the structure of the programme in order to accommodate the number of patients within the resources available (for example, availability of the gym and physiotherapist sessions); this may mean, for instance, holding sessions once rather than twice weekly, or the course lasting for four rather than eight weeks
- *Patient selection*—to provide guidelines agreed with consultant colleagues to identify high risk groups; this may require the coordination and reporting of exercise tests
- *Education*—to agree with consultant colleagues a uniform approach to risk factor modification and to supervise the written and audiovisual material used
- *Audit*—to monitor all adverse events and regularly audit performance, particularly the drop-out rate.

The role of the coordinator is equally crucial.[13] The management of myocardial infarction in the first three months encompasses the transition between intensive hospital care and the gradual resumption of normal activities at home. The nurse with experience in cardiac care is well equipped to cope with the various problems that may arise in the different stages of recovery. When a patient is faced with so many health professionals in a short hospital stay, the coordinator can provide the single face to which the patient and family can relate and through whom the educational and preventive aspects of the programme can be channelled. Regular contact with individual patients and partners is maintained through the rehabilitation sessions and, where necessary, patients can be contacted or visited at home. Duties of the coordinator should involve:

- *Inpatient programme*—to contact the patient and partner and identify problems prior to discharge; to advise on activity following discharge; to provide educational material and answer early queries; to provide a contact for patients and partners prior to the first follow up appointment or the start of the rehabilitation programme
- *Exercise tests*—to coordinate the post-infarction exercise test prior to entering the programme and to ensure that high risk patients have been identified
- *Education/counselling*—to participate in and coordinate educational sessions for patients and partners; to liaise with consultants, dietitians, psychologists, and other health care professionals to provide further sessions; to provide counselling for individuals or couples, where required
- *Non-attenders*—to identify problems that may prevent attendance; these may include social problems, difficulty with transport, or psychological problems
- *Tailoring programmes*—to provide if necessary, special provision for women, and liaison with ethnic minorities, and accommodate the needs of the older patient
- *Self help patient groups*—to provide support and liaison with the hospital based service
- *Audit*—to monitor activity in relation to nationally or locally agreed guidelines

The coordinator may also be able to maintain links with those who, for various reasons, can not or will not attend the formal rehabilitation session and ensure that they too receive adequate counselling and education.

In summary, setting up a hospital based programme is not difficult. It requires agreement between the consultant group that such a facility is needed, negotiation with the physiotherapy department for the sessions, and the establishment of either a part-time or full-time nurse coordinator. Bearing in mind the numbers of patients who are likely to require this service in most district hospitals, the overall costs are relatively small (estimated by the working party report as £5.00–15.00 per patient session at 1989 prices). The cost depends largely on whether there is a nurse coordinator, the number of physiotherapists and other staff involved in each session, the number of patients treated in each session, the number of sessions each week, and the duration of the course for each patient. There needs to be only a small reduction in patient readmission rate to more than cover the cost of such a programme.[14]

Phase I—Inpatient care

With the advent of thrombolysis most patients with myocardial infarction are now treated in designated cardiac care units, but their stay there is relatively short and there follows a period of three to seven days in the general ward before discharge home. This period offers a number of opportunities for education and counselling, and the problem is often one of too much rather than too little advice—patients and their relatives being showered with pamphlets, diet sheets, and other educational material. For patients with no previous cardiac symptoms this can be bewildering, and one of the prime roles of the coordinator is to ensure that there is a consistent approach both in terms of advice and educational material. It is probably sensible to agree to just one or two advice leaflets at this early stage. Such material should be attractively designed and easy to read, and it should make the important points simply. There is plenty of opportunity for providing more detailed educational literature in the following weeks, and the choice of material can then be tailored to suit the patient's needs.

During the inpatient phase there is little real need for active physiotherapy, early ambulation being sufficient for the short period in hospital. It is, however, an opportunity for the physiotherapists who will be involved subsequently in the rehabilitation programme to visit the patient and explain what is involved, both in terms of the exercises that will be undertaken, and the ultimate goals that can be achieved. Specific needs, such as those of patients whose work is manual, can be anticipated.

The period of inpatient care offers the opportunity for the nurse coordinator to have preliminary discussions with the patient and partner and outline the scope of the rehabilitation service in terms of not just the physical activity involved but also the other changes of lifestyle which are important to prevent a recurrence. The most immediate and important of these is to stop smoking. Almost all patients stop when they are admitted and many hospitals now have a no smoking policy so that temptation does not arise until they are discharged. Specific advice and counselling on smoking is more important at this stage than discussions about other lifestyle changes such as diet and stress management. Indeed, this is a good opportunity for the partner and the rest of the household to stop smoking and to help prevent a relapse.

Perhaps the most important aspect of the rehabilitation programme during the inpatient phase is the need to prepare for the first few weeks at home. This hiatus is a very vulnerable time for both patients and their partners, and a failure to understand what is to be expected can lead to many unnecessary readmissions. Advice about everyday activities around the house is important, as well as some encouragement to undertake increasing amounts of light exercise such as walking outside. Failure to give specific advice can often lead to overprotection by the partner and a pattern of invalid behaviour which is difficult to reverse at a later stage. Although most doctors and health care professionals are now aware of the importance of a positive approach in these early weeks, there is still sometimes a conflict between advice given by the hospital and by the patient's own general practitioner, who may not be aware of the current change towards active rehabilitation. A brief advice sheet outlining the essential goals of rehabilitation is essential in these early weeks so that both the general practitioner and the patient can see what advice has been given. Perhaps the most important thing the patient should leave hospital with is a contact number for the nurse coordinator so that questions are not left unanswered until the patient attends the first rehabilitation session.

Phase II—recovery after discharge

Unlike other countries, such as Germany and Italy, prolonged inpatient rehabilitation does not exist in the United Kingdom, the only exception being the intensive course run by the British Army. Instead rehabilitation programmes have been centred on regular exercise sessions spread over the first three to four months of the recovery period. The British Cardiac Society survey in 1989, and more recently in 1992,[4] has shown the pattern to be remarkably similar throughout the United Kingdom. The number of patients now being treated in the United Kingdom has been estimated at over 25 000 per year.[4] Courses start two to six weeks after the myocardial infarction and generally continue for 4-12 weeks (figs 7.3 and 7.4). The British Cardiac Society survey in 1989 showed that the typical centre held classes twice weekly with between five and 10 patients at each session, with sessions of one to two hours, but there were some who managed to hold more and some less, presumably reflecting local conditions such as the availability of personnel and the gym and the number of patients requiring the programme (figs 7.5 to 7.7).

The structure of the rehabilitation session is also fairly consistent and follows the low level programme advocated by Goble et al[15] from Melbourne, rather than the high intensity programmes seen in North America. Exercise is generally in a form of a circuit, consisting mainly of dynamic exercises, in which the pulse is monitored as a means of regulating the exercise level attained. Staff usually spend time with individual patients on their first session, going through the exercises and stressing the importance of a warming up period, but thereafter patients undertake the exercise in the gym, self monitoring their activity. Exercises will usually include treadmill or an exercise bicycle, items that may have to be purchased specially for the rehabilitation programme, often through

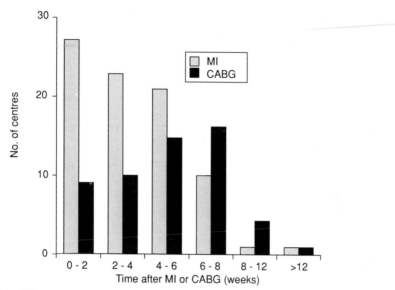

Figure 7.3   Time of commencing cardiac rehabilitation outpatient programmes: comparison of patients after myocardial infarction (MI) and coronary artery bypass grafting (CABG) (source: British Cardiac Society survey of 89 rehabilitation programmes, 1989).

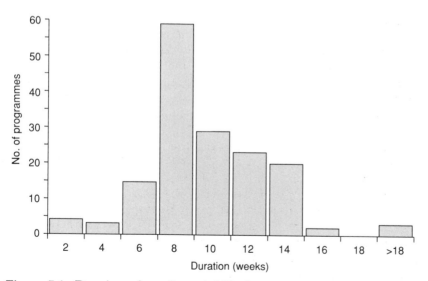

Figure 7.4   Duration of cardiac rehabilitation programmes in the United Kingdom (source: British Cardiac Society survey, 1992).

153

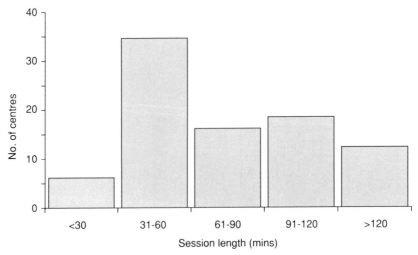

Figure 7.5 Duration of cardiac rehabilitation sessions (source: British Cardiac Society survey of 89 rehabilitation programmes, 1989).

funds raised by the patients themselves. In the initial assessment, physiotherapists take note of other physical disabilities, such as arthritis, back problems, and chest disease, which may limit the degree to which a particular patient may be able to participate.

One important aspect of the rehabilitation class is the fact that it does

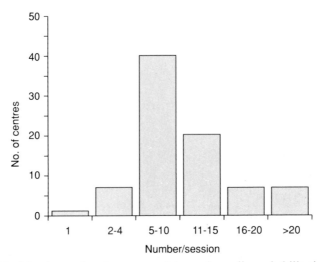

Figure 7.6 Numbers of patients treated in each cardiac rehabilitation session (source: British Cardiac Society survey of 89 rehabilitation programmes, 1989).

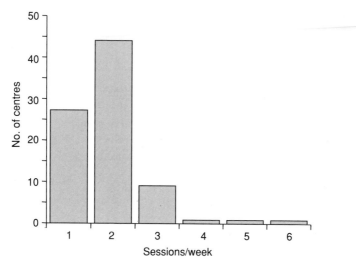

Figure 7.7 Number of sessions per week in cardiac rehabilitation programmes (source: British Cardiac Society survey of 89 rehabilitation programmes, 1989).

represent group activity, unlike many other areas of rehabilitation. Although there will be small cohorts of patients entering the programme who had their heart attack or surgery at about the same time, they will inevitably be taking part with others who are at various stages of recovery. Seeing patients in the later stages of the programme gives a great boost in

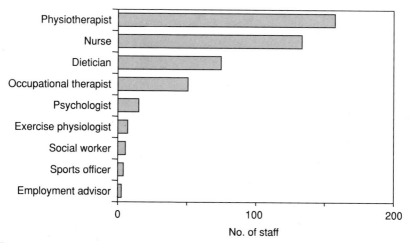

Figure 7.8 Paramedic involvement (number of staff) in cardiac rehabilitation programmes in the United Kingdom (source: British Cardiac Society survey, 1992).

155

confidence to those who are still frightened about exercising after a heart attack. Moreover, when partners attend with patients they have an opportunity to see what can be achieved and to discuss their experiences with other partners. Some groups even encourage partners themselves to take part in the exercise.

Although exercise has both physiological benefits and improves patients' self esteem, other aspects of rehabilitation are equally important and should be scheduled into the session, often as part of the cooling down period. At this stage, some time after the event itself, patients and their partners are often more receptive to educational material, and the disease process can be discussed in some detail to allow a greater understanding of how the heart attack may have occurred and what can be done to prevent recurrence. This is an opportunity to give patients more detailed leaflets and audiovisual material and, increasingly nowadays, make use of educational video tapes. Such educational aids are, however, of little value unless backed up by question and answer sessions with health professionals themselves.

Many questions about heart disease and its treatment can be answered by the cardiac nurse, but a doctor should be available once a month so that at some period in the programme everyone will have an opportunity to discuss medical issues more specifically. In the early stages, too, there are usually questions about diet, and dietitian sessions can be very valuable in terms of both group discussion and individual counselling. Finally, a clinical psychologist can be valuable in helping to identify and treat the small proportion of patients with significant problems in coming to terms with their illness, many of whom can be identified early on after the heart attack itself. Such sessions are not widely available but may prevent much long term morbidity. Discussions with the clinical psychologist will usually be on an individual rather than a group basis, though in many centres some form of group relaxation therapy is practised. The extent of participation of these other health professionals in current programmes is shown in figure 7.8.

Phase III—long term rehabilitation

In Europe and North America most rehabilitation programmes offer long term supervised exercise but this is not the practice in the United Kingdom. What have developed, although on an *ad hoc* basis, are patient support groups in which regular exercise may play a part in their activities. These support groups have been facilitated by the British Heart Foundation and the Chest, Heart and Stroke Association. Because of the way in which they have developed the groups are very different in style,

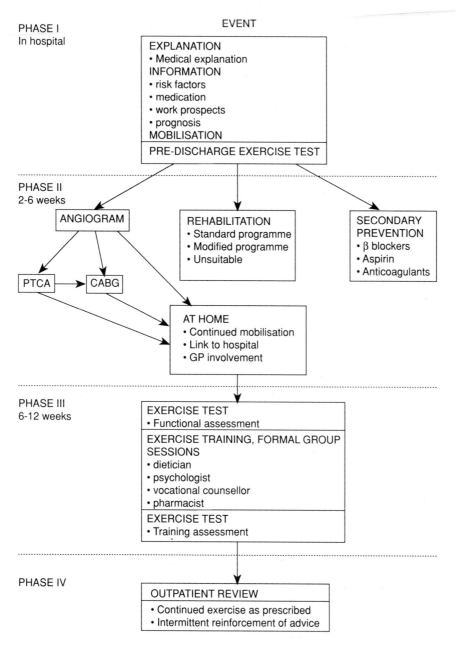

Figure 7.9 Suggested scheme for the assessment of patients recovering from a heart attack (adapted from Horgan et al,[3] with permission).

some concentrating more on social and supportive activities and some focusing largely on long term exercise.

One of the criticisms of the current rehabilitation programmes in the United Kingdom is that whilst behavioural change can be achieved over a short term period, patients often return to their "bad" habits over the next year or two unless further reinforcement is provided. Moreover, in a meta-analysis[7] of controlled trials in cardiac rehabilitation the mortality benefit seemed to be more pronounced in the long term rehabilitation programmes than in the short term ones, and although this was not statistically significant it would make sense in terms of the physiology of training and the pathophysiology of coronary disease.

Setting up a patient self help group is usually not difficult. There are many patients who feel, after a period of active rehabilitation, that they would like to continue supervised exercise, though not necessarily in the hospital environment. Once a few interested patients get together with the support and encouragement of the consultant and programme coordinator, such a self help group can easily be established. The British Heart Foundation provides a format for a constitution as well as offering limited liability insurance for group meetings. Further exercise sessions can be arranged in the hospital gym, but psychologically it is probably better for them to be held in a community sports centre under the supervision of a trained physiotherapist or other sports professional. During phase II each patient has already established the level of exercise with which he is comfortable, and this level can be gradually increased providing the patient does not have any adverse prognostic factors. These patients are relatively low risk and defibrillation equipment is probably not required, provided a prompt ambulance response can be relied on. It is essential, however, that the supervising physiotherapist or gymnast is trained in cardiopulmonary resuscitation.

The critism of many patient self help groups is that they become inward looking and disease orientated, which is the very opposite of what the rehabilitation process is intended to achieve. For this reason it is important that there is support from the outset by the patients' consultant and the cardiac rehabilitation coordinator. Once established such groups often fulfil a valuable function not only for themselves in continuing the beneficial effects of rehabilitation but also in offering a group that can provide support to other patients in phase I and phase II of the rehabilitation programme. A fit patient who has continued to exercise for six months after his myocardial infarction can often help to relieve the anxieties of patients in the early phase of recovery more than any amount of medical discussions and audiovisual material. A self help group can also offer great support to partners in the early stages after myocardial infarction or bypass surgery, and these are resources which should not be ignored.

Cardiac assessment during rehabilitation

One of the vital functions of the supervising physician or cardiologist is to select patients who are going to benefit most from rehabilitation. At present most programmes operate some selection even if this is not necessarily formalised; heart failure, continuing angina, or arrhythmias are the usual exclusions. However, like all interventions in ischaemic heart disease, the patients who benefit most may be those who are at highest risk.[16] As we shall see, patients with cardiac failure, for example, may benefit considerably, but their programmes do need to be tailored individually and they must be monitored carefully.

The recommendations of the working party were that patients should be formally assessed during the period of rehabilitation to see whether they are candidates for coronary angiography and re-vascularisation procedures. The recommendations, which are summarised in figure 7.9, emphasise the importance of exercise testing both before and after a period of cardiac rehabilitation. Many cardiologists would go further and suggest that all patients with myocardial infarction in whom re-vascularisation is an option should have an exercise test before leaving hospital.

This ideal scheme is rarely achieved even in well staffed cardiothoracic centres and the main reason for this is the lack of availability of junior medical staff to supervise the exercise testing sessions. If the 1989 survey is respresentative (table 7.1), then less than a third of hospitals undertake routine exercise tests prior to rehabilitation, and it is unlikely that the remainder have any formal policy for selecting patients suitable for coronary angiography. Reductions in junior doctors' hours of work are likely to aggravate this problem further, and the British Cardiac Society's recent recommendations on exercise testing are therefore very timely(see box).[17] These endorse the practice of senior physiological measurement technicians undertaking exercise tests without the supervision of a doctor, provided they are fully trained in cardiopulmonary resuscitation and provided medical help is immediately available if necessary. Although this should improve matters considerably, there are many parts of the country where there are inadequate numbers of senior technicians available to undertake such testing, and in this situation the experienced nurse coordinator could provide valuable additional help.

The British Cardiac Society report showed that, at least with the patients currently being selected for cardiac rehabilitation, the risks of cardiac events during a rehabilitation programme are very small, so exercise testing before entering such a progranmme is probably not mandatory. If, however, we accept that some stratification of risk is to be attempted in the recovery period after a myocardial infarction, an exercise test will need to be done at some stage and this is probably best arranged

---

Summary of the British Cardiac Society guidelines for exercise testing where no doctor is present

- *Exercise test room*: close to outpatients or cardiac ward; adequate size to allow full resuscitation procedures with cardiac arrest alarm to summon medical help

- *Resuscitation equipment*: full equipment, which should be checked regularly

- *Technicians*: test to be supervised by two senior grade technicians competent in resuscitation and approved by consultant/head of department

- *Physician cover*: a designated physician must be responsible for each test and be in the vicinity to respond to calls for help; the physician must have examined the patient and seen the resting ECG, and confirm that it is safe to proceed with the test by signing a statement on the request form

- *High risk tests*: in cases of unstable angina or recent myocardial infraction, aortic stenosis, hypertrophic cardiomyopathy, and where malignant arrhythmias are possible, all high risk tests *must* be supervised by a doctor

---

in the first four to six weeks. The cardiac rehabilitation coordinator is ideally situated to coordinate such an approach and, if necessary, could supervise the exercise tests with the senior physiological measurement technician. Patients with chronic stable angina and heart failure should *all* be assessed formally with an exercise test before entering the programmes so that exercise levels can be properly prescribed. The number of these patients is, however, quite small and in the total throughput of a cardiology service would not add greatly to the workload.

Tailoring programmes to include a wider range of patients

Most patients who have sustained a myocardial infarction are suitable for phase I and phase II cardiac rehabilitation programmes. However, there are groups of patients who do not fit neatly into the "standard package" and these may be overlooked by the system.

In setting up a cardiac rehabilitation programme most centres concentrate initially on the relatively low risk good prognosis group, and this is important in giving all concerned sufficient experience. Classically, the target group has been the largest—that is, middle aged white men. However, the needs of women, the elderly, and patients from the ethnic minorities do have to be considered soon after the programme has become established. Further development to accommodate the high risk patient will depend upon the level of experience of those involved and the time available.

Post-cardiac surgery

Although many cardiac surgery centres offer rehabilitation, patients can often attend a local programme much more easily, and it is logical that they do so bearing in mind that admission will take place locally if there are any complications. In the British Cardiac Society 1992 survey, 163 out of 186 rehabilitation programmes could accommodate patients after coronary artery bypass grafting (CABG), and these formed about 17% of the patients treated. After surgery the patients' needs are slightly different from those after myocardial infarction; they usually start the programme a week or two later (fig 7.3), and the emphasis will be towards more dynamic exercise (for example, bicycle, or treadmill) than floor exercise because of pain from sternal and leg wounds. On the whole, CABG patients can increase their exercise levels more quickly and three or four weeks may be sufficient, particularly if they have already had rehabilitation following earlier myocardial infarction. Cardiac rehabilitation may also be valuable in the much smaller numbers of patients who have had valve replacement, though patients will need to be assessed on an individual basis as many are elderly. The transplant patient also has special needs, but rehabilitation may well be undertaken in the cardiac centre, which the patient visits frequently in the early stages of recovery.

Women

Several studies have shown that the standard exercise based programme may be relatively poorly attended by women.[18,19] This is partly due to the fact that the age range of female patients is higher, but even in younger women lack of domestic support may prevent attendance. Some women have also expressed embarrassment in undertaking exercise in a group in which the majority is men, and they often prefer different forms of exercise, such as aerobics. If there are sufficient numbers of female patients passing through the cardiac care unit it may be necessary to design specific sessions in which there may be less focus on exercise and more on diet and prevention.

Older patients

In the early days of cardiac rehabilitation the main focus was on returning the working man to his job and patients over retirement age were not usually considered for cardiac rehabilitation. In population terms more than half of patients suffering a heart attack are over 65. With the increasing use of thrombolysis in the elderly population these patients are now passing through the cardiac care unit where once they may have been cared for in general ward or their home and, as such, they may become eligible for rehabilitation programmes. The recent British Cardiac Society enquiry (1992) showed that 38 of 176 programmes still operated an age related policy, though the level at which the age limit was set was not indicated. Where resources are limited, this may be inevitable, but there are many elderly people who would benefit from aspects of the rehabilitation programme.[20,21] Even if the focus on exercise is less important, their needs should be accommodated by special sessions that are more specifically tailored to the other disabilites they may have.

Ethnic minorities

Many conurbations in the United Kingdom now have large Asian and Afro-Caribbean minority groups, and Asians from the Indian subcontinent are particularly subject to premature coronary disease. Unlike most European cultures, Asian culture does not give exercise a regular place, and many Asians are unwilling to attend exercise sessions. Such groups should be identified and a special programme designed (which might involve other techniques such as yoga) with the help of community leaders where possible. Provision may need to be made for dietary and other health advice to be available in several Asian languages.

"High risk" patients

There is increasing evidence that patients with stable angina and heart failure may benefit from controlled exercise by improvement in exercise tolerance, perhaps coming about by changes in the peripheral circulation.[22] Whatever the mechanism, patients who remain symptomatic and limited in their activities should be considered for cardiac rehabilitation with a view to continuing this as a long term (phase III) activity. In the early stages, however, there is need for close supervision and before entering the programme, such patients should be screened with a suitable exercise test to determine the exercise level to be prescribed. If the patient is liable to arrhythmias, telemetric monitoring may need to be considered.

Non-attenders—What to do about them

A significant number of patients who could benefit from cardiac rehabilitation fail to attend even well established and popular programmes, and non-attenders are probably at higher than average risk.[23] There is no doubt that patients self select for an exercise based programme, with female sex, obesity, smoking, low income, and old age being important factors.[24,25] In the case of the elderly, early drop out tends to be for medical reasons, and in contrast to the younger patient, late defaulting is uncommon.[20] In the British Cardiac Society 1989 survey the drop-out rate was estimated to be less than 10% in the majority of centres (60 out of 76 responding). In 10 centres it was 10–20% in four centres 20–30%, and in two centres it was thought to be more than 30%. There was no correlation between the drop-out rate and the length of the programme or the number of patients treated each year. Motivation, transport, medical problems, and interference with returning to work were all regarded as important reasons for non-attendance. It was clear, however, that few if any centres were monitoring drop-out rates formally, and the figures available are probably a considerable underestimate, as indicated from the total numbers of patients with myocardial infarction per district as a proportion of the numbers attending cardiac rehabilitation.

Whilst patients should not be dragooned into a rehabilitation programme against their wishes, it is important that there is a sufficiently flexible approach to accommodate most people who would benefit. This requires positive action by the programme coordinator to identify the problem areas: difficulties in transport, adequate support from the partner (particularly in the case of women), social support in low income households, and individualised or small group sessions for patients who do not wish to participate in the exercise sessions. It is also important that the programme does not actually interfere with the patient returning to work two to three months after myocardial infarction. A continual review of programmes is essential, seeking patient opinion where appropriate, to ensure that the right balance is maintained and that the programme does attract the widest possible group of potential patients.

Evaluation and audit

In the working party survey of established programmes in 1989, audit was almost non-existent. No centres had a standard reporting format for adverse events or had any arrangement for formal follow up to assess the efficacy of the physical and educational aspects of the programme in the long term. The working party concluded that a standard form of audit was highly desirable, but as yet there has been no initiative establishing this.

Outcome measures in cardiac rehabilitation have been recently reviewed,[26] but many are more suited to research than for everyday use. A more practical scheme for auditing cardiac rehabilitation programmes is shown in the box. Some aspects of the programme need to be monitored continuously, particularly safety, and every significant adverse event should be reviewed in detail by the consultant in charge. In the case of a cardiac arrest important questions need to be answered: Was this a random event or could it have been predicted? Did the patient have an exercise test prior to the programme and did he fall into a high or low risk group? Was he being monitored adequately during the period of exercise?

163

⊃uggested scheme for auditing an established cardiac rehabilitation programme

Continuous assessment:

- *Safety*: any adverse events during sessions; consultant to identify whether these were avoidable; a nationally agreed format for reporting events is desirable

- *Numbers*: needed to monitor resources; age and gender valuable to provide trends

- *Non-complicance*: monitor numbers unable or unwilling to attend; identify correctable problems hindering attendance

Periodic review: Interval follow up of patients completing programme to assess:

- *Cardiac status*: angina, cardiac failure, re-infarction, hospitalisation

- *Risk factor modification*: smoking status, weight, exercise level

- *Quality of life*: work status, outlook, anxiety about health

---

Were resuscitation facilities adequate? Were the personnel present adequately trained in cardiopulmonary resuscitation?

These events and basic demographic details about the numbers attending the programme and those who did not do so are essential for finding the resources needed for the programme and should be continuously monitored. From time to time, however, it is essential to undertake an in-depth audit of a sample of unselected patients, both participating and not participating in the programme, to assess whether the emphasis should be changed, as in a recent study reported by Bertie *et al* in Plymouth.[27] They found that the quality of life measures as well as the patients' perception of their illness was not as favourable as they would have expected, and they proposed changes in the programme to remedy this. The importance of preventive measures, such as stopping smoking and achieving optimum weight, are also crucial to the efficacy of a rehabilitation programme. Failure to achieve satisfactory targets suggests that the measures employed should be changed.

One of the earliest measures of effective cardiac rehabilitation was return to work, but in the current economic climate this has become a much less useful measure of the patients resuming their normal activities. In a recent survey we, like others,[28] found that the rate of return to work was disappointingly low and that many people in middle life take early retirement if in a financial position to do so.

Audit activity is central to the role of the coordinator of the rehabilitation programme and is a strong argument for employment of a dedicated member of staff rather than *ad hoc* arrangements with senior nurses or physiotherapists. Close liaison between the coordinator and the consultant in charge is essential and any investigations carried out by them should be submitted to peer review by the other physicians and professionals involved.

The Future

Cardiac rehabilitation programmes are now becoming an accepted service commitment and are in place in the majority of district hospitals in the United Kingdom. However, almost half these programmes are in their infancy, having only been established in the last three years. Some national coordination to provide training and education is clearly needed, and the formation of the British Association for Cardiac Rehabilitation in 1992 may be very important in this respect. This body, the British Cardiac Society, and the British Heart Foundation must now draw up accepted standards of practice, with guidelines for evaluation and audit by which all cardiac rehabilitation programmes can be properly assessed. A coordinated approach would offer an immensely powerful tool in further innovation and research.

References

1 Hellerstein HK, Ford AB. Rehabilitation of the cardiac patient. *JAMA* 1957; **164**: 225–31.
2 Gottheiner V. Long range strenuous sports training for cardiac reconditioning and rehabilitation. *Am J Cardiol* 1968; **22**: 426–35.
3 Horgan J, Bethell H, Carson P, Davidson C, Julian D, Mayou RA, *et al.* Working Party Report on Cardiac Rehabilitation. *Br Heart J* 1992; **67**: 412–18.
4 Davidson C, Revell K, Chamberlain DAC, Parker J. Cardiac Rehabilitation Services 1992. *Br Heart J* 1995; **73**: 201–2.
5 Carson P, Phillips R, Lloyd M, Tucker H, Neophytou M, Buch NJ, *et al.* Exercise after myocardial infarction: a controlled trial. *J R Coll Physicians Lond* 1982; **16**: 147–51.
6 O'Connor GT, Buring JE, Yusuf S, Joldhager SZ, Olmstead EM, Paffenbarger RS, *et al.* An overview of randomized trials of rehabilitation with exercise after myocardial infarction. *Circulation* 1989; **80**: 234–44.
7 Oldridge NB, Guyatt GH, Fischer MD, Rimm AA. Cardiac rehabilitation after myocardial infarction: combined experience of randomized clinical trials. *JAMA* 1988; **260**: 945–50.
8 Jugdutt BI, Michorowski BL, Kappagoda CT. Exercise training after anterior Q wave myocardial infarction. *J Am Coll Cardiol* 1988; **12**: 362–72.
9 Haskell WL. Cardiovascular complications during exercise training for cardiac patients. *Circulation* 1978; **57**: 920–4.
10 Van Camp SP, Peterson RA. Cardiovascular complications of out-patient cardiac rehabilitation programmes. *JAMA* 1986; **256**(1): 160–3.
11 Bethell HJN, Mullee ME. A controlled trial of community based coronary rehabilitation. *Br Heart J* 1990; **64**: 370–5.

12 Kellerman JJ. Long-term comprehensive cardiac care—the perspectives and tasks of cardiac rehabilitation. *Eur Heart J* 1993; **14**: 1441–4.

13 Todd IC, Wosornu D, Stewart I, Wild T. Cardiac rehabilitation following myocardial infarction. *Sports Med* 1992; **14**: 243–59.

14 Ades PA, Huang D, Weaver SO. Cardiac rehabilitation participation predicts lower rehospitalisation costs. *Am Heart J* 1992; **123**: 916–21.

15 Goble AJ, Hare DL, Macdonald PS, Oliver RG, Reid MA, Worcester M. Effect of early programmes of high and low intensity exercise on physical performance after transmural acute myocardial infarction. *Br Heart J* 1991; **65**: 126–31.

16 Pashkow FJ. Issues in contemporary cardiac rehabilitation: a historical perspective. *J Am Coll Cardiol* 1993; **21**: 822–34.

17 Medical Practice Committee of the British Cardiac Society. Clinical guidelines for exercise testing. *Br Heart J* 1993; **70**: 488.

18 Oldridge NB, Lasalle D, Jones NL. Exercise rehabilitation of female patients with coronary artery disease. *Am Heart J* 1980; **100**: 755–7.

19 McGee HM, Horgan JH. Cardiac rehabilitation programmes: are women less likely to attend? *BMJ* 1992; **305**: 283–4.

20 Siddiqui MA. Cardiac Rehabilitation in elderly patients. *Age Ageing* 1992; **21**: 157–9.

21 Ades PA, Harrison PA, Gunther PGS, Tonini RP. Exercise conditioning in the elderly coronary patient. *J Am Ger Soc* 1987; **35**: 121–4.

22 Coats AJS, Adamopoulos S, Meyer TE, Conway J, Sleight P. The effects of physical training in chronic heart failure. *Lancet* 1990; **335**: 63–6.

23 Kavanagh T, Shephard RT, Chisholm AW, Quereshi S, Kennedy J. Prognostic indexes for patients with ischaemic heart disease enrolled in an exercise centred rehabilitation programme. *Am J Cardiol* 1979; **44**: 1230–40.

24 Oldridge NB, Donner AP, Buck C, *et al.* Predictors of dropout from cardiac exercise rehabilitation. *Am J Cardiol* 1983; **51**: 70–4.

25 Tooth L, McKenna K, Colquhuon D. Prediction of compliance with post-myocardial infarction home based walking programme. *Aust Occup Ther J* 1993; **40**: 17–22.

26 Michel TH. Outcome assessment in cardiac rehabilitation. *Int J Tech Assess Health Care* 1992; **8(1)**: 76–84.

27 Bertie J, King A, Reed N, Marshall AJ, Ricketts C. Benefits and weaknesses of a cardiac rehabilitation programme. *J R Coll Phys London* 1992; **26**: 147–51.

28 Hedback B, Perk J, Engvall J. Predictive factors for return to work after coronary by-pass grafting: the role of cardiac rehabilitation. *Int J Rehabil Res* 1992; **15**: 148–53.

8 Community based cardiac rehabilitation

HUGH JN BETHELL

Introduction

There is much to be said for community based cardiac rehabilitation. Being away from hospital it seems less like treatment than would a regular trip back to the physiotherapy department—it is recreation, normal physical activity, fun, something which is more likely to be incorporated into the daily life of the patient; indeed, the "patient" can rapidly become integrated into the normal exercising population and stop being a patient at all. The ideal venue is the community sports centre. This is equipped with all the expensive exercise training equipment that is needed for the endeavour. It does, however, lack some of the necessary medical hardware such as a defibrillator and intubation equipment, but it is not difficult to "scrounge" these from the hospital or raise money for them through local charitable organisations. An interested general practitioner is also the ideal person to supervise the rehabilitation programme. Few hospitals will have a physician or cardiologist who would wish to devote much time to the programme but each district has several hundred general practitioners from whom to choose a suitable person. He is likely to be around for many years (unlike a junior hospital doctor), to develop the programme and his own skills. He is also relatively cheap to employ.

The Basingstoke and Alton cardiac rehabilitation unit provides a model of such a cardiac rehabilitation programme, and is the basis of this chapter. It was established in Alton sports centre by a general practitioner and a sports officer. Over the first two years of operation we provided exercise training for 25 coronary patients from my own practice list and from the lists of other local general practitioners. After two years we offered the services of the unit to Basingstoke District Hospital, and since 1978 we have provided routine aftercare for patients discharged from the Basingstoke coronary care unit. Initially we ran an exercise only programme, but over the years it has evolved and developed into its present form. The aim is to provide integrated care from the hospital (phase I) to the stage when the patient should be living a fully active and healthy life (phase IV).

Phase I: In hospital

In hospital the patient receives the standard care and education which is provided by most coronary care units.

Education. One-to-one talks, small groups, and videos are used to give useful information and reassurance. At this time the patient, having survived a brush with death, is usually anxious and, being concerned about the effect of the attack on future activities, easily becomes depressed.[1-4] A positive approach is needed with much reassurance that he will recover and return to a way of life which is as active—or more so— as the pre-infarction condition. The patient cannot be expected to remember much of what is taught at this stage, but an optimistic attitude can be instilled and smokers can be persuaded as strongly as possible to use this opportunity to give up the habit—to avoid going back to cigarettes after the enforced period of nonsmoking in the coronary care unit. Simple dietary advice should be given to the patient and spouse. Since the greatest risk of death will be shortly after discharge this is the ideal time to teach the spouse cardiopulmonary resuscitation.

Mobilisation. The physiotherapist is the correct person to guide the patient's increasing exertions—starting with simple movement exercise and walking, progressing to stair climbing by the end of the hospital stay.

Risk assessment and medication. Appropriate medication is important for reducing post-hospital morbidity and mortality. Future dangers are greatest for those with evidence of extensive cardiac damage and of residual ischaemia.[5,6] Severe left ventricular damage is most likely to be present with second and subsequent infarctions, anterior infarctions, widespread electrocardiographic (ECG) changes, high enzyme rises, and signs of left ventricular failure or cardiogenic shock at the time of infarction. Supplementary evidence can be gleaned from the echocardiogram. Both β blockade[7,8] and angiotensin converting enzyme (ACE) inhibition[9,10] improve prognosis for some patients when they are prescribed the appropriate drug. All patients in whom it is not contraindicated are sent home on a small daily dose of aspirin.[11]

Before discharge the patient is visited by the programme coordinator, told about the rehabilitation programme, and given a folder which includes a brief summary of the admission (date, site of infarction, enzyme levels,

Advice sheet given to patients on leaving hospital

GOING HOME

Here is a programme which will suit most people going home after a *heart attack*. This is a general guide and young people, after small heart attacks, may be able to speed the programme up. Older patients, and those with problems after the attack, may need to slow it down. The staff on the *coronary care unit* will advise you if necessary

- *Week 1*: stay indoors, but get dressed. You may climb stairs, slowly, up to four times a day. A daily bath is fine, but not too hot. Simple household chores such as washing up and laying tables are okay, but do not hoover, make beds, or carry heavy objects. Most of your time will be spent at rest, reading, watching TV, talking (but not too heatedly!), and playing cards

- *Week 2*: start going out for short walks, initially taking a stroll in the garden, followed by going slowly down the street. Cooking and light housework may be started

- *Week 3 and 4*: the daily walks can now be built up, starting with about half a mile and increasing over the next fortnight to two miles. You may go out in a car, but do not drive yet (see below). By the end of week 3 light gardening, such as weeding can commence

- *Week 5 and onwards*: After this time gradual resumption of full activity is a matter of common sense. The daily walk, which need not exceed two miles, can be gradually speeded up—always avoiding undue tiredness, breathlessness, or chest pain

OTHER ACTIVITIES

- *Sexual intercourse*: by three weeks after discharge sex should present no problems for you. The energy used is roughly the same as climbing two flights of stairs. If doing this brings on chest pain or other worrying symptoms, you should avoid sex until you have discussed it with your doctor

- *Driving*: you are not allowed to drive for the first four weeks after the attack. After that you may drive if it causes you no problems. You do not need to inform the DVLA, but you should inform your insurance company.

- *Air travel*: it is perfectly safe to travel by air any time from six weeks after the attack, unless you are very short of breath with exercise or are getting chest pain with small amounts of exercise. If in doubt, ask your doctor

SYMPTOMS

When you get home you may well get some symptoms which worry you. The common ones are niggling and sharp left sided chest pain, tiredness, light-headedness, and occasional missed beats or extra beats. All of these symptoms are quite normal and can be completely ignored

continued

The following symptoms *may* be more serious:

- A tight central chest pain, or a pain similar to the heart attack pain, brought on by exercise and settling with rest (angina). A similar pain coming on at rest and unrelieved by using *glyceryl trinitrate* (see below)

- Being very breathless with small exertions, and particularly being woken at night by breathlessness

- Rapid thumping in the chest, particularly if it makes you feel faint

If you get any of these symptoms, (fortunately very few people do!), you should let your doctor know

USING GLYCERYL TRINITRATE (GTN, TRINITRIN NITROLIN-GUAL, CORO-NITRO)

- *Angina*: glyceryl trinitrate tablets or spray are designed to relieve angina. This is a tight central chest pain, sometimes going up into the throat or down into the arm, which comes with exercise and settles when you stop. Sometimes it comes on at rest

- *How to take them*: if you get such a pain, place a glyceryl trinitrate tablet or a puff of spray under your tongue. The drug takes effect very quickly and the chest pain is usually relieved within a few minutes. If your chest pain is not relieved within five minutes of taking the first tablet or spray, take a second. If again the pain is still present after five minutes take a third tablet or spray. If this does not remove your pain after another five minutes you should call your doctor. If you regularly get chest pains with exercise (*i.e. walking up a slope*) try taking a glyceryl trinitrate before starting

- *Side effects*: some people get a thumping headache with glyceryl trinitrate—spit out the tablet if this happens

- *Looking after the tablets*: Keep them in the *brown* bottle they come in, with the top screwed on tight. After two months they start to "*go-off*" and should be replaced. The spray has a two year life span

BLOOD TEST AT THREE MONTHS

You are encouraged to have a blood test, to measure your cholesterol and blood fat levels, at three months after the attack. You will be given the appropriate form with instructions at the rehabilitation centre or in outpatients

---

complications, treatment, and discharge medication) and the pre-discharge ECG. An appointment is made for three to four weeks hence to be seen at Alton Health Centre. Most importantly the folder contains a two page summary of advice including recommendations for physical activities, guidance on when to resume sex and car driving, and when it is safe to travel by air. The advice sheet also includes information about likely physical and emotional problems and a warning of dangerous symptoms that warrant calling the doctor. The use of glyceryl trinitrate if needed is described (see box).

Phase II: At home

Most patients and their partners identify the first few days at home as the worst time of all after a heart attack.[12] Leaving the protective womb of the hospital can be an intensely anxious experience for them both—and there is usually very little support for them in the community. They can be helped in the following ways.

Leaflets. Clear, written guidance in a language and style which patients can understand, as described above, should be provided. The programme coordinator or a nurse should go through this document with the patient and spouse before discharge and they should be encouraged to refer to it at home.

A hospital helpline. Some coronary care units give patients a telephone number to ring if they have any worries or queries. Also a nurse from the coronary care unit can arrange to telephone the patient at an interval after discharge.

A home visit from a nurse, either hospital or community based, or a health visitor. This may be the nurse involved with phase III of the rehabilitation programme. If community staff are used they need training for the task. The visiting nurse can give further education and guidance and assess problems that have arisen since discharge. She can also encourage the patient to continue with gradually increasing activities about the house and with a progressive walking programme.

A home visit from the general practitioner. Only a minority of patients receive a spontaneous home visit from their general practitioner (unpublished observations). This is a pity because at this time the patient and partner are usually bursting with anxiety, and with questions about symptoms and queries about the future which are not always easy for a nurse to answer. They can be strongly reassured about the tiredness, lightheadedness, missed beats, and niggling left-sided chest pains so common at this stage. A minority of patients, however, suffer more sinister symptoms such as angina on minor exertion (indicating severe residual coronary narrowing), breathlessness on minor effort or in bed (indicating left ventricular failure), or sustained palpitations perhaps accompanied by faintness (possibly indicating ventricular tachycardia—a precursor of ventricular fibrillation and sudden death.[13]) In any of these cases, the general practitioner will need to modify medication or refer the patient back to hospital.

A home visit by a "graduate" of the cardiac rehabilitation programme. This can be a boost to the patient's morale. We have introduced a training course for "graduates" (former patients who have been through rehabilitation) who wish to take up this task, teaching them listening skills, how to empathise with the new patient, and the basic knowledge to help them to give suitable advice. It is important, however, that the lay visitor does not try to adopt a "medical" role.

Whoever contacts the patient during the first week or two after discharge should continue to offer reassurance, encourage progressive increase in activities and plan entry into phase III of the rehabilitation programme and a return to a normal life. Lifestyle advice, particularly the dangers of restarting smoking and including dietary education, should be continued.

Phase III: Exercise, etc

Initial consultation

At about four weeks after the attack (and at about six weeks for heart surgery patients) the programme coordinator and I see the patient at Alton Health Centre, take a history, including an assessment of psychological wellbeing and mental health, examine the heart and lungs, and explain the rehabilitation programme.

At this consultation, some patients are found to be suffering from problems such as heart failure or progressive angina which have developed since their discharge from hospital. They are referred back to their physician for appropriate treatment before they join the programme.

For the vast majority who are judged fit to proceed the following are added to their folders: a medical summary, a description of the exercise course, instructions for taking the pulse rate, a Borg score sheet for perceived exertion rating, guidance on the use of a two mile walk (or walk/jog) to increase fitness, a description of warm-up exercises and home exercises using dumb-bells, home exercise recording sheets, details of the education and stress management course, and a low fat diet sheet. Arrangements are made for a fasting blood test at three months after the acute event to measure total cholesterol, triglycerides, T4 and sugar.

Exercise test

An exercise test at this stage is essential and serves the following purposes:

- *To detect residual coronary narrowing*: the finding of exertional ST segment depression, whether or not accompanied by chest pain, is usually an indication for coronary angiography and may require a change in medication.[14] A positive test need not prevent the patient entering the programme.
- *To detect high grade exercise-induced ventricular arrhythmias* such as multifocal ventricular ectopics or runs of ventricular tachycardia[13]: such

arrhythmias must be treated and the test repeated before the patient can start exercising.

- *To establish appropriate training heart rates*: the rates usually recommended for increasing physical fitness are between 70 and 85% of predicted maximum heart rate,[15] but maximum heart rate may be considerably lowered by drugs, particularly β blockers, ACE inhibitors, and some calcium channel blockers. Some patients have lower than normal heart rate responses to exercise—so-called chronotropic incompetence. If a maximum test is performed, the target exercise heart rate can be set at between 70 and 85% of the heart rate achieved. Alternatively, a submaximum test can be performed using the Borg scale of perceived exertion.[16] The appropriate heart rates lie between three and five for the "new" scale (table 8.1). Patients who develop reversible ischaemia should have their targets decided from the heart rate at which they develop either angina or ST segment depression.

- *To assess the fitness level of the patient*: the time on the treadmill or the load on the bicycle can be used to assess physical fitness, which is expressed either as peak oxygen consumption achieved or as metabolic equivalents (METs: 1 MET = 3·5 ml O_2/min/kg body weight[17]). For a submaximal test this will usually be between 10 and 30 ml/min/kg (about 3–8 METs). This figure will help to plan initial exercise loads and provides a level against which to measure subsequent progress. A low initial score is a poor prognostic feature.[18]

- *To detect exercise-induced hypotension*: this may be caused by drugs but is also a sign of poor left ventricular function.[19] Patients with this reponse need careful handling during physical training and are at risk

Table 8.1 The Borg perceived exertion scales (from Borg,[17] with permission).

Original scale	Verbal expression	New scale
	Nothing at all	0
7	Very, very light	0·5
	(just noticeable)	
8		
9	Very light	1
10		
11	Light.	2
12		
13	Moderate.	3
14	Somewhat heavy.	4
15	Heavy.	5
16		6
17	Very heavy.	7
		8
18		9
19	Very, very heavy	10

for developing severe and prolonged hypotension after vigorous exertion, particularly during hot weather.

Rehabilitation programmes that do not have the facilities for performing exercise tests must ensure that their patients have tests before joining the course and must know the results and be able to interpret them. It is a great help to have free and rapid access to re-testing for those patients who develop problems during the course.

For most patients the exercise course starts after an exercise test at five to six weeks after the infarction, but older patients and those who are judged to have suffered serious cardiac damage (those with more than one previous infarction, with large anterior infarctions, with evidence of cardiac failure in the coronary care unit) are set a walking programme for a few weeks before attending the sports centre.

The exercise test is performed by myself during an exercise session thus involving the patient in the course from the beginning. This has the added advantage of ensuring a doctor's presence at all sessions (frequently called upon to answer patients' concerns and worries), to assess new or changing symptoms, to check medication and adjust it if necessary and to redo the exercise test if this seems appropriate.

The exercise test is performed on a mechanically braked bicycle ergometer with continuous 12 lead ECG monitoring. The bicycle is used because patients find it less daunting than the treadmill—they can just stop pedalling if they feel they have done enough—and it allows much easier measurement of blood pressure. If a patient cannot reach a high enough heart rate on the bicycle and a more vigorous test is deemed necessary, this is performed on the treadmill later.

The patient starts cycling at 25, 50, or 75 W, depending on age, frailty, symptoms, and cardiac damage, and the load is increased by 25 W every three minutes. The aim is to reach the end point within six to nine minutes. The predetermined end points are:

- Angina pectoris with 2 mm ST segment depression
- ST segment depression of 3 mm or more without pain (silent ischaemia)
- A heart rate of 85% predicted maximum (195 minus age)
- Borg score of 6 or more
- High grade ventricular arrhythmia: this includes multifocal ventricular ectopics, repeated ventricular couplets, a run of three or more ventricular beats
- A fall of 20 mm or more of systolic blood pressure.

These end points are guides rather than absolute limits. Much can be learned from the patient's demeanour and from his reactions to the test. Some patients are comfortable to continue to heart rates above 85%

maximum; others who have no apparent cardiac defect are quite unable to reach one of the stated end points without feeling ill or frightened.

The ECG is retained by the patient in the rehabilitation folder. This saves storage and ensures that it is available to any doctor who is involved in the patient's management. Some hospital doctors remove the ECGs from the patient's folder and place them in the hospital notes!

Patients with significant angina or silent ischaemia are usually referred for coronary angiography. Unless they have very severe disease they are enrolled on the exercise course, after any necessary adjustment of medication, while they await investigation. Those with minor symptoms or ECG changes are not referred at this stage—as the course progresses it may become clear that they are having increasing symptoms, in which case they are referred later, as are those whose post-course exercise test shows deterioration. One of the main benefits of including exercise testing facilities in the programme is the ability to repeat the test at a moment's notice if difficulties are encountered, allowing reassurance when appropriate or change in treatment if this is indicated from the result. There is a problem with patients on β blockade. The exercise test data *on* medication is needed for the physical training course but this test may miss important ischaemic changes. Such patients should be re-tested *off* their blockers at some stage of the course, but this does stretch resources.

Patients with dangerous arrhythmias have their drug treatment altered to control the problem—since we do not have access to electrophysiological testing this has to be done by a process of trial and error and may require the performance of two or three further exercise tests.

Each patient has a record card, which consists of a database and flow chart. The database includes age, weight, cardiac and other history, drugs, and exercise test results. From the latter are derived and recorded the peak $\dot{V}O_2$ at the end of the test, the target heart rates, and the risk category of the patient—from A, which is low risk, through B, which is intermediate risk (that is, mild to moderately positive test, moderate sized infarction), to C, which is high risk (large infarction, cardiac failure or shock in the coronary care unit, strongly positive test or dangerous arrhythmias). The flow chart includes pre-exercise heart rate and blood pressure, exercise repetitions, time and load on the bicycle, post-exercise heart rates, Borg score, and blood pressure, and columns for weight and comments.

The exercise course

Exercise takes a central place in most cardiac rehabilitation programmes because it helps the patient back to normal life and also plays an important

175

part in secondary prevention. Some of the benefits of exercise for the post-infarction patient include:

- *Increased physical fitness*:[20–22] most heart attack victims have low levels of fitness because very few are regular exercisers, the period of post-infarction rest further reduces fitness, and the infarction reduces cardiac performance. Recovery of the damaged myocardium leads to a spontaneous improvement in exercise tolerance over the next three months or so,[23] and this can be enhanced by physical training, which improves muscle performance and peripheral circulatory adjustments to effort.[24] Only if physical training is continued for a year or more is cardiac performance likely to improve, with increases in both ejection fraction and ventricular contraction.[25–27] The initial effects of exercise programmes are, therefore, specific to the exercises performed—hence the advantage of circuit training, which exercises many different muscle groups.
- *Reduced angina*:[28] improved fitness means a lowered demand on the heart for any activity. This is an extremely important result for angina sufferers. Most will notice a significant reduction in the symptom as they become fitter and some will lose it altogether.
- *Enhanced coronary blood flow*: although there have been no trials which show an increase in collaterals after exercise training, there is indirect evidence to suggest that coronary blood flow *is* improved,[29] and this is supported by thallium perfusion studies.[30]
- *Reduced arrhythmias*: high grade ventricular ectopic activity is reduced by physical training after myocardial infarction.[31] This may explain some of the improved prognostic effect of this treatment.[32]
- *Improved lipid profiles*: regular vigorous exercise increases high density lipoprotein and reduces total cholesterol.[33] The level of exercise needs to be high and partly depends upon associated weight loss.[34]
- *Lowered blood pressure*: exercise lowers the blood pressure in hypertensive subjects and in mild hypertension may obviate the need for drug treatment.[35]
- *Improved fibrinolysis*: a high level of plasma fibrinogen and low fibrinolytic activity are powerful risk factors for coronary disease.[36] Both post-infarction and CABG patients have been shown to have increased fibrinolytic activity after exercise training.[37,38]
- *Restoration of confidence*: teaching the patient and partner that it is safe to exercise is a useful tool for restoring the confidence and self reliance which are so important for recovery. Depression is reduced and wellbeing increased.[21,39]
- *Improved survival*: several meta-analyses of controlled trials of cardiac rehabilitation have shown a reduction in mortality of over 20% in the treated groups.[40–42]

Most cardiac rehabilitation centres in the UK use circuit training—an easy way to supervise a number of patients in a limited area—as the basis for their exercise.[43] A few centres use a single exercise such as walking, walk/jogging or cycling.[44,45] The guidelines are shown in the box.

Guidelines for exercise

- *Frequency:* to increase physical fitness requires more than one session per week—ideally three or four; more frequent sessions can produce small further benefits but bring an increased risk of musculoskeletal injuries[15]

- *Duration:* between 20 and 30 minutes each session is ideal; shorter sessions are ineffective, while longer sessions also increase the risk of musculoskeletal problems[15]

- *Intensity:* the optimal increase in fitness is achieved by exercising to between 70 and 85% of maximum heart rate (MHR);[16] for the patient with normal cardiovascular responses who is not taking heart rate slowing drugs, predicted MHR (PMHR) is approximately 220 minus age:

$$85\% \ PMHR = 195 - age$$
$$70\% \ PMHR = 170 - age$$

Exercise in our programme starts with two induction sessions, each lasting two hours, at which the patients are taught in groups how to perform the warm up and stretching exercises and how to cool down thoroughly. They are also taught the home exercise circuits, which employ a pair of dumb-bells, the staircase, and an ergometer. These circuits are designed to simulate the supervised circuits as closely as possible.

The patient is then prescribed exercise every day—circuit training on Monday, Wednesday, and Friday, and walking on Tuesday, Thursday, Saturday, and Sunday. Low and intermediate risk patients perform one of the circuit sessions at the sports centre and the rest of their exercise at home. High risk patients perform two of the circuit sessions under supervision at the sports centre. All patients are set home circuits so that they become used to exercising without supervision. If they do not do this they tend to give it up as soon as the course ends.

The procedure for circuit training is the same whether it is performed at the sports centre or at home, though the home circuits are kept slightly less demanding than the centre circuits. The patient measures and reports or records the initial pulse rate and at the centre has his blood pressure taken. Stretching and progressive warm ups start each session and are followed by cycling on an ergometer, a sitting leg press, a bench press, jogging on a trampoline or on the spot, an arm curl, a squat lift, an overhead pull, and a two step climb. At the end of each circuit the pulse rate and the Borg score are checked. The circuits are repeated three times, after which the patient cools down on either the bicycle or the treadmill or simply by walking round the room. Initially the patient bicycles for one minute at the highest load for which three minutes was completed at the initial test and then repeats each of the circuit exercises three to 10 times, depending upon the fitness level. The weights are chosen to suit the sex, age, and strength of the patient. The pulse rate is checked and the result used to determine the number of repetitions at each station for the second circuit. This routine is repeated for the third circuit, after which the pulse rate is taken and the patient cools down for a few minutes before the final blood pressure is taken. At each sports centre attendance the number of repetitions and the load on the bicycle are gradually increased to ensure that the patient exercises to the target pulse rate as he becomes fitter. The home exercise circuits are prescribed in the exercise folder, to a level which is slightly lighter than the supervised session, and the patient records the pulse rate before starting and at the end of each circuit and the finishing Borg score.

On the remaining four days of the week the patient is set a two mile walk, also prescribed and recorded in the folder. He is encouraged gradually to increase the speed of the walk to reach the target heart rate. Some younger individuals can start jogging to reach this target—they are advised to begin by adding 15 seconds of slow jog at the end of each five minutes walk and to progress by increasing this by 15 seconds every week until the whole distance is taken at a jog. After this they may increase the distance but are cautioned to stay within their target pulse rates.

The education course

The exercise course is the centrepiece of the rehabilitation programme since it serves the dual aims of returning the patient to a normal life and providing long term reduction of risk. However, exercise on its own is insufficient to give maximum protection, and a number of other measures are needed to improve prognosis and quality of life:

Education. An understanding of the nature of coronary disease, its syptoms, the effects of treatment, the risk factors and how to reduce them all help patients to comply with treatment and advice and to take the steps necessary for their long term health. Education sessions should cover the following topics, and in our programme are taken by one of our nurses or the programme coordinator, who is a physiotherapist:

- The nature of coronary disease and its symptoms
- The risk factors for coronary disease and how to reduce them
- The drugs used in coronary disease—their effects and side effects
- Cholesterol, diet, and coronary disease—practical cooking demonstrations would be very helpful.

Other suitable educators are the community dietitian and the hospital pharmacist.

Relaxation and stress management. Behaviour, stress, anxiety, depression, and life events have all been found to play a part in coronary disease. They may be partly responsible for causing the disease, they may aggravate its symptoms, they may accelerate its progression, and they may worsen its prognosis. In addition, the results of excessive stress and of anxiety and depression are unpleasant for the patient and retard his recovery. Stress management tuition and training in relaxation techniques can be very valuable for the post-infarction patient for all these reasons, not least because the effect of the attack will have aggravated any pre-existing emotional problem.[46] We use two simple tests of psychological status at the initial consultation, to identify those with most to gain from this part of the programme. The sessions are conducted by a stress management consultant.

Risk factor monitoring

The main reversible risk factors are:

- *Cigarette smoking*: most smokers succeed in giving up while in the coronary care unit. They must be very strongly cautioned about the dangers of relapse. Persistent smokers are very difficult to help but every attempt to do so must be made since continued smoking is associated with twice the risk of future infarction.[47] Community Look After Your Heart (LAYH) tutors are well trained to run stopping smoking courses to which post-infarction patients can be referred.
- *High blood pressure*: blood pressure tends to fall after myocardial infarction but may rise to hypertensive levels over the subsequent few months, and it should be checked regularly and treated if it becomes persistently raised. Treatment of hypertension has a small but definite effect on the risk of recurrence, but before embarking on drug therapy patients should be encouraged to keep their blood pressures as low as possible by non-pharmacological means. These include weight reduction, low salt intake, low alcohol intake, regular exercise, and avoidance of stressful reactions, particularly anger, irritation, and frustration.
- *Raised cholesterol*: the blood cholesterol level falls within 24 to 48 hours of myocardial infarction or of major surgery and then takes about three months to recover.[48] If the blood lipids have not been measured very soon after the attack, blood should be taken at about three months for this purpose. All patients should be encouraged to keep their level as low as possible by eating a diet low in animal fat, by keeping their weight down, by taking regular exercise, and by avoiding aggressive behaviour. The aim should be to keep the level below 5·2 mmol/l with

179

as high density to low density lipoprotein ratio as possible—preferably 25% or more.[49] The use of lipid lowering drugs, which have been shown to produce regression of coronary atheroma, should be considered in treating raised blood cholesterols that are only slightly above the recommended level.

- *Obesity*: being overweight is only a weak independent risk factor for coronary disease but it does increase blood pressure and blood cholesterol. The cholesterol lowering effect of exercise depends partly on concomitant weight loss. Patients should be given a weight target and then every encouragement to reach it.

After approximately three months the bicycle test is repeated to measure the change in fitness level. An exercise circuit is performed at the end of the course and a "graduation" certificate presented to thunderous applause from the rest of the "undergraduates".

Final consultation

It is necessary to meet the patient one more time in the peace of the health centre to review progress, symptoms, and risk factors, and to plan future exercise and clarify follow up arrangements. The patient is strongly encouraged to continue with regular exercise and a low fat diet. Follow up and treatment of risk factors such as raised blood pressure and blood cholesterol is handed over to the general practitioner. Patients with known residual ischaemia which is not thought to warrant surgery are offered repeat exercise testing after a year.

Phase IV: The long term

Patients who have sustained a myocardial infarction or been treated by CABG have a chronic progressive disease from which most of them will sooner or later die.[50] Long term follow up to ensure compliance with preventive advice and to monitor, and if necessary treat, risk factors should reduce the recurrence of coronary events. Until recently there was no system for the surveillance of coronary patients—following their acute illness they returned to their previous life with a wish and a prayer that this might be led rather more healthily than before. The new system of paying general practitioners for health promotion and chronic disease management, however, does include under Band 2 the requirement to set up regular follow up of patients with coronary disease. They should receive some guidance from the cardiac rehabilitation programme about which aspects of their patients' care need particular attention. The following are the main aims of the chronic management of coronary patients.

To reinforce the secondary prevention message. The impact of the heart attack is a powerful incentive to adopt new and healthy ways of living.

Unfortunately this incentive fades with time and patients benefit from periodic reinforcement of advice to maintain regular exercise, low fat eating, stress-free living, and permanent abstinence from cigarettes. It is extremely helpful if the rehabilitation programme can be followed on by a self help group with exercise facilities, which the graduates of the programme can join. We have three such groups in different parts of the district as well as three other exercise locations. The graduates often appreciate having continued contact with the friends whom they have made during their time on the course, and the contact helps to keep them on the straight and narrow.

To check on risk factors. This applies particularly to return to or persistence of smoking, weight, blood pressure, and blood cholesterol.

To assess symptoms. At least half of those who die from coronary disease have the condition diagnosed *before* the episode which kills them. A regular check on the symptoms of those who are known to have coronary disease will, in a proportion, detect progression of old symptoms or the development of new ones. The acquisition or worsening of angina particularly should lead to referral for further investigation. At present, re-vascularisation improves the prognosis only of those with three vessel disease, but as procedures and techniques improve the number of patients who can benefit from intervention will increase.

To review medication. Low dose aspirin should be continued for ever—reducing long term mortality by over 20%.[51] β Blockers have a protective effect for at least two years after infarction, but it is uncertain whether they are helpful beyond this time.[8] It is possible that the lipid raising effects of these drugs eventually overcomes their benefits. Some other medications which were started in hospital may not be necessary in the long term—that is diuretics and long acting nitrates. Other new drugs may become available that can improve the prognosis of coronary patients—as in the case of ACE inhibitors for those with low ejection fractions. Only regular planned review of coronary patients can ensure that they benefit from advances in knowledge and in drug treatment.

To detect asymptomatic progression of coronary disease. Serial ECGs may give evidence of further problems such as silent infarction, but resting ECGs can only reveal fairly gross changes. The only practical way of uncovering increasing coronary narrowing is by serial exercise testing, and at present the NHS does not have the capacity to do this for more than a very small minority of coronary patients. Our rehabilitation unit offers repeated testing to those who have residual disease which is not felt to be severe enough to require re-vascularisation at the time. Progression of the exercise—induced ischaemic changes allows such patients to be re-evaluated and treated if and when it become appropriate.

References

1 Cay E, Philip A, Dugard P. Psychological reactions to a coronary care unit. *J Psychosom Res* 1972; **16**: 437–47.
2 Cassem N, Hackett T. Psychiatric consultation in a coronary care unit. *Ann Intern Med* 1971; **75**: 9–14.
3 Schliefer S, Macari-Hinson H, Coyle D, *et al.* The nature and course of depression following myocardial infarction. *Arch Intern Med* 1989; **149**: 1785–9.
4 Mayou R. Prediction of emotional and social outcome after a heart attack. *J Psychosom Res* 1984; **28**: 17–25.
5 Moss A. Prognosis after myocardial infarction. *Am J Cardiol* 1983; **52**: 667–9.
6 Bigger J, Fleiss J, Kleiger R, *et al.* The relationships among ventricular arrhythmias, left ventricular dysfunction and mortality in the two years after myocardial infarction. *Circulation* 1984; **69**: 250–8.
7 Beta-Blocker Heart Attack Trial Research Group. A randomised trial of propranolol in patients with acute myocardial infarction. *JAMA* 1982; **247**: 1707–14.
8 Olssen G, Wikstrand J, Warnold I, *et al.* Metoprolol induced reduction in post-infarction mortality: pooled results from five double blind randomised trials. *Eur Heart J* 1992; **13**: 28–32.
9 Yusuf S, Pepone C, Garces C, *et al.* Effect of enalapril on myocardial infarction and unstable angina in patients with low ejection fraction. *Lancet* 1992; **340**: 1173–8.
10 Editorial. From cardiac to vascular protection: the next chapter. *Lancet* 1992; **340**: 1197–8.
11 Isis 2 Collaborative Group. Randomised trial of intravenous streptokinase, oral aspirin, both, or neither among 17,187 cases of suspected acute myocardial infarction: Isis 2. *Lancet* 1988; **i**: 349–60.
12 Hackett T, Cassem N. Psychological adaptation to convalescence in myocardial infarction patients. In: Naughton J, Hellerstein K, editors. *Exercise testing and exercise training in coronary heart disease.* New York: Academic Press, 1973.
13 Federman J, Whitford J, Anderson S, *et al.* Incidence of arrhythmias in first year after acute myocardial infarction. *Br Heart J* 1978; **40**: 1243–50.
14 Theroux P, Waters D, Halphen C, *et al.* Prognostic value of exercise testing soon after myocardial infarction. *New Engl J Med* 1979; **301**: 341–6.
15 Hellerstein H, Hirsch E, Ader R, *et al.* Principles of exercise testing for normals and cardiac subjects. In: Naughton J, Hellerstein H, editors. *Exercise testing and exercise training in coronary heart disease.* New York: Academic Press, 1973.
16 Borg G, Psycho-physical bases of perceived exertion. *Med Sci Sports Exerc* 1982; **14**: 377–9.
17 Jette M, Sidney K, Blumchen G. Metabolic equivalents (METs) in exercise testing, exercise prescription and evaluation of functional capacity. *Clin Cardiol* 1990; **13**: 555–65.
18 Madsden G, Gilpin E, Staffan A, *et al.* Prediction of functional capacity and use of exercise testing for predicting risk after acute myocardial infarction. *Am J Cardiol* 1985; **56**: 834–45.
19 Hetherington M, Haennel R, Teo K, *et al.* Importance of considering ventricular function when prescribing exercise after acute myocardial infarction. *Am J Cardiol* 1986; **58**: 891–5.
20 Carson P, Phillips R, Lloyd M, *et al.* Exercise after myocardial infarction: a controlled trial. *J Roy Coll Physicians* 1982; **16**: 147–51.
21 Bethell H, Mullee M. A controlled trial of community based coronary rehabilitation. *Br Heart J* 1990; **64**: 370–5.
22 Froelicher V, Jensen J, Genter F, *et al.* A randomised trial of exercise training in patients with coronary disease. *JAMA* 1984; **252**: 1291–7.
23 Haskell W, de Busk R. Cardiovascular responses to repeated treadmill exercise testing soon after myocardial infarction. *Circulation* 1979; **60**: 1247–51.
24 Clausen J. Circulatory adjustments to dynamic exercise and effect of physical training in normal subjects and in patients with coronary artery disease. *Prog Cardiovasc Dis* 1976; **18**: 459–95.
25 Martin W, Heath G, Coyle E, *et al.* Effect of prolonged intense endurance training on systolic time intervals in patients with coronary disease. *Am Heart J* 1984; **107**: 75–81.

26 Ehsani A, Biello D, Schultz J, *et al*. Improvement of left ventricular contractile function by exercise training in patients with coronary artery disease. *Circulation* 1986; 74: 350–5.

27 Kellerman J, Shemesh J, Fisman E, *et al*. Arm exercise training in the rehabilitation of patients with impaired ventricular function and heart failure. *Cardiology* 1990; 77: 130–8.

28 Dressendorfer R, Smith J, Amsterdam, *et al*. Reduction of submaximal exercise myocardial oxygen demand post-walk training program in coronary patients due to improved physical work efficiency. *Am Heart J* 1982; 103: 358–62.

29 Franklin B. Exercise training and coronary collateral circulation. *Med Sci Sport Exerc* 1991; 23: 648–53.

30 Doba N, Shukuya M, Yoshida H, *et al*. Physical training of the patients with coronary heart disease: non-invasive strategies for the evaluation of its effects on the oxygen transport system and myocardial ischaemia. *J Circ J* 1990; 54: 1409–18.

31 Hertzeanu H, Shemish J, Aron A, *et al*. Ventricular arrhythmias in rehabilitated and non-rehabilitated post-myocardial infarction patients with left ventricular dysfunction. *Am J Cardiol* 1993; 71: 24–7.

32 La Rovere M, Mortara A, Sandgrove G, Lombard F. Autonomic nervous system adaptations to short term exercise training. *Chest* 1992; 101 (suppl): 299–303.

33 Heath G, Ehsani A, Hagberg J, *et al*. Exercise training improves lipoprotein lipid profiles in patients with coronary artery disease. *Am Heart J* 1983; 105: 889–95.

34 Haskell W. The influence of exercise training on plasma lipids and lipoproteins in health and disease. *Acta Med Scand* 1986; (suppl) 711: 25–37.

35 World Hypertension League. Physical exercise in the management of hypertension: a consensus statement. *J Hypertension* 1991; 9: 283–7.

36 Meade T, Ruddock V, Stirling Y, *et al*. Fibrinolytic activity, clotting factors and long term incidence of ischaemic heart disease in the Northwick Park Heart Study. *Lancet* 1993; 342: 1076–9.

37 Estelles A, Aznar J, Tormo G, *et al*. Influence of a rehabilitation sports programme on the fibrinolytic activity of patients after myocardial infarction. *Thromb Res* 1989; 55: 203–12.

38 Wosornu D, Allardyce W, Ballantyne D, Tansey P. Influence of power and aerobic exercise training on haemostatic factors after coronary artery surgery. *Br Heart J* 1992; 68: 181–6.

39 Oldridge N, LaSalle D, Jones N. Exercise rehabilitation of female patients with coronary disease. *Am Heart J* 1980; 100: 755–6.

40 Shephard R. The value of exercise in ischaemic heart disease: accumulative analysis. *J Cardiac Rehabil* 1983; 3: 294–8.

41 Oldridge N, Guyatt G, Fischer M, *et al*. Cardiac rehabilitation after myocardial infarction. Combined experience of randomised clinical trials. *JAMA* 1988; 260: 945–50.

42 O'Connor G, Buring J, Yusuf S, *et al*. An overview of randomised trials of rehabilitation with exercise after myocardial infarction. *Circulation* 1989; 80: 234–44.

43 Horgan J, Bethell H, Carson P, *et al*. British Cardiac Society working party report on cardiac rehabilitation. *Br Heart J* 1992; 67: 412–18.

44 Wenger N. Rehabilitation after myocardial infarction. *Postgrad Med J* 1979; 66: 128–43.

45 Kavanagh T, Shephard R. Conditioning of post-coronary patients: comparison of continuous and interval training. *Arch Phys Med Rehabil* 1975; 56: 72–6.

46 Theorell T. Psychosocial intervention as a part of the rehabilitation after a myocardial infarction. *Int Rehabil Med* 1983; 5: 185–8.

47 Mulcahy R, Graham I, MacAirt J. Factors affecting the 5 year survival rate of men following acute coronary heart disease. *Am Heart J* 1977; 93: 556–9.

48 Rose G, Shipley M. Plasma cholesterol concentration and death from coronary artery disease: 10 year results of the Whitehall study. *BMJ* 1986; 293: 306–7.

49 Betteridge D, Dodson P, Durrington P, *et al*. Management of hyperlipidaemia: guidelines of the British Hyperlipidaemia Association. *Postgrad Med J* 1993; 69: 359–69.

50 Squires R, Gau G, Miller T, *et al*. Cardiovascular rehabilitation: status 1990. *Mayo Clin Proc* 1990; 65: 731–55.

51 Antiplatelet Trialists' Collaboration. Collaborative overview of randomised trials of antiplatelet therapy—I: Prevention of death, myocardial infarction, and stroke by prolonged antiplatelet therapy in various categories of patient. *BMJ* 1994; 308: 81–106.

183

9 Evaluation of rehabilitation programmes

ROBERT WEST

Introduction

This chapter reviews evaluation of rehabilitation and discusses methodological issues in assessment of effectiveness. The need for rehabilitation, the objectives or goals of rehabilitation, and the historical development of comprehensive rehabilitation programmes for patients after acute myocardial infarction and for patients with other cardiac conditions have been covered in earlier chapters. Nevertheless, some recapitulation is relevant in order to put evaluation into context. In 1964 the World Health Organisation (WHO) defined cardiac rehabilitation as "the sum of activity to ensure them the best possible physical, mental and social conditions so that they by their own efforts regain as normal as possible a place in the community and lead an active productive life".[1] This definition highlights three important points: that rehabilitation is about enabling patients to help themselves, rather than treating patients or training patients to perform certain tasks; that rehabilitation is multi-disciplinary, which recognises the diversity of patients' needs and relevance of different therapists; and that the goal is for patients to regain optimum quality of life as nearly as possible, which is not necessarily synonymous with the wishes of therapists.

The distinction between enabling and treating is not always clear cut but, for purposes of reviewing the literature on effectiveness of rehabilitation, it is useful to limit what is included. Rehabilitation is generally understood to be the outpatient activity, following the acute period in hospital, initiating and facilitating the recuperative period at home. The hospital inpatient period is primarily characterised by therapeutic activity and patient dependency, and the convalescent period is primarily one of self care, adjustment and "by their own efforts regaining as normal a place as possible". While accepting that some rehabilitative activities may be initiated relatively early in the acute phase and that some professional guidance may continue months or even years after discharge, the thrust of rehabilitation is to help patients over the bridge from the acute phase to the recuperative phase. For practical purposes of limiting the scope of this evaluation, this working definition of rehabilitation also excludes long term therapies (by β blocker, diuretic, aspirin, etc), the effectiveness of which have been reviewed extensively elsewhere.

The rationale for rehabilitation may be described as physical, psychological, educational, and social, and the individual needs of individual patients may vary significantly in any one of these dimensions. The principal components or modalities of rehabilitation are designed to address these perceived needs and programmes may include physical, psychological, and educational components, or combinations of these. In evaluating effectiveness it is necessary to appreciate that a programme that concentrates on one of the above modalities (for example, physical) may achieve pre-defined objectives in that dimension (for example, improved exerise tolerance) and may at the same time benefit another dimension (for example, reduced social isolation) but may achieve the pre-defined objective at the expense of another dimension (perhaps, for example, increased anxiety). Before discussing the issue of multiple end points and selecting relevant end points that satisfy the overall objective of rehabilitation, it is appropriate to consider whose overall objective is to be satisfied. This inevitably invokes patients' autonomy. While many therapists consider extended survival following exercise training as excellent evidence of benefit, many people including cardiac patients with different value systems, calculate that every hour of life extension is bought at the expense of an hour (or more) on the treadmill. While some may enjoy physical exercise, others clearly do not and would not consider such fitness as "regaining as normal as possible a place in the community", their former and preferred status quo.

End points for assessing rehabilitation

The plurality of aims and objectives of rehabilitation is justification for use of more than one end point in assessing effectiveness of intervention strategies. In current parlance, rehabilitation may "add life to years as well as years to life". There are several dimensions to quality of life that may not add, at least not on a simple linear scale. Benefits in one dimension may be accompanied by benefits in another for some patients and not for

185

others, and may not be appreciated as benefits at all by others again. Despite using these arguments to justify more than one end point in the evaluation of rehabilitation programmes, therapists should be aware of the potential misuse of multiple end points: if enough variables are studied one end point may be shown to benefit through chance alone.

Survival

Survival (or its inverse, mortality) has been seen as the hard statistic by clinicians, epidemiologists, and the lay public for generations; mortality statistics, if available, have tended to dominate evaluation in many fields of medical endeavour. A well known example in cardiology is evaluation of coronary artery bypass graft surgery. While the technique was introduced for relief of longstanding angina intractable to medication, three randomised controlled trials demonstrated reduced total mortality in those patients most severely compromised (those with disease of left main stem or disease in three principal vessels). Since publication of the results of those trials the operation has been seen as life saving and so firmly believed to be life saving that many have extrapolated survival benefits beyond the range of experimental evidence to include patients with few symptoms and occlusion in only one vessel. Survival is clearly one end point by which rehabilitation interventions may be evaluated.

Quality of life

Quality of life is more ephemeral and its measurement is more ambiguous—since individuals value aspects of their lives differently. Many scales have been developed over the years for the measurement of various aspects of health status, but few have attempted to measure directly patients' perceptions of improvement in level of performance and satisfaction with level of health, although it is these which largely determine whether patients consider themselves to be recovered or in need of further care or treatment.[2] Many scales measure aspects of health, including functional ability, psychological wellbeing, social support, and health status, each of which may contribute to patients' perceived quality of life. These scales may well be relevant to patients' total health status and to whether patients see themselves as recovered. However, it should be appreciated that these scales measure different features of health and that patients may be recovered and well on one scale and at the same time sick and in need of further treatment on another.

Return to work

One measurement, that has been used to evaluate effectiveness of rehabilitation in many studies, has been "return to work". This has been measurable in a relatively clear cut manner (as for mortality) and has been seen as removing some of the perceived subjectivity of health status scales.

It has been pointed out in Chapter 2 that in its applicability this simple measure is limited to young men in areas of generally high employment. With widening eligibility for rehabilitation to include more women and more retired patients, and with the changed social circumstances of widespread unemployment, this simple measure of "regaining a normal place in the community" has become less relevant as a measure of effectiveness of rehabilitation.

Physical function

A further class of measures has been widely used to demonstrate effectiveness of rehabilitative interventions. These are measurements of physical function and include, for example, resting heart rate, blood pressure, exercise time, maximum heart rate, and rate pressure product. It is fairly clear that these have a direct relevance to monitoring physical training and fitness, and they are conveniently measurable. Rehabilitationists should be cautious against over-reliance on such measures or overinterpreting change in these measures. While they may be very direct measures of physical functions, the physical functions themselves are not necessarily representative of quality of life or successful rehabilitation.

"Natural history" of adoption and evaluation of new therapies

A "natural history" of the adoption of medical technologies has been described by several observers, where the term "medical technology" has been used quite generally to include therapies and health care programmes, such as cardiac rehabilitation.[3] The principal phases are (1) the theoretical phase, when someone formulates the idea, based on observations in related areas or in animal experiments; (2) the initiation phase, when the idea is tested on the first "guinea pigs"; (3) the development phase, when methods are refined and tested on larger numbers (in "centres of excellence"); (4) the marketing phase, when the technique is taken into regular practice (in district hospitals); and (5) the establishment phase, when regular practice becomes routine. It has been noted that routine practice is often overtaken by the next technology, unless unchallengeable through "unquestionable merit" or protected by "protocols". The history of cardiac rehabilitation may possibly be fitted into this model. It is fairly clear from earlier chapters that cardiac rehabilitation is in different phases in different countries. In Britain, cardiac rehabilitation may be moving from the third to the fourth phase, with programmes recently introduced into many district general hospitals, largely as a consequence of the Chest, Heart and Stroke Association and British Heart Foundation "pump-priming" grants. At the same time it is clear that rehabilitation is well established in parts of America and Canada, and in parts of Northern Europe rehabilitation hospitals see themselves as being "overtaken by the times" (of thrombolysis?).

There is a natural history of evaluation that accompanies this natural history of development of a therapeutic practice. In these days of mega trials,[4,5] and of statistical overviews of large trials,[6] statisticians have turned attention away from the importance of early "phase 1" and even "phase 0" trials. Where there is no knowledge of the effect of a proposed new therapy or intervention, the first ($n=1$) experiment is highly significant. Of course in advancing science the investigator never really starts from absolutely zero knowledge: there is always some expectation of the consequences of following the existing therapy (or lack of therapy) and there is usually some comparable experience or animal experiment relevant to the proposed new therapy, on which to base an expectation of using it for the first time. The logical first ($n=1$) experiment is the longitudinal study of the first "guinea pig". Because of biological variation and statistical chance, a good (or bad) outcome in one may or may not suggest a good (or bad) outcome in 10 and hence the second logical experiment is the longitudinal study of a small group of patients given the innovative treatment. At this stage, if initial promise is maintained and the new treatment appears to offer an improved time course in the measured functions, parameters, or variables, it is necessary to undertake controlled experiments to compare the temporal improvements under the innovative therapy with possibly comparable improvements under the existing therapy (or no therapy). While early ($n=1$) experiments and early "uncontrolled" experiments on small numbers have their role in the evolution of a new scientific theory, they do not justify claims of effectiveness based on series of "uncontrolled" observations because without a fairly matched comparison group, such "uncontrolled" observations could be reflecting nothing more than the natural resolution of morbidity following myocardial infarction.

Causality

Epidemiologists have suggested a hierarchy of evidence for judging causality of association in medicine, ranging from personal clinical observation, through structured case control and cohort (observational) studies to randomised controlled trials and, where possible, randomised crossover trials.[7] This hierarchy is perhaps better recognised by cardiologists than by any other medical specialty, which is quite possibly what lies behind the cautious acceptance of rehabilitation programmes in this country.[8] Thus in assessing the effectiveness of rehabilitation in this chapter, evidence is drawn principally from the randomised controlled trial literature.

Therapists surrounded by patients who appear to be clearly recovering from myocardial infarction may find this detached objectivity unduly negative. But they should appreciate that their perspective is naturally biased: patients who continue to attend rehabilitation programmes are those who progress, those who drop out have reasons for so doing and these reasons often include failure to progress. In the extreme, patients who drop out include those who relapse with further myocardial infarction, experience a stroke, or die. Secondly, therapists surrounded by grateful patients progressing weekly further through the exercise circuit do not have comparable experience of witnessing the weekly process of "natural rehabilitation" of patients who are not attending rehabilitation programmes. The only fair assessment of relative advantage of rehabilitation to patients is comparison of the progress of similar patients with and without rehabilitation programmes by independent assessors and using independent measures.

The relevance of independent assessors and independent measures to fair comparison is often overlooked and may be quite an important consideration in evaluation of function and quality of life in cardiac rehabilitation. It is not uncommon for physical function to be measured on the same machine as that on which the patient trained (for example bicycle ergometer). In such situations there may be some difficulty in distinguishing between specialist training for that particular activity and training *per se* and its associated improvement in general fitness. Patients trained for a particular activity on a particular machine clearly have the advantage of familiarity in repeated tests over untrained controls, recuperating naturally, who remain unfamiliar with and possibly apprehensive about the machine, the test, the result, and the consequences of the result. Furthermore, patients perform differently for familiar therapists (physiotherapist, nurse, psychologist) compared with unfamiliar examiners. These phenomena are well recognised even for quite objective measures, such as blood pressure and heart rate, and for performance among healthy normals and athletes, let alone anxious or depressed, apprehensive, or dependent patients after the life threatening crisis of myocardial infarction.

Evolution of rehabilitation trials

The evolution of rehabilitation programmes based on physical training or retraining from "armchair treatment",[9] through early mobilisation,[10,11] supervised exercise,[12-14] to expert committee recommendations[15,16] has been described in other chapters. Here it is intended to review the evolution of the accompanying evidence for physical rehabilitation, where, as indicated above, rehabilitation is defined operationally as an outpatient activity designed to follow discharge from acute care in hospital and to facilitate long term rehabilitation at home.

With memories of classic advice of Heberden (1750)[17] and Stokes (1854),[18] more recent reports of the safety of armchair treatment[9] and evidence from animal experiments and epidemiological studies that showed inverse associations between exercise and cardiovascular disease,[19,20] physicians in Israel and parts of north America began exercising selected patients after myocardial infarction.[21-24] For several years the primary evidence of effectiveness of these exercise programmes was of improved cardiac performance among compliant volunteer patients after a period of (re)training compared with the period prior to (re)training. A sample comparison is given in table 9.1.

Table 9.1 Improvement of rate pressure product (heart rate × systolic blood pressure) after exercise training programmes.

Study	Year	Number of patients	Rate pressure product	
			Before training	After training
Frick and Katila[25]	1968	7	262	242
Hellerstein[26]	1968	100	248	193
Clausen et al[27]	1969	9	204	166
Kasch and Boyer[28]	1969	11	163	156
Detry et al[29]	1971	12	116	94

These findings suggest that, at different levels of exercise testing, improvements of 10–20% in rate pressure product (heart rate × blood pressure) might be attributed to exercise training. Few studies made comparisons with controls (not enrolled in rehabilitation programmes), whose performance might have improved comparably with the passage of time after myocardial infarction or with familiarity with the testing procedure. An exception was the study by Rechnitzer et al[22] who compared eight exercised cardiac patients with eight cardiac controls and also eight exercised normals with eight non-exercised normals.

Controlled trials

Controlled trials of exercise rehabilitation programmes emanated from Scandinavia.[30-32] Two of these suggested a reduction in mortality following rehabilitation but, because numbers were relatively small, possible reductions were not statistically significant. Table 9.2 shows the relative risk of death for exercised patients compared with non-exercised patients in these trials and the approximate probability that such relative risks of death could have been observed under the null hypothesis that programme and control samples were drawn from the same populations

Table 9.2 Mortality following exercise based rehabilitation.

| Trial | Year | Deaths/patients | | Relative risk | p |
		Programme	Controls		
Kentala[30]	1972	11/77	11/81	1·05	>0·9
Sanne[31]	1973	25/158	30/147	0·83	0·5
Palatsi[32]	1976	18/180	28/200	0·71	0·2

(with the same mortality experiences). While a relative risk of death of 0·83 might represent a 17% reduction in (all cause) mortality, such trial results could have arisen by chance.

Several more trials of exercise based rehabilitation have been reported since.[33–39] Others might be added to this list except that they included other components of rehabilitation (risk factor modification, psychological therapy or counselling) and will be considered under Comprehensive rehabilitation (see later). Several of the 10 trials suggest possible reductions in (all cause) mortality but none was statistically significant.

Trial size

Statisticians can advise on the size of a trial needed to demonstrate a mortality reduction (of say 15%) when the expected mortality in the follow up period is reliably estimated (say 10%), which is tantamount to seeking a comparison of 8·5% with 10%, at a predetermined level of significance (usually $p < 0.05$) and power (usually 80 or 90%). In planning the national exercise heart disease project, the power calculation asked for 4 300 patients.[40] In practice the study yielded 651, so that even the largest of these trials was unlikely to obtain a significant result with reasonable starting assumptions.

Clinicians and health service managers need to make decisions on the basis of available information, in this case decisions on prescribing exercise rehabilitation or on setting up exercise rehabilitation programmes on the basis of a number of randomised trials, each of which was too small to provide a satisfactory answer either way. Rehabilitation is a typical example of many clinical or health service management decisions and demands a carefully considered review or overview of the relevant available evidence.

Reviews and statistical overviews

In the past reviews tended to be written by the senior authority on the subject (usually anonymously as an occasional editorial) and consensus evolved informally, often permeating from centres of excellence and the anonymous reviewers. Following the explosion of scientific activity, literature, and journals, statisticians have taken a lead in formalising the review process. Reviewing has moved some way from being an art to being a science, with the fairly widespread use of the statistical overview (or meta-analysis). Editorials have become much more numerous so that, in many journals, each new trial (or original paper) is accompanied by an editorial, designed to help place the trial in context. Editorials often do little more than rearrange the words of the original paper's discussion, and it is not uncommon for a journal to carry contradictory editorials only a year or so apart on the "state of the art" in a given subject. However, since editorials are now more often named it is easier than previously to identify the source of prevalent views and of dissident views.

The statistical overview has largely replaced the past occasional editorial in summarising the state of knowledge in many developing research areas. While such a role for the statistical overview is clearly established,[6] it needs to be undertaken properly and its findings still need to be interpreted, in an "editorial of editorials". An accompanying though not necessarily related trend has been the formalising of consensus development, through consensus conferences or expert committees.

A source of overviewing

Before applying the methods of a statistical overview to 10 exercise-based rehabilitation trials, it is relevant to consider briefly a few cautions on use of the technique.[41] These may be considered under five headings: representativeness, homogeneity, statistical, publication bias, and *post hoc* enquiry bias or inevitable prejudice.[42] All the recommendations of critical appraisal of the scientific (medical) literature are relevant in assessing the "truth" behind a paper.[7,43] In any reading of the scientific literature and interpretation of the findings, readers must appreciate that they are not really told what happened, they have only the word of the author(s) and often a very abbreviated account. Frequently, several years have passed between project design or completion and final submission of the paper, and often the paper has passed through many editorial stages between researcher and publication. While redrafting and editorial revision may be designed to achieve "conformity", they may "improve reality". Peto[6] has stressed the need to include all trials in statistical overviews and there are clear examples of the effect of publication bias in fields in which trial registration is practiced.[45] Begg and Berlin presented an example in which the pooled effect of published trials was significant, while at the same time the pooled effect of registered trials was not.[44] Homogeneity considerations include for example: Were the patient populations similar: were they all confirmed myocardial infarctions or have some trials included patients after cardiac surgery? Were the interventions similar: have all trials compared formal exercise with no exercise, have some compared a lot of exercise with a little exercise, or have some included significant amounts of risk factor reduction advice or counselling? Were end points comparable: was two year total mortality used, have some trials compared six month or five year mortality, or have some compared fatal and non-fatal cardiac events together?

Publication bias

Publication bias is popularly attributed to journal editors, behaving to some degree as purveyors of scientific news or interesting stories and preferring papers with results to those without. There have been several proposals for a journal of negative results, and proposals that journals should accept papers on the basis of introducion, methods, and discussion, with perhaps blank tables of results (to show layout and comparisons), but the practicalities of writing a discussion that does not give away the result are rather daunting. Many readers of the scientific literature do not appear to fully appreciate how many may contribute to 'non-publication'. Studies that fail to produce the anticipated answer are often abandoned before completion, possibly because funding is not continued and temporary research staff move on to their next short term project and junior medical staff move on to their next training post. Studies may even be abandoned quite early and staff redirected towards testing a different hypothesis. It has been reported that more negative studies are withdrawn by their authors than are rejected by editors.[45] Publication bias is not "black or white", publish or reject: papers may be accepted after editor and referee feedback, which is often directed towards helping mould the "unacceptable" into the prevailing consensus.

Post hoc analysis

The most important criticism of statistical overviews is that they contravene one of the hallowed principles of science, "first the hypothesis, then the test".[46] By its very nature the statistical overview is *post hoc*; the reviewer starts with a set of results (in this case trials that compare mortality of exercise trained patients after myocardial infarction with mortality of the untrained) and then selects from these results those that suit his purpose. He should be and may attempt to be as detached and as dispassionate as possible and select trials on the basis of methodology, size, duration of intervention, etc, but it is rare for the reviewer to be truly blind as to the result and the effect of its inclusion (or exclusion) on the pooled overall estimate. It is much more common that he starts with the answer (in the abstract or even in the title) and learns about the methodology, problems encountered, or errors committed on closer reading or by further interrogation of the authors.

Some statistical overviews have described a "scientific" process of selecting and including trials, which requires a team (a) to read articles and transcribe them into a results-free format, (b) to judge eligibility criteria and weighting of papers selected for inclusion, (c) to pool the findings of the selected papers, and (d) to interpret the pooled findings in the light of other relevant knowledge. Doing it properly requires several people, at least one of whom should be well informed methodologically and totally ignorant of the subject of study, a very unlikely combination, and doing it properly requires considerable time. One statistical overview of exercise based rehabilitation found considerable inter-rater differences in what the programmes actually included (for example, in how many weeks of exercise, and how many times per week) and what outcome measure the trials compared (for example, comparing deaths after discharge, randomisation, or start of rehabilitation).[47] Comparison of statistical overviews reveals that different reviewers have interpreted and reported results of the same papers differently.[42,47,48]

Statistical overviews of controlled trials

Physical rehabilitation

Mortality comparison of 10 trials of exercise based rehabilitation are summarised in figure 9.1. In five of these trials the mortality appeared to be reduced after physical training programmes but in none was the benefit over controls statistically significant. In the other five trials mortality after physical training programmes appeared to be very comparable with that of

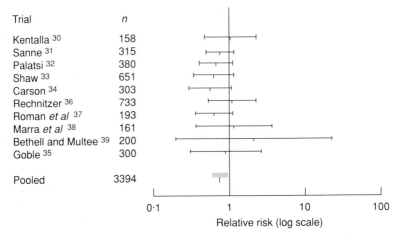

Figure 9.1 Mortality following exercise based rehabilitation: estimated relative risk of death in medium term among myocardial infarction patients offered rehabilitation, compared with controls, in 10 individual trials and in a pooled estimate of all 10 trials (bars show 95% confidence intervals).

controls. Overall, the pooled results of the 10 trials suggest a mortality reduction of approximately 22%, that is statistically significant (relative risk 0·78, 95% confidence interval 0·63–0·96). However, this pooled result should be interpreted with caution, since the trials differed in a number of respects. For example, Kentala[30] compared two hospitals, one with rehabilitation, one without (rather than randomised patients), Rechnitzer et al[36] compared a supervised moderate exercise training programme with light exercise advice (rather than with no exercise), and Bethell and Mullee[39] reported mortality after only three months and hence contributed very few deaths to the pooled results (compared with other trials that reported mortality after up to three years). Furthermore, without registration of rehabilitation trials, we do not know how many negative trials were left unfinished or unpublished. For example, the Southern Ontario trial[49] the largest single exercise-based trial ($n = 733$) was cited by May et al[50] as showing 36 deaths among exercised patients compared with 26 among controls, which suggested a mortality disadvantage to exercised patients. The trial reported only fatal re-infarctions (15 versus 13) and non-fatal re-infarctions (39 versus 33).[36]

Comprehensive rehabilitation

Comprehensive rehabilitation programmes were evaluated in the WHO European collaborative trial.[51] Some reviews have described these programmes as "exercise plus" rehabilitation. Since this was a collaborative study, with a coordinating committee, there was more homogeneity between centres than in the individual exercise trials discussed above. Nevertheless, the report excluded seven of the original collaborating centres, and some subsequent reviewers have chosen to exclude further centres on grounds of comparison group selection or loss to follow up.[48]

Three year mortality was summarised in the WHO report as one centre (of 17) showing a significantly reduced mortality among rehabilitation patients, balanced by one other centre showing a significantly increased mortality among rehabilitation patients. The relative risks (and 95% confidence intervals) of each of the 17 centres and of all 17 centres combined are summarised in figure 9.2. Overall, this suggests that the European collaborative rehabilitation programmes may have reduced three year mortality by about 14% (relative risk 0·86, 95% confidence interval 0·72–1·03), on the basis of 17 centres and 2 602 patients. It would be interesting to know the outcomes of the 582 patients in the seven centres that were originally enrolled but were omitted from the report. Other trials have evaluated multidisciplinary rehabilitation since the WHO collaborative trial, but with relatively small numbers these add little new information on relative mortality.

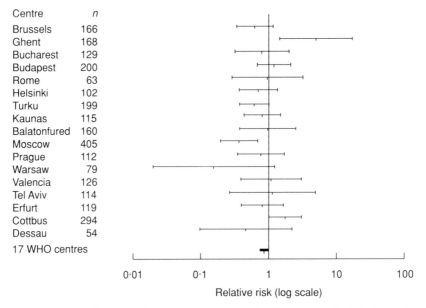

Centre	n
Brussels	166
Ghent	168
Bucharest	129
Budapest	200
Rome	63
Helsinki	102
Turku	199
Kaunas	115
Balatonfured	160
Moscow	405
Prague	112
Warsaw	79
Valencia	126
Tel Aviv	114
Erfurt	119
Cottbus	294
Dessau	54
17 WHO centres	

Relative risk (log scale)

Figure 9.2 Mortality following comprehensive rehabilitation in the World Health Organisation European collaborative trial:[51] relative risk of death at three years among myocardial infarction patients offered rehabilitation, compared with controls, in 17 individual centres and in a pooled estimate of all 17 centres (bars show 95% confidence intervals).

Psychological rehabilitation

Rehabilitation programmes based on psychological therapy and counselling evolved in parallel with those based on physical training and a number of trials reported on their effectiveness in parallel with those mentioned above. Ibrahim et al[52] were the first to report on mortality, Friedman et al[53] compared a long course of type A behaviour modification and cardiologic counselling (health education) with cardiologic counselling alone, Rahe et al[54] compared a programme of psycho-educational sessions with controls, Stern et al[55] compared group counselling with exercise training and with controls, and Frasure-Smith and Prince[56] compared a counselling service activated by regular telephone enquiries. All of these suggested some mortality benefit of psychological rehabilitation, although each trial was too small individually to provide statistically significant results. In Britain, Naismith et al[57] and Mayou et al[58] did not report mortality benefit.

The mortality outcomes of trials of psychologically based rehabilitation are summarised in figure 9.3. Overall, the pooled results of these trials suggest that mortality may be reduced by as much as 28%. However, this

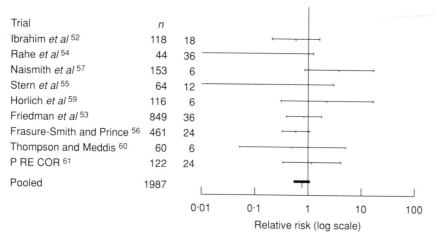

Trial	n	
Ibrahim et al [52]	118	18
Rahe et al [54]	44	36
Naismith et al [57]	153	6
Stern et al [55]	64	12
Horlich et al [59]	116	6
Friedman et al [53]	849	36
Frasure-Smith and Prince [56]	461	24
Thompson and Meddis [60]	60	6
P RE COR [61]	122	24
Pooled	1987	

Relative risk (log scale)

Figure 9.3 Mortality following psychological rehabilitation: relative risk of death in the medium term among myocardial infarction patients offered rehabilitation, compared with controls, in nine individual trials and in a pooled estimate of all nine trials (bars show 95% confidence intervals).

finding should be interpreted cautiously, since there is considerable heterogeneity between programmes as to what psychological support was provided and in duration of follow up or the time after enrolment that mortality was compared. One of the larger trials reported cardiac deaths rather than all deaths (deaths due to all causes).[56] The only trial sufficiently large to detect a mortality benefit of this order recruited patients six months or more after myocardial infarction and was far from achieving a statistically significant result.[53]

The three groups of trials reviewed above suggest a possible reduction in medium term mortality among patients included in rehabilitation programmes. However, because most trials were small with inadequate power to confirm or refute mortality differences of the order of 20%, because of heterogeneity between programme contents and between trial outcomes, and because of the spectre of publication bias, conservative cardiologists have been reluctant to view these results as comparable with mortality reductions following, for example, early thrombolysis[62] or long term aspirin.[63]

Pooling morbidity findings

Important though a possible mortality reduction might be, the principal rationale for rehabilitation is to facilitate patients' recovery and achieve the best possible quality of life. It is relevant therefore to review the effects of rehabilitation programmes on morbidity while bearing in mind that many morbidity measures may be poor proxies for quality of life.

Heterogeneity between trials in morbidity measures is considerably greater than heterogeneity between trials in mortality comparisons. Many trials have reported non-fatal myocardial infarction as a significant and measurable end point. The national exercise and heart disease project, for example, reported 15 non-fatal infarctions among 323 exercised patients compared with 11 among 328 control patients (or 18 compared with 13, if suspected infarctions were included).[33]

These findings almost balance the reported reduction in cardiovascular deaths: 14 compared with 20. A few trials added fatal and non-fatal as "hard cardiovascular end points" (and in some cases referred to these as "cardiovascular deaths"). One overview reported 223/2202 non-fatal re-infarctions among exercised patients compared with 191/2145 controls in nine trials plus 11 centres of the WHO european trial.[47] The pooled relative risk for non-fatal infarction (1·15, 95% confidence interval 0·93 = 1·42) was not significant but appeared to be in the opposite direction from the pooled relative risk for total mortality of both exercise based and comprehensive rehabilitation trials.

Several exercise trials have compared prevalence of angina. For example, Carson et al[34] reported angina of effort among 23% of rehabilitation patients compared with 38% of controls, and Marra et al[38] reported stable angina among 30% of patients and 38% of controls. Because of the relative subjectivity of angina reporting, many exercise based trials and many trials of programmes that include exercise as an important component have reported at least one measure of physical performance. Carson et al[34] for example, compared mean cycling time and showed that trained patients were able to maintain exercise for significantly longer than the untrained (mean 17·5 v 13·0 minutes) at the end of the training programme, although the difference lessened over time so that it was not significant at the end of three years (14·5 v 13·0 minutes). The WHO[51] collaborative study showed that maximum workload remained higher at three years among young men (700 v 620 kp.m/min among those aged under 50) but not among older men (500 v 490 kp.m/min among those aged 60–65).

Most trials of psychologically based rehabilitation have compared some form of psychological morbidity but various scales of measurement have been used. Comparisons have been reported in terms of "caseness" in some trials and with distributions of scores in others. For example Rahe et al[54] reported clinically significant depression, in the judgment of a psychiatrist, for three of 22 rehabilitation patients compared with five of 22 controls after three years. Thompson and Meddis[60] reported both anxiety and depression at one, three, and six months follow up on the hospital anxiety and depression (HAD) scale in their trial of in-hospital counselling. Treatment significantly reduced both anxiety and depression compared with controls in all but the six month follow up. Stern et al[55] used a battery of scales including the Taylor manifest anxiety scale,[52] Zung self rating depression scale and the National Institutes of Mental Health self report mood scale. They reported improvements, for example in depression on the Zung scale, from 34·1 at baseline to 31·5 at three months among 31 counselled patients, compared with 37·3 and 38·3, respectively, among 27 controls.

The variety of measures of psychological morbidity reported in psychological trials makes difficulties for pooling of the treatment effect which allows the advocate of rehabilitation to select favourable results from trials and create estimates of "treatment effect" and then perhaps add "standardised treatment effects" of different outcome measures in different trials. However, it also allows the critic to question the objectivity of reports and question the ability of treatment to produce meaningful clinical benefit. Several psychological trials have reported angina (for example, Friedman et al[53] reported angina in 48% of cases compared with 59% in controls at three years), which allows comparison of a measure of morbidity with exercise based trials (see earlier).

For many years return to work has been used as an overall measure of success in rehabilitation and has been reported as an end point in many rehabilitation trials. The WHO European collaborative study[51] tabulated return to work by age (< 60 years) at three and six months, and one, two, and three years. There was considerable inter-centre variation, with 56–100% of rehabilitation patients and 34–96% of controls returned to full time or part time work within three years. In most centres more rehabilitation patients than controls returned to work; on average about 12% more. As discussed earlier, in more recent years return to work has become less relevant as a measure of effectiveness of rehabilitation. Furthermore, because many comprehensive programmes facilitate return to work as part of the rehabilitation package, return to work remains less than ideally objective. Thus, as with other proxy measures of morbidity, some caution is needed in the interpretation of the modest benefits in return to work reported in several trials.

Overall, heterogeneity in content of rehabilitation programmes — in design of randomised trials to evaluate programmes and in end points or outcome measures by which trials are judged — makes statistical overview quite impracticable for morbidity comparisons. The reviewer is left therefore with a wide series of comparisons of a variety of different measures and a series of value judgments as to which to include in his pooling and what weight to give to each in his estimation of overall effect. The apparent possible mortality reduction in exercise based, psychologically based, and comprehensive programmes (of borderline statistical significance in the statistical overviews; see figs 9.1–9.3, gives credibility to the possibility of modest morbidity benefits of a comparable magnitude, as selectively reported in trials.

Representativeness

Although trials have reported comparable benefits from a number of countries in the past 20 years, one further important consideration remains before pooled results of these trials are interpreted as unequivocally supportive of rehabilitation. Many trials included only men (for example, see WHO[51]) and those few trials that did include women included only very modest numbers (for example, 35/315[31]). Thus the trial experience is almost wholly limited to men, although approximately 30% of myocardial infarction patients are women. Secondly, most trials included age as an admission criteria, so that in the reported trial results barely 2% of patients were aged over 65 years, yet more than 40% of myocardial infarction patients are over 65 years. Considerable caution should be exercised in extrapolating results reported in trials of young men to the total patient population. It may be that the needs for rehabilitation among women or among older patients are different and that goals should be adjusted accordingly. It may be that appropriate rehabilitation is as effective in older patients as in younger men or it may be that objective benefits are fewer (work capacity among 60–65 year olds showed little benefit in the WHO collaborative study[51]). Rehabilitation for women and for older patients has yet to be formally evaluated.

Furthermore, many programmes (and many trials) operated further exclusion criteria (for example concomitant disease, second infarction, residence too far from base hospital) so that possibly as little as 10% of the total patient population have been studied and reported. In some trials this non-representativeness has been reported and/or discussed: for example, Shaw[33] found total mortality to be only one third of that expected. It is quite possible that selection criteria were "appropriate" or that, in clinical situations, experienced therapists (informally) select those patients most amenable to treatment. It might then follow that comparable benefits would not be expected among all patients. Effectiveness of rehabilitation "at the margin", to borrow an economist's term, is largely untested. These points should be borne in mind as rehabilitation programmes undergo expansion from initially including only selected patients treated by enthusiastic experts in specialist centres to the broad service commitment of providing a basic programme for all (or most) in every acute general hospital.

Health education and secondary prevention

Health education and secondary prevention are included in many rehabilitation programmes but evidence for these is not reviewed in the same depth as exercise training and psychological therapy. The reasons for this are principally because (a) health education (and heart disease prevention) is widely recognised as a free-standing activity and has been discussed and reviewed extensively; (b) it is not synonymous with rehabilitation—it is not aimed at returning a patient to his former self but is undertaken opportunistically (usually with the best motives and intentions) to entice the patient into a "better than former self"; and (c) it has not been separated out from exercise training and/or psychological therapy in most trials—indeed several trials have provided a core of health education (or "cardiologic counselling") to both rehabilitation (by exercise training and/or psychological therapy) and control groups.

A minimum of information on simple anatomy, physiology, and pathology of the heart, and on epidemiology, manifestations, and sequelae of heart disease seem eminently relevant for all patients, to add to their understanding of what happened, how they were treated in hospital, how to anticipate and minimise angina, and how to reduce risks of further myocardial infarction. Programmes vary greatly in how much information is supplied, how thoroughly it is taught, how often it is reinforced, and how much assistance in seeking change is offered. The three principal controllable risk factors for heart disease are well known and the aims for addressing these are outlined in Chapter 1.

Smoking

The principal external and controllable risk factor is undoubtedly smoking. Observational studies of patients after myocardial infarction suggest that those who give up smoking experience extended survival (and postponement of subsequent infarction).[64] Interestingly, there is little experimental evidence of the effect of giving up smoking as an active component of rehabilitation.[65] It is therefore largely on the basis of observational studies and particularly on the many large classic observational studies (cohort studies) of primary risk factors that doctors strongly advocate giving up smoking. The recommendation is almost universal, and the advice is usually given in hospital (when the patients cannot get access to cigarettes) and before referral to rehabilitation. The majority of smokers do give up after the shattering experience of myocardial infarction.[66] Quite possibly many of those who do not give up may wish to. Thus the rehabilitation counsellor can help in advising, facilitating, and encouraging those who wish to give up but have difficulty in doing so.

Blood pressure

High blood pressure is a well known primary risk factor for heart disease and its contribution as a secondary risk factor is discussed in other chapters. Its control is principally pharmacological and hence falls within the responsibility of physician, cardiologist, or general practitioner, and outside the remit of most rehabilitation therapists and of most health promoters. The effectiveness of blood pressure reduction on mortality and cardiac morbidity has been evaluated in many trials and is extensively reviewed elsewhere. Blood pressure has been suggested as a mechanism by which relaxation training (for example by progressive muscle relaxation or hypnosis or yoga) might contribute to reduced risk of subsequent infarction and death. However, the main trials of rehabilitation that include relaxation training as an important element have presented little data on blood pressure change. A few trials, mostly of exercise based rehabilitation or comprehensive rehabilitation, have reported significant blood pressure reduction.[67]

Body weight, diet and cholesterol

The risk factor that lies most clearly within the health education area is excess body weight (or obesity). The relationship between standardised weight (or ponderal index) and mortality has been known for many years, since the detailed tables of the New York Metropolitan Life Insurance Company[68] were published in 1960.[69] Overweight is the consequence of metabolic imbalance, so in health education there are two ways of reducing weight: increasing exercise (the evidence for which has been reviewed above) or reducing intake of calories. Most trials that have reported on weight showed no significant difference between patients on rehabilitation programmes and controls. The prime target within diet is fat, but most attention has been directed at cholesterol specifically, because of its very strong association with heart disease mortality.

While no rehabilitation trial has focused exclusively on dietary intervention, there are many trials of cholesterol reduction. Many of these were primary prevention trials and statistical overviews suggest that the overall effects on total mortality were negligible. Cholesterol reduction appeared to reduce heart disease mortality by between 10 and 20% but this benefit was balanced by increases in mortality from all other causes combined so that total mortality was unchanged.[43,70] Secondary prevention trials and overviews have shown that patients at high initial risk of heart disease may experience net overall reduction on mortality.[70] These trial results are compatible with the epidemiological observations: the same classic cohort studies, that showed strong associations with heart disease mortality, showed nearly equally strong inverse associations with mortality from all other causes combined, so that overall the relationship between cholesterol and mortality is gently U shaped.[71] The literature on cholesterol and cholesterol-lowering is extensive and interested readers may wish to refer elsewhere but it would seem that cholesterol-lowering may be more effective in secondary prevention than in primary prevention.[72]

Self motivation

While evidence for effectiveness of health education as a component of rehabilitation remains equivocal, rehabilitation therapists may be interested to know that lifestyle changes occur after myocardial infarction, even without targeted education programmes. Nearly 20 years ago, well before the introduction of the major health promotion campaigns, many myocardial infarction survivors quit smoking (30%), reduced dietary fat (36%), increased consumption of vegetables and salads (30%), and reduced weight (50%), all significantly more than age- and sex-matched controls.[66] This would imply that people are conscious of the principal cardiac risk factors and that myocardial infarction jolts patients into acting on that knowledge. It would seem therefore that the principal role for health education in rehabilitation is facilitative, to advise on how to quit (or reduce) smoking, how and where to get more appropriate food, and how to reduce weight (without incurring too much misery). Rehabilitation therapists will be aware of the differing needs of individuals.

Summary

Statistical overviews of the effectiveness of rehabilitation in exercise based, psychologically based, and comprehensive rehabilitation programmes suggest mortality benefits comparable with those reported for several pharmacological interventions.[62,63] However, since overall statistical significance has been only marginal, since no individual trial has had sufficient power to demonstrate mortality difference of these magnitudes, and since there has been considerable between-trial heterogeneity in patient selection, programme content, and end point comparison, the possible benefits should be viewed with caution. The morbidity comparisons reported are subject to the same caveats plus further heterogeneity between trials of measurements compared. While poolings of "standardised relative effect" of rehabilitation shown in several morbidity measures suggest benefits of comparable order to those reported for morbidity, these poolings should be viewed more cautiously than those for mortality. Larger trials are needed to detect benefit in both mortality and morbidity with statistical significance, and more representative trials are needed to detect benefit in the wider patient population currently being offered rehabilitation. Large numbers are available and much larger numbers have been recruited to trials of the major pharmacological interventions. "Open" trials of a prolonged health care intervention like rehabilitation are more difficult to conduct than "double-blind" drug trials, but they are necessary if clinicians and health service managers are to be given comparable information on which to judge the effectiveness of these programmes.

References

1 World Health Organisation. Rehabilitation of patients with cardiovascular disease: report of WHO expert committee. *WHO Tech Rep Series* 1969; **270**

2 Bowling A. *Measuring health: review of quality of life measurement scales.* Milton Keynes: Open University Press, 1992.

3 Council for Science and Society. *Expensive medical techniques: report of a working party.* London: Council for Science and Society, 1982.

4 ISIS 2 Collaborative group. Randomized trial of intravenous streptokinase, aspirin, both or neither in 17,187 cases of suspected acute myocardial infarction. ISIS 2. *Lancet* 1988; **ii**: 349–60.

5 GISSI 2. Factorial randomised trial of alteplase versus streptokinase and heparin versus no heparin among 12,490 patients with acute myocardial infarction. GISSI. *Lancet* 1990; **336**: 65–71.

6 Peto R. Clinical trial methodology. *Biomedicine* 1978; **28** (special issue): 24–36.

7 Elwood JM. *Causal relationships in medicine.* Oxford: Oxford University Press, 1988.

8 deBono D, Hopkins A. Management of acute myocardial infarction guidelines and audit standards (report of workshops). *J Roy Coll Phys* 1994; **28**: 312–17.

9 Levine SA, Lown B. Armchair treatment of acute coronary thrombosis. *JAMA* 1952; **148**: 1365–9.

10 Groden BM, Allison A, Shaw GB. Management of myocardial infarction. *Scot Med J* 1967; **12**: 435–40.

11 West RR, Henderson AH. Randomised multi-centre trial of early mobilisation after uncomplicated myocardial infarction. *Br Heart J* 1979; **42**: 381–5.

12 Kellerman JJ, Levy M, Feldman S, Kariv I. Rehabilitation of coronary patients. *J Chron Dis* 1967; **20**: 815–21.

13 Kavanagh T, Shephard RT. Importance of physical activity in post coronary rehabilitation. *Am J Phys Med* 1973; **52**: 304–13.

14 Bethell HJN. Rehabilitation of coronary patients. *Practitioner* 1982; **226**: 477–82.

15 Horgan J, Bethell H, Carson P, *et al.* Working party report on cardiac rehabilitation. *Br Heart J* 1992 **67**: 412–18.

16 Task force on cardiac rehabilitation of European Society of Cardiology Cardiac rehabilitation. *Eur Heart J* 1992; **13(suppl C)**: 1–45.

17 Heberden W. Commentaries on the history and cure of disease. London, T Payne, 1802. In: Willins FA, Keys TW, editors. *Classics in cardiology.* Vol 1. New York: Dover, 1961.

18 Stokes W. *Diseases of the heart and aorta.* Dublin, 1854.

19 Morris JN, Chave SPW, Adam C, *et al.* Vigorous exercise in leisure and incidence of coronary heart disease. *Lancet* 1973; **i**: 333–9.

20 Paffenbarger RS, Wing AL, Hyde RT. Physical activity as an index of heart attack risk in college alumni. *Am J Epidemiol* 1978; **108**: 161–75.

21 Hellerstein HK, Ford AB. Rehabilitation of the cardiac patient. *JAMA* 1957; **164**: 225–31.

22 Rechnitzer PA, Yuhasz MS, Paivio A, *et al.* Effects of 24 week exercise programme on normal adults and patients with previous myocardial infarction. *BMJ* 1967; **ii**: 734–5.

23 Gottheiner V. Long range strenuous sports training for cardiac rehabilitation. *Am J Cardiol* 1968; **22**: 426–35.

24 Wenger NK. Early ambulation after myocardial infarction: rationale, programme components and results. In: Wenger NK, Hellerstein HK, editors. *Rehabilitation of the coronary patient.* New York: John Wiley, 1978.

25 Frick MH, Katila M. Hemodynamic consequences of physical training after myocardial infarction. *Circulation* 1968; **37**: 192–202.

26 Hellerstein HK. Exercise therapy in coronary disease. *Bull N Y Acad Med* 1968; **44**: 1028–47.

27 Clausen JP, Larson OA, Trap-Jensen J. Physical training in the management of coronary artery disease. *Circulation* 1969; **40**: 143–54.

28 Kasch FW, Boyer JL. Changes in maximum work capacity resulting from six months' training in patients with ischaemic heart disease. *Med Sci Sports* 1969; **i**: 156–9.

29 Detry JMR, Rousseau M, Vandenbroucke G, *et al.* Increased arteriovenous oxygen difference after physical training in coronary heart disease. *Circulation* 1971; **44**: 109–18.

30 Kentala E. Physical fitness and feasibility of physical rehabilitation after myocardial infarction in men of working age. *Ann Clin Res* 1972; **4** (suppl 9): 1–84.

31 Sanne H. Exercise tolerance and physical training of non-selected patients after myocardial infarction. *Acta Med Scand* 1973; (suppl 551): 1–124.

32. Palatsi I. Feasibility of physical training after myocardial infarction and its effect on return to work, morbidity and mortality. *Acta Med Scand* 1976; (suppl 599): 4–84.

33 Shaw LW. Effects of a prescribed supervised exercise program on mortality and cardiovascular morbidity in patients after a myocardial infarction. The National Exercise and Heart Disease Project. *Am J Cardiol* 1981; **48**: 39–46.

34 Carson P, Phillips R, Lloyd M, *et al.* Exercise after myocardial infarction: a controlled trial. *J R Coll Phys* 1982; **16**: 147–51.

35 Goble AJ, Hare DL, Macdonald PS, *et al.* Effect of early programmes of high and low intensity exercise on physical performance after transmural acute myocardial infarction. *Br Heart J* 1991; **54**: 126–31.

36 Rechnitzer P, Cunningham DA, Andrew GM, *et al.* Relation of exercise to the recurrence rate of myocardial infarction in men. Ontario exercise-heart collaborative study. *Am J Cardiol* 1983; **51**: 65–9.

37 Roman O, Guitierrez M, Luksie I, *et al.* Cardiac rehabilitation after myocardial infarction: nine year controlled follow up study. *Cardiology* 1983; **70**: 223–31.

38 Marra S, Paolillo V, Spadaccini F, Angelino PF. Long-term follow-up after a controlled randomized post-myocardial infarction rehabilitation programme: effects on morbidity and mortality. *Eur Heart J* 1985; **6**: 656–63.

39 Bethell HJN, Mullee MA. Controlled trial of comunity-based coronary rehabilitation. *Br Heart J* 1990; **64**: 370–5.

40 Naughton J, *et al.* National exercise and heart disease project. *Cardiology* 1978; **63**: 352–67.

41 Thompson SG, Pocock SJ. Can meta-analyis be trusted? *Lancet* 1991; **337**: 1127–30.

42 West RR. A look at the statistical overview (or meta-analysis). *J R Coll Phys* 1993; **27**: 111–15.

43 Gehlbach SH. *Interpreting the medical literature: a clinician's guide.* Lexington: Collamore Press, 1982.

44 Begg CB, Berlin JA. Publication bias: a problem in interpreting medical data. *J R Statist Soc* 1988; **151**: 419–63.

45 Dickersin K, Yuan IM, Curtis LM. Factors influencing publication of research results: follow-up of applications submitted to two institutional review boards. *JAMA* 1992; **267**: 379–88.

46 West RR. Assessment of evidence versus consensus or prejudice. *J Epidemiol Community Health* 1992; **46**: 321–2.

47 Oldridge NB, Guyatt GH, Fischer MD, Rimm AA. Cardiac rehabilitation after myocardial infarction: combined experience of randomised clinical trials. *JAMA* 1988; **260**: 945–50.

48 O'Connor GT, Buring JE, Jusuf E, *et al.* Overview of randomised trials of rehabilitation after myocardial infarction. *Circulation* 1989; **80**: 234–44.

49 Rechnitzer PA, Sangal S, Cunningham DA, *et al.* Randomized controlled prospective study of effect of endurance training on recurrence rate of myocardial infarction: description of experimental design. *Am J Epidemiol* 1975; **102**: 358–65.

50 May GS, Eberlin KA, Furberg CD, *et al.* Secondary prevention after myocardial infarction: a review of long-term trials. *Prog Cardiovasc Dis* 1982; **24**: 331–52.

51 World Health Organisation. Rehabilitation and comprehensive secondary prevention after acute myocardial infarction. Copenhagen: World Health Organisation, 1983. (EURO report 84.)

52 Ibrahim MA, Feldman JG, Sultz HA, *et al.* Management after myocardial infarction: a controlled trial of the effect of group psychotherapy. *Int J Psychiatry Med* 1974; **5**: 253–67.

53 Friedman M, Thorenson CE, Gill JJ, *et al.* Alteration of type A behaviour and reduction in cardiac recurrences in post-myocardial infarction patients. *Am Heart J* 1984; **108**: 237–48.

54 Rahe RH, Ward HW, Hayes V. Brief group therapy in myocardial infarction rehabilitation: three-to-four-year follow-up of a controlled trial. *Psychosom Med* 1979; **41**: 229–41.
55 Stern MJ, Gorman PA, Kaslow L. The group counselling vs exercise therapy study: a controlled intervention with subjects following myocardial infarction. *Arch Intern Med* 1983; **143**: 1719–25.
56 Frasure-Smith N, Prince R. Long-term follow-up of the ischaemic heart disease life stress monitoring program. *Psychosom Med* 1989; **51**: 485–513.
57 Naismith LD, Robinson JF, Shaw GB, MacIntyre MMJ. Psychosocial rehabilitation after myocardial infarction. *BMJ* 1979; **1**: 439–46.
58 Mayou R, Macmahon D, Sleight P, Florencio MJ. Early rehabilitation after myocardial infarction. *Lancet* 1981; **ii**: 1399–401.
59 Horlich L, Cameron R, Firor W, *et al*. Effects of education and group discussion in post myocardial infarction patients. *J Psychosom Res* 1989; **28**: 485–92.
60 Thompson DL, Meddis R. Prospective evaluation of in-hospital counselling for first time myocardial infarction. *J Psychosom Res* 1990; **34**: 237–48.
61 P RE COR. Comparison of rehabilitation programme, counselling programme and usual care after acute myocardial infarction: results of a long-term randomized trial. *Eur Heart J* 1991; **12**: 612–16.
62 GISSI. Effectiveness of intravenous thrombolytic treatment in acute myocardial infarction. *Lancet* 1986; **i**: 397–402.
63 Elwood PC, Cochrane AL, Burr ML, *et al*, Randomized controlled trial of acetyl salicylic acid in secondary prevention of mortality from myocardial infarction. *BMJ* 1974; **i**: 436–40.
64 Mulchay R. Influence of cigarette smoking on morbidity and mortality after myocardial infarction. *Br Heart J* 1983; **49**: 410–15.
65 Wenger NK, Hellerstein HK. *Rehabilitation of the coronary patient*. New York: John Wiley, 1978.
66 West RR, Evans DA. Lifestyle changes in long-term survivors of acute myocardial infarction. *J Epidemiol Community Health* 1986; **40**: 103–9.
67 Kallio V, Hamalainen H, Hakkila J, Luturila OJ. Reduction in sudden death by a multifactorial intervention programme after acute myocardial infarction. *Lancet* 1979; **ii**: 1091–4.
68 Metropolitan Life Insurance New York. Mortality among overweight men and women. *Statist Bull* 1960; **41**(Feb).
69 Royal College of Physicians. Obesity: report (Black D, chair). *J R Coll Phys* 1983; **17**: 5–16.
70 Smith GD, Song F, Sheldon TA. Cholesterol lowering and mortality: importance of considering initial level of risk. *BMJ* 1993; **306**: 1367–73.
71 West RR. Cholesterol reduction: trials corroborate epidemiological evidence on total and case specific mortality. *Br Heart J* 1993; **69** (suppl 5): 37.
72 British Hyperlipidaemia Association Symposium (Laker M, Neil A, Wood C, editors). *Cholesterol lowering trials: advice for the British Physician*. London: Royal College of Physicians, 1993.

10 A multi-centre randomised controlled trial of psychological rehabilitation

DEE JONES AND ROBERT WEST

Introduction

History

Since the 1960s there have been many changes and developments in the rehabilitation of patients who have suffered a myocardial infarction. The '60s saw the introduction of early ambulation and the recognition of the benefits of exercise (see Chapters 1 and 3). Early ambulation is seen by many as having been the nemesis of cardiac rehabilitation and with the demonstration of the benefits of early exercise came the development of exercise-based rehabilitation programmes. In those early days rehabilitation was almost synonymous with exercise training: the primary goal of rehabilitation was return to paid employment and exercise training was seen as enabling patients to become "fit" for work. However, there were others who recognised the psychological sequelae of myocardial infarction and who laid the foundations of psychological rehabilitation[1,2] (see also Chapters 2 and 4).

The '80s saw significant improvements in survival following myocardial infarction, in both the acute and later stages, and decreases in the pathophysiological consequences, so that fewer survivors were suffering physical disability than previously.[3] This decade also saw the emergence of quality of life as a health care issue, which may be attributed to the increasing prevalence of chronic illness and increasing awareness of chronic disease in society generally. Quality of life, or the manner in which an illness impacts upon a person's life and wellbeing, includes physical, sexual, emotional, social, and intellectual functioning. The philosophy and thinking surrounding rehabilitation thus progressed from early mobilisation and physical training to include social and psychological perspectives, and the goals of rehabilitation broadened from return to work to encompass social and psychological dimensions, including participation in valued activities in the home and community and improved adjustment. This broader approach was reflected in the development of multi-component programmes or "comprehensive rehabilitation".[3]

The growth of knowledge of and interest in risk factors for coronary heart disease led to the introduction and development of a further objective in rehabilitation, that of secondary prevention to reduce recurrences of myocardial infarction and improve function by encouraging appropriate lifestyle alterations. The most relevant lifestyle alterations include cessation of smoking, reduction of alcohol consumption and dietary changes, for example reduction of fat and increase of fibre and fresh fruit and vegetables. Consequently rehabilitation programmes became more eclectic in their approach and incorporated advice on smoking cessation, alcohol reduction, and dietary changes, as well as exercise training, although for most the central component remained exercise training.

Since the '70s there have been many reports of psychosocial adjustment after myocardial infarction. Although many studies were rather small and of selected populations and although they used different methods and measures, they reported broadly similar findings: that the psychosocial adjustment of a substantial proportion of post-myocardial patients was not as good as expected.[4] Patients' quality of life was found to be impaired up to eight years after the event,[5] and the deleterious effect of myocardial infarction on quality of life was not necessarily proportional to the severity of the myocardial infarction.[6,7]

Myocardial infarction is usually a sudden, unexpected event, which is life threatening and causes great distress and fear. A crisis of this nature requires a major psychological and social readjustment. Following infarction, patients tend to pass through several stages—fear, anger, denial, anxiety, and depression—but there is considerable variation in response. These stages are discussed in more detail in Chapter 11. This pattern has been seen as a normal process of successful adaptation following a life threatening event, but for some a prolonged level of morbidity ensues and prolonged anxiety and depression may prevent patients from implementing recommended lifestyle changes.[8]

A life threatening event such as myocardial infarction also has a profound impact on principal carers, often greater than the impact on patients themselves. Initially there is fear of imminent death of the patient and subsequently fear of recurrence of infarction. For some carers these high levels of fear and associated anxiety can remain in the long term. While spouses, partners, or carers may have much to contribute to patients' rehabilitation and adjustment and many may considerably assist these processes, long term fear and anxiety among carers may have a deleterious effect on patients' rehabilitation. This impact of myocardial infarction on spouses and their role in rehabilitation is discussed in more detail in Chapter 11. As a result of the expanding literature on the difficulties that a substantial number of cardiac patients and their carers face, the need for a psychosocial component in rehabilitation has been increasingly acknowledged. The content of this component has variously included education, counselling, relaxation, training, stress management, and anger management. Some programmes have also involved spouses and partners, to a lesser or greater degree.

During the '80s cardiac rehabilitation developed further in several parts of North America and Europe, and many of these programmes were 'comprehensive' and adopted a multidisciplinary approach, involving clinician, nurse, psychologist, social worker, dietitian, physiotherapist, and exercise physiologist. The development of cardiac rehabilitation programmes has been much slower in the United Kingdom; those few that developed focused mostly on exercise training.[9,10] The multidisciplinary team model, developed in North America and Europe (particularly Scandinavia) was inevitably a more costly approach than one offering only exercise training and perhaps exercise training in large classes with relatively little supervision. In the UK it seemed unlikely in the mid-80s that, in a time of "economic stringency", the NHS would welcome the establishment of "comprehensive" rehabilitation programmes involving several professions, particularly if the benefits were not demonstrably better than cheaper less intensive programmes. At that time there were few established programmes in England[11] (see also Chapter 7) and no rehabilitation programmes in Wales.

Background to the trial

There was, despite the absence of any Welsh rehabilitation programmes, a receptive climate for rehabilitation and for practical evaluation of a new service. Many physicians and cardiologists in Wales were supportive of Archie Cochrane's exhortation to test each medical intervention by a randomised controlled trial[12] and 13 Welsh hospitals had taken part in a randomised controlled trial of duration of bed rest following myocardial infarction.[13] Furthermore, there were clinical psychologists in Wales with interest and experience in the use of psychological approaches to treating acute and physical conditions.

At that time in the mid-1980s the evidence of effectiveness of rehabilitation was relatively sparse. Several trials of exercise training had shown improvements in physiological parameters, but few reported on effectiveness in improving quality of life and all were too small to achieve statistical significance in reduced mortality (Chapter 9). While statistical overviews had yet to be published, clinical consensus was moving in the direction that benefits were comparable to those shown in the World Health Organization trial of "comprehensive" rehabilitation.[14] Little was known of what contribution the components of comprehensive rehabilitation made to the possible overall benefit. The psychological approach to rehabilitation had not been evaluated in sufficiently large numbers of patients across several centres. A few trials had reported evaluation of a psychological approach to the rehabilitation of myocardial infarction patients, with rather equivocal or disappointing results.[15,16] Larger trials with more promising results and with continuing programme evolution had been reported in America.[17,18] In the United Kingdom, more promising results had been reported from programmes based on a psychological approach to the treatment of both hypertension and chronic stable angina,[19–21] providing some insight into possible mechanisms and, more practically, giving some clinical psychologists first hand clinical experience with cardiovascular disease patients. Most studies evaluating rehabilitation programmes had excluded women of all ages and excluded men in the older age group (Chapter 9). Almost half of myocardial infarction patients are classified as "elderly", and there seemed to be no evidence to justify excluding half the myocardial infarction patients from rehabilitation.

The study described in this chapter therefore sought to evaluate the benefits or otherwise of a cardiac rehabilitation programme based on a psychological intervention in a large sample of unselected myocardial infarction patients and their carers in six district general hospitals, where no programmes had previously existed. It was considered that a multi-centre randomised controlled trial could ethically be undertaken as no service was currently provided to post-myocardial infarction patients and their carers. The following section describes the setting up of six new rehabilitation programmes and their evaluation.

Establishing psychological rehabilitation programmes

Recruitment of centres

At the time of initiating this study there were no known formalised, outpatient rehabilitation programmes in Wales for myocardial infarction patients. Several district general hospitals in Wales and the borders were invited to participate in the trial to evaluate a rehabilitation programme with an agreed format. These centres were asked to accommodate, administer, and resource their own programmes. Referring physicians were asked to include post-myocardial infarction patients of both genders and all ages. While in the past most programmes in England and Scotland selected patients on the basis of age and/or gender, there appeared to be no rational basis for excluding patients from psychological rehabilitation on either of these grounds. There was no evidence that older people would suffer or that they would not benefit from such a programme, so it was considered unethical to exclude them. Some centres wished to exclude patients aged 65 years and over and declined to join the study because of this open approach. One centre preferred to initiate an exercise programme and so chose not to join the study. Six centres agreed to participate, two in the borders and four in South Wales; in total three district health authorities were involved, and ethical approval was sought and granted for the study in each district.

Development of programmes

In collaboration with clinical psychologists, nurses, health visitors, physicians, and experts from overseas, information was gathered from other programmes about their content and how well they worked. A standard form of rehabilitation programme was developed and agreed by all collaborating centres. On the basis of advice from established programmes, mostly overseas, and on the grounds of costs, a seven-week programme was designed for groups of up to 15 patients, all of whom started on the same day. The programme consisted of seven half-day sessions held on the same day each week. Spouses or partners were invited to the first two sessions and to the last session. Sessions were held in quiet comfortable informal rooms on district general hospital sites except for one, which was held in a health centre, because a new district general hospital was under construction. Each programme was run by a clinical psychologist and a health visitor, each of whom had experience of working with groups. The half-day sessions were usually divided into two parts with a coffee break between. Medical cover was provided in each setting, in case of emergency.

The overall aims of the programmes were to enable myocardial infarction patients and their spouses to adjust optimally and to return to the best possible quality of life. The programmes were based on psychological rehabilitation and the principal objectives of the programmes were:

- To provide information about the normal functioning of the heart, myocardial infarction, treatment and management of myocardial infarction and the natural recovery process
- To discuss anger, fears and anxiety in both patients and spouses and develop skills for reducing these

- To inform patients and spouses about stress and its effect upon the body
- To instruct patients and spouses in relaxation methods
- To teach stress management techniques
- To enable modification of type A behaviour.

Time was allocated for informal discussion, when patients were encouraged to express and share their fears, anxieties, and problems with the group. Time was also allocated for patients to consult either the clinical psychologist or the health visitor in private. Spouses were provided with opportunities to discuss their experiences, fears, anxieties, and coping strategies with the health visitor and with other spouses in a separate room, whilst patients underwent relaxation training.

For the reasons already discussed, the programmes were unifactorial; they were psychologically based and did not include physical exercise, nor did they attempt to change smoking, drinking, or diet. Patients who requested information or advice outside the agreed programme including medical advice were advised and were encouraged to consult their general practitioner.

Each rehabilitation team attended "training sessions" to establish a standard approach to the programmes and, despite minor differences of opinion among the teams, all agreed to standardise their practice for the duration of the trial. Having agreed on the content of the seven session programme, the teams met regularly to share and evaluate their experiences in order to maintain conformity and enthusiasm. Also, the principal investigators periodically participated in programmes as "patient" or "spouse" to monitor standardisation.

Key features of the trial

- Multi-centre randomised controlled trial
- Both sexes and all ages were included
- One intervention (the psychological approach) was evaluated
- Intervention was standardised in all centres
- Baseline and outcome measures were made by independent observers

---

Evaluation of psychological rehabilitation programmes

Patients

A consecutive series of confirmed myocardial infarction patients of both sexes and all ages from the six participating centres was included in the study. Patients who remained in hospital after 28 days from admission, or were discharged to residential or nursing homes, were excluded. Patients were randomised to intervention or control groups; those in the intervention group were invited to the next rehabilitation session and those in the control group received the advice and management they would normally have received. As none of the centres had previously provided a rehabilitation programme, this advice usually took the form of a one-page set of instructions or guidelines provided on discharge from hospital or verbal advice at an outpatient appointment, or neither. Patients were randomised by the research team and invitations were mailed to the intervention group on behalf of their consultants, inviting the patients and their spouses to attend the next rehabilitation session.

Data collection: baseline

Brief clinical summaries were recorded by junior medical staff and in some cases by senior coronary care unit nursing staff on structured pro formas, as soon as the information was available after admission. The first clinical pro forma included the usual patient identification and a sufficient minimum information to confirm diagnosis and estimate prognosis.[22]

Baseline information was obtained soon after discharge, by trained interviewers seeing all patients independently in their own homes, using structured interview schedules. The experienced and specially trained interviewers were not aware of the randomisation status of the respondents. The patient interview included several previously used and validated questionnaires to measure disability,[23] angina,[24] anxiety and depression,[25] state and trait anxiety,[26] social network and support, and sexual activity; and to measure smoking,[27] drinking,[28] diet,[29] exercise,[30] as potential confounders.

Spouses were also interviewed separately using different structured interview schedules. The shorter spouse interview schedule included the usual sociodemographic factors but also used standardised questionnaires to measure aspects of their quality of life: distress,[31] anxiety and depression,[25] and state and trait anxiety.[26] Other topics covered included the patients' myocardial infarction, hospitalisation, attitudes to the infarction, future expectations, and sexual activity.

Data collection: outcome

In order to measure health outcomes, all patients and their spouses were re-interviewed six months later, again independently in their own homes. The second interview schedule was very similar to the first and used the same standard measures and also included a new section at the end of the interview, which explored programme attenders' views of the rehabilitation programme. The interviewers were again unaware of the study status of the patients, whether they were members of the intervention or control group, until the end of the second interview.

The second spouse interview at six months after discharge was the same as the first except that it also had a supplementary section at the end for those who attended a programme, to explore their opinions of the programme.

Participating physicians generously agreed to conduct an outpatient follow up as part of the trial. Twelve months after discharge all patients were invited by their physicians to attend a follow up outpatient appointment and the clinical outcome information was recorded on structured pro formas to standardise the data collected. Some hospitals chose to run special clinics to follow up trial patients, while others chose to include patients in routine outpatient clinics. The twelve month follow up clinical examination included blood pressure, ECG, exercise stress test (where possible), serum cholesterol (where possible), cardiac complications, further myocardial infarctions, cardiac surgery, and cerebrovascular accidents. For those patients who had relocated to another part of the country, the clinical information was sought from general practitioners.

Mortality data were sought at six months, if patients were not available for interview, and at twelve months, if not available for clinical follow up, by examining medical records, contacting general practitioners, and subsequently by contacting the NHS central registry. The central registry provided copies of death certificates of patients who had died.

Analysis

The principal analyses were undertaken on an "intention to treat" basis for the trial as a whole. The results were also analysed by centres to investigate possible differences between centres. Analyses were undertaken subsequently on a "dose" basis by subdividing the intervention group into non-attenders, low attenders, and high attenders, as attendance at the progammes was adversely affected by prolonged ambulance strikes which prevented some patients who wished to attend from doing so.

Practical problems

It is worth mentioning some of the problems that arose in initiating and implementing the programmes and in the evaluation. Some clinicians continued to have doubts about including patients aged 65 years and over in the programmes and expressed the view that older people would not benefit. Even when exclusion criteria have been agreed in advance, some, such as severe frailty and confusion, may be somewhat subjective as criteria. Exclusion before randomisation does not affect internal validity of the trial but any selective exclusion of patients randomised to the rehabilitation group would introduce bias. The trial was "single blind" in the sense that clinicians referring patients to the research team were unaware of which group individual patients would join; furthermore, there were few exclusions.

Some teams experienced difficulty in managing groups that were very heterogeneous in terms of age and disability. Severe disability and hearing impairment were considered to be the most common cause of problems, not only for the individuals concerned but also for others in the group. Relaxation training was undertaken in some sessions with patients lying on the floor and some patients found this difficult. Some teams would have liked to have developed their programmes in different ways, for example by giving advice on smoking, drinking, and diet, or by using different techniques, for example by using self-hypnosis, and they found conforming to a standardised programme restrictive.

In some hospitals there were difficulties in completing the first clinical forms and some forms were very delayed in reaching the research team. Completion and forwarding of forms were most successful when senior coronary care nurses coordinated these activities. There were delays and difficulties in completing clinical follow up in some hospitals, particularly when trial patients were included in routine outpatient clinics. The most efficient 12 month follow up was in those hospitals that chose to organise special outpatient clinics for this trial. The usual delays were experienced in obtaining follow up information on patients who had relocated to another part of the country or emigrated, and in confirming date and cause of death.

Findings of the trial

All physicians, except one, in the six collaborating hospitals referred their acute myocardial infarction patients to the trial coordination centre. In all, 2287 were entered into the randomised control trial of psychological rehabilitation. All patients discharged home within 28 days were included and only those who were still in hospital, discharged to long term care, severely frail, or confused were considered ineligible. Patient numbers divided almost equally between those invited to attend rehabilitation (cases) and those discharged home without being referred to rehabilitation (controls). Randomisation yielded similar age and sex distribution of cases and controls: small differences were not statistically significant. Cases and controls were very similar with respect to history, site and size of infarct, and complications, and with regard to smoking, drinking, and physical exercise prior to myocardial infarction.

Nearly three quarters of patients reported angina according to the Medical Research Council questionnaire at the six months follow up interview.[24] Cases and controls reported prevalences of 73 and 75% respectively, and the very modest advantage to cases was not statistically significant ($\chi^2 = 1.6$, NS). Very similar numbers reported anginal episodes during the previous week (41%): the average number of episodes per week was possibly lower among cases, 6·0 episodes compared with 6·9 among controls, but again this small difference was not statistically significant ($t = 1.5$, NS). Similar modest differences were evident in the use of glyceryl trinitrate (GTN) spray and tablets; 38% of cases estimated using these, compared with 42% of controls ($\chi^2 = 2.9$, NS), and among users the reported frequency of use in the previous week was slightly less among cases (average 7·8 uses per week compared with 8·9 among controls; ($t = 1.8$ NS).

Anxiety, deemed clinically significant (DSSI/sAD (Delusion Symptom State Inventory/State Anxiety and Depression) score 4+),[25] was evident among 34% of cases and 31% of controls ($\chi^2 = 1.8$, NS). These prevalences were almost the same as those recorded at discharge before referral to rehabilitation. An American scale of state anxiety[26] similarly indicated no significant difference. Clinically significant depression (DSSI/sAD score 4+)[25] was found among 19% of both cases and controls, and this prevalence was unchanged from that assessed at discharge. It would appear that neither anxiety nor depression prevalences changed between discharge and six month follow up in either the control group or the intervention group.

Some functional disability[23] was found among 76% of cases and 79% of controls at six months. Half of these reported only mild disability, but 33% of cases and 38% of controls were classified as moderately or severely disabled ($\chi^2 = 5.9$, df = 3, NS). These prevalences of moderate or severe disability were somewhat lower than those reported at discharge: 45 and 47%, respectively.

Smoking, drinking, diet, and exercise were measured not as outcomes but because they were potential confounders. In other words, some change might have occurred in these habits among cases compared with controls, possibly as a consequence of some health education getting into the rehabilitation programme. A change in one or more of these relative to controls might have affected the outcome and, if such change affected outcome, might have masked any effect of psychological therapy. At the six month follow up interview 23% of both cases and controls smoked, which was significantly fewer than the 53% who smoked before their myocardial infarction. At six months 32% of cases and 34% of controls reported drinking no alcohol or drinking only occasionally, which showed little change from the 30% who reported no drinking or only occasional drinking before their myocardial infarction. At six month follow up the average exercise scores on the Minnesota leisure time inventory[30] were 126 for cases and 116 for controls ($t = 1.4$, NS), which was significantly lower than their pre-infarction scores (161 for both cases and controls). The weight distributions of cases and controls were very similar at follow

Table 10.1 Employment status at six months: percentage of all patients and of those in paid employment before myocardial infarction

	Cases		Controls	
	All (n = 1063)	Previously in work (n = 433)	All (n = 1069)	Previously in work (n = 405)
Retired	60	30	63	31
Unemployed	12	9	9	7
Sick leave	11	20	11	20
Employed ("returned to work")	17	41	16	42

up, with means of 78 and 77 kg, respectively. These findings of little or no difference in these potential confounders suggest that there was little or no differential health education effect. The small non-significant benefit to cases in terms of exercise was of the same order as modest and non-significant reduction in the prevalence of moderate or severe disability.

Comparison of "return to work" showed that, overall, 17% of cases and 16% of controls had returned to work within six months (table 10.1). Since nearly half of the total patient population were over retirement age and quite a few of those under retirement age were not in paid employment at the time of their myocardial infarction, the table also shows the comparison of those who were in paid employment before their myocardial infarction: 41% of previously employed cases and 42% of controls had returned to work. Similar numbers reported that they had retired because of their myocardial infarction (20% of the cases and 19% of the controls who had been in work before their myocardial infarction). Also similar numbers reported finding work moderately or severely stressful (20% of those cases and 23% of those controls who had returned to work). Thus the rehabilitation programme appeared to have no effect on "return to work".

Patients' and carers' opinions

Nearly three quarters of patients randomised to rehabilitation attended (783/1072) and nearly 60% of those attended six or seven sessions (see later for the reasons for non-attendance and dropping out). Seventy one per cent of attenders reported that they found the programme helpful, particularly for relaxation, release of tension, awareness of tension, breathing, and sleeping patterns. Those who considered the programme unhelpful gave as their main reasons "no need for relaxation training", "too difficult to understand/learn", "difficult to relax in public" and "knew it already". Seventy per cent reported that they still practised

217

relaxation at the six month follow up. Nearly 80% found the information provided in the rehabilitation sessions helpful. The relatively small number who considered the information they were given unhelpful gave as their reasons that "they knew it already" or that "it was frightening to be told too much". Seventy two per cent considered that the group discussions were helpful, particularly sharing experiences with others and learning that they "were not alone". A few criticisms were voiced by those who preferred "not to discuss personal subjects with strangers". Patients who attended rehabilitation programmes were asked to rate the programmes overall: 30% awarded ratings of 10/10 and 50% awarded ratings of 8/10 or 9/10. A variety of possible improvements were suggested, including more sessions, longer sessions, and follow up meetings. A few suggested more individual attention or availability of a doctor for consultation. Rather more suggestions were of an "external" nature and not related to the content of the programmes, particularly better transport and better venue.

Those who did not attend or those who gave up after only one or two sessions gave as their main reasons for non-attendance "being too unwell", "back in hospital", "difficulty in obtaining transport", "returned to work", and second myocardial infarction, with the implication that there was "little more to learn". An ambulance strike significantly affected attendance rates in three hospitals.

Interpretation of findings

Rehabilitation based on psychological therapy, relaxation training, and counselling might reasonably be expected to show its principal benefit in the psychometric measures of anxiety and depression. Direct comparison of cases with controls at six months, a trial end point chosen in advance, showed no statistical difference. As previous smaller trials have reported benefit of psychological rehabilitation, it behoves us to consider possible reasons for the non-significant findings of the present trial. Because anxiety and depression were measured at discharge prior to rehabilitation as well as at six months, it is possible to examine trends over time. Comparison between discharge and six month follow up shows the same prevalence of both anxiety (33 and 31% among cases and controls, respectively) and depression (19% among both cases and controls). This suggests that six month follow up might be too early to detect recovery. Since this trial was designed, some studies have suggested that rehabilitation might take longer to establish its effect on patients and that outcome measurements at 12 months might be more appropriate.[32]

The benefits of the different components of rehabilitation—physical, psychological, and educational—do not always appear to act monotonically on the corresponding dimensions of quality of life and physical, psychological, and risk factors. There has been discussion among cardiac rehabilitation experts on possible interaction, for example whether exercise training improves psychometric measures, anxiety, and depression, as well as physical performance, and whether psychological therapy and counselling might improve physical performance as well as psychological wellbeing. The modest advantage experienced by cases in disability score and the moderately higher exercise score support the possibility that psychological therapy and counselling may help physical rehabilitation.

Tailoring rehabilitation and selecting patients

It is possible that the rehabilitation "package", offered in the programmes and standardised for the trial, suited some patients and not others and hence benefited some patients and not others. As discussed in other chapters, many rehabilitation programmes have been available only to selected patients and most trials have reported benefits for quite highly selected series of patients. While current expansions of rehabilitation are designed to include all who might benefit,[11,33,34] it may be that at least some of the previously practised selection successfully identified those patients most likely to benefit, and hence it is possible that benefits shown in those selected patient series will not be sustained in wider and unselected patient populations.

There is some evidence from the present trial to suggest the view that the programmes suited some patients less well than others. The possible slight disadvantage to cases in anxiety at the six month follow up (statistically non-significant) concentrated to some extent among younger men, those aged under 65, although the disadvantage, even in this group, was not statistically significant. Also between-hospital comparison demonstrated differences in response, and in one hospital in particular there was more anxiety among cases than controls at the six month follow up. These two results together suggest the possibility that psychological programmes, in the absence of physical exercise training programmes, may not suit younger male patients. Some trials have reported on psychological therapy as an adjunct to exercise training[35] and it may be that, particularly for young men, exercise training is the more appropriate primary vehicle for rehabilitation. Therapists will be aware of the case for tailoring rehabilitation to individual needs and offering patients exercise training, psychological therapy, and counselling, or a combination, as considered appropriate.

Programme length and intensity

Another possible explanation for the finding obtained in this trial may be the shortness of the programme, since several of the trials that have reported reduced morbidity were of programmes that lasted for a year or more (for example, see Friedman et al[17]). The programme duration in this trial was chosen as a practical minimum to meet clinical need and to suit staff and space availability, funding, and patient acceptability. In a publicly funded NHS providing free care ("at the point of delivery") resources for a new service are limited. At the time of setting up this trial, expert clinical opinion considered that a seven week programme should be sufficiently long and thorough to start patients on their rehabilitation, to help those in greatest need and yet not develop dependency or keep patients from helping themselves on the road to recovery. Not all previous trial programmes have been intensive: Frasure-Smith and Prince[18] merely kept in touch with their patients by telephone and counselled only those in need. That was effectively another form of patient selection, with some patients receiving no counselling and others receiving periodic *ad hoc* counselling possibly for years. Such selected or targeted provision may be a more effective way of employing scarce resources.

Therapist experience

Further possible explanations for the apparent difference between the findings of this trial and of several reported previously deserve some consideration. One is that this was almost a pragmatic trial of a new service provision, while most of the early trials involved specialist centres evaluating established therapies provided by enthusiastic experts. In many therapies there is a "learning curve" and better results are obtained with experience. It is also recognised that, even with experience, better results may be obtained by experts in specialist centres than by generalists who spend only part of their working week with these patients. Thirdly, many would acknowledge a "green fingers" effect of some individual enthusiasts, whether it be in teaching the piano, training an Olympic athlete, or rehabilitating depressed patients.

Objectivity of evaluation

Several of the small pioneering trials have been "self evaluations", in which psychiatrists, psychologists, or nurse counsellors led their patients through the rehabilitation programme and compared some before and after measurements, or compared some measurements in their patients with measurements in a control group. Some loss of objectivity can creep into self evaluations, even if therapists are not consciously trying to demonstrate effectiveness of their methods. School children can be taught how to answer IQ tests and hence prepared for school entrance exams, and cardiac patients can be taught to extend their exercise times on a particular machine by training on the same machine. It may be possible similarly to teach patients to improve their score on a particular psychometric measure by "training" on that psychometric measure. The present trial employed

---

Possible reasons for non-significant finding of the trial

- Six month follow up may be too early to detect psychological recovery

- Programmes may need to be longer and more intensive

- Programmes may need to be more tailored to individual patients' needs

- Psychological intervention may only benefit selected patients

- Therapists may need greater experience before achieving results

- Psychological intervention may be more effective combined with physical training and health education

- 'True' effect may be modest: reports of previous trials may have been affected by publication bias and selective reporting

---

"blind" interviewers, who were not connected in any way with the rehabilitation team or the rehabilitation programme, and outcome comparisons were based on measurement scales that were not part of the therapeutic programme.

Publication bias

Publication bias is discussed more fully in Chapter 9. There is evidence to suggest that selective reporting may be due more to investigators and authors than to editors,[36] and that biased reporting of studies with positive findings may tend to overestimate the therapeutic effects in counselling and psychotherapy.[37] An example of reporting depression in the results of psychological rehabilitation trials serves to illustrate this point. Four trials have reported comparisons between patients in rehabilitation programmes and controls of prevalence of depression or depression scores (table 10.2). A few other trials have reported comparisons of "mental state" or "psychological function", which included a depression component. Several more trials have indicated that they measured depression but did not report their findings, and only a few of these indicated that differences were slight. The larger trials have presented no data on depression, although this measure of morbidity must be regarded as

Table 10.2 Depression after psychological rehabilitation: prevalences or scores

	Rehabilitation patients	Control patients	Trial	Year
Prevalence (or "caseness")	3/22	5/22	Rahe et al[38]	1979
	3/31	10/27	Stern et al[39]	1983
Mean score and no of patients (n)	3·1(30)	4·2(30)	Thompson and Meddis[40]	1990
	2·6(78)	2·7(81)	Oldridge et al[41]	1991

important for psychological rehabilitation. Three of the four trials that have reported depression outcome data suggested quite impressive benefits of psychological rehabilitation programmes on depression. However, the fourth trial included as many patients as the other three combined and showed no benefit. It would appear that there has been some selective reporting of this outcome in the literature: the absent results of the larger trials may be important, particularly in the light of our results (the same prevalence of depression among cases and controls: 19%).

Pragmatism in health-care evaluation

In evaluations of health-care activities like cardiac rehabilitation, there is potential for conflict between professional judgment and programme standardisation. Therapists may well wish to exercise to the full their professional judgment, gained over many years of specialist training, to help patients in the best way they know and perhaps also to tailor therapies to individual patients. Scientists, evaluating health care seek to standardise treatment in trials so that, when outcome of intervention and control groups are compared, it is clear what may have caused any differences.[42] The "ideal" clinical trial is typified by the single dose pharmacological trial, in which all other medications, surgical, nursing, and dietary factors are strictly controlled. It is clear that such ideal trials are impracticable in many health-care evaluations. A compromise has to be struck between allowing therapists "clinical freedom" within very loosely defined aims of "providing psychological support as needed" and being "ultra-prescriptive" in, for example, "introducing the biofeedback monitor in the fourth—not the third or the fifth—physical relaxation training session". It is important that both therapist as practitioner and scientist as evaluator appreciate this practical reality. Psychological therapy following myocardial infarction cannot be distilled down into a single action like administering streptokinase; nor for that matter can exercise training. Yet if therapists do not agree to standardise and evaluate component by component we shall never learn how effective psychological therapy is, what effect is has, and what elements and methods are more effective.

Two aspects of standardisation in this trial may be used as examples to illustrate the point. The chosen primary psychological method for relaxation training was progressive muscle tension–relaxation and this was taught and practised first lying down, then seated and finally in "live" situations. The choice was on the basis of clinical experience of senior clinical psychologists, mostly with hypertensive patients and following review of the literature, at the time of designing the trial. Some clinical psychologists find a role for self hypnosis and may prefer self hypnosis in certain situations. However, in the interests of making the trial as "pure" as reasonably possible (as like a simple single dose pharmacological trial as possible), clinical psychologists agreed to standardise on progressive muscle tension–relaxation as the lead technique for inducing relaxation.

The second example of standardisation in this trial was of standardising on the exclusion of health education on the classic risk factors of smoking, drinking, diet, and exercise. As all of these were potential confounders, the trial sought to provide no more health education to cases than to controls. It was therefore quite important that the nurse member of the team refrained from providing advice on, for example, reducing smoking or reducing dietary fat. This might not have come naturally to health visitors, many of whom have been teaching along these lines for several years. However, for the sake of the trial and in order to give psychological therapy as fair a test as practically possible, the health visitors agreed and the results demonstrated that smoking, drinking, diet, and exercise habits were indistinguishable between cases and controls at six months. An alternative trial methodology would have been to compare psychological therapy plus health education (for cases) with health education alone (for controls) as did Friedman et al.[17]

Health visitors were chosen as the nurse members of the rehabilitation team in this trial for a number of reasons, centring on their post-qualification training and experience in educating normal healthy people (often mothers of young children) rather than caring for patients, working with groups, and working in non-hospital (non-clinical) settings. Additionally, health visitors are accustomed to working in ordinary civilian clothing, which helps to convey a non-clinical atmosphere more conducive to rehabilitation.

Trials remain essential to the advancement of scientific knowledge. Whilst respecting clinical judgment and clinical autonomy, it is important to appreciate that these can lead to clinical dogmatism without directly relevant evidence. This is in part the justification for doctors being expected to engage in some research, during their training years before obtaining their consultant posts. The theory is that by taking part in research they become more aware that many questions remain unanswered and more aware of the methods researchers use to address these questions. The practice remains that too many learn by their own mistakes, too many engage in poorly supervised research, much medical research is ill-coordinated, many studies and trials are too small, and hence many of the answers remain inconclusive. Therapists in professions allied to medicine could usefully learn from the doctors' experience. It is likely to be a valuable experience to collaborate with researchers, particularly during the later specialist training years, but it is likely to be a more valuable training experience if the collaboration is with well-found research.

By their very nature, health-care evaluation trials are more complex than parmacological trials. Although we may emulate the "double-blind placebo controlled trial" in overall design, we cannot achieve it in practice. A programme of cardiac rehabilitation takes time and involves several therapists, and its evaluation is of necessity "open". Nevertheless, such "open" trials should be rigorous and should follow so far as is reasonably possible the principles of fair and unbiased comparison and of evaluating one standardised intervention at a time. Despite "standardisation", trials of health-care interventions remain multifactorial by comparison with drug trials. Aspirin is aspirin in England (ISIS) or Italy (GISSI), and statisticians analysing the results of drug trials can reasonably infer that any differences in outcome between cases and controls may be attributed to the experimental drug. In health-care evaluations many factors combine to form the prescribed "intervention" (for example, therapist, therapy, one feature of the therapy, "Hawthorn" effect) and therefore it is the combined effects of these factors that is compared between case and control groups. The "multifactorial" nature of the prescribed intervention leads to dilution of the "pure" effect in the experimental evaluation. Differences or lack of differences in outcome between case and control groups may be attributable to any of the factors that combine to make up the programme and to interactions with pre-randomisation patient characteristics. While it would make little difference to an aspirin trial if there were an imbalance between hospitals in the sex ratio of case and control groups if overall the sex ratios were similar, such imbalance could have quite a marked effect in a rehabilitation trial if the programme were more successful with men than women in one hospital with an atypical sex ratio. This apparent untidiness of health-care evaluation trials, by comparison with drug trials, means that they justify analysis more comparable with that of observational studies. One of the main differences therefore between these trials and the ideal double-blind placebo-controlled trial is that health-care evaluation trials require more data and more detailed analysis than the simple "toss of a coin" and straightforward comparison of one end point.

Conclusions

Randomised controlled trials in health-care evaluations are no easy option (although their design may look deceptively simple in outline) but they are a necessary option. Archie Cochrane in *Effectiveness and efficiency* stressed the importance of the randomised controlled trial in evaluating medical care[12] and exhorted clinicians "to randomise until it hurts—the clinicians" (A.L. Cochrane, personal communication, 1973). The present trial may have included as many patients as all previous psychological trials combined, but it does not close the book on psychological rehabilitation trials. Rather, there is need for further carefully designed collaborative randomised controlled trials of standardised rehabilitation programmes, and following those there is likely to be a continuing need for pragmatic trials to evaluate progressively evolving rehabilitation strategies.

References

1 Adset CA, Bruhn JG. Short-term group psychotherapy for post myocardial infarction patients and their carers. *Can Med Assoc J* 1968; **99**: 577–84.
2 Ibrahim MA, Feldman JG, Sultz HA, *et al*. Management after myocardial infarction: a controlled trial of the effect of group psychotherapy. *Int J Psychiatry Med* 1974; 5: 253–68.
3 Wenger NK. Quality of life: why the burgeoning interest in the clinical and research cardiology committees. In: Walter PJ, editor. *Quality of life after open heart surgery*. Dordrecht: Kluwer, 1992.
4 Byrne DG. Psychological aspects of outcomes and interventions following heart attack. In: Byrne DG, Roseman RH, editors. *Anxiety and the heart*. New York: Hemisphere, 1990.
5 Croog SH, Levine SL. *Life after a heart attack*. New York: Human Science Press, 1982.
6 Stern MJ, Pascale L, McLoone JB. Psychosocial adaptation following an acute myocardial infarction. *J Chronic Dis* 1976; **29**: 513–26.
7 Mayou R. Prediction of emotions and social outcome after a heart attack. *J Psychosom Res* 1984; **28**: 17–25.
8 Krantz DS. Cognitive processes and recovery from heart attack: a review and theoretical analysis. *J Human Stress* 1980; **6**: 27–38.
9 Carson P, Neophytou, Tucker H, Simpson T. Exercise programme after myocardial infarction. *BMJ* 1973; **iv**: 213–16.
10 Bethell HJN, Larvan A, Turner SC. Coronary rehabilitation in the community. *J R Coll Gen Pract* 1983; **33**: 285–91.
11 Horgan J, Bethell H, Carson P, *et al*. Working party report on cardiac rehabilitation. *Br Heart J* 1992; **67**: 412–18.
12 Cochrane AL. *Effectiveness and efficiency: random reflections on health services*. London: Nuffield Provincial Hospital Trust, 1972.
13 West RR, Henderson AH. Randomised multi-centre trial of early mobilisation after uncomplicated myocardial infarction. *Br Heart J* 1979; **42**: 381–5.
14 World Health Organization. *Rehabilitation and comprehensive secondary prevention after acute myocardial infarction*. Copenhagen: WHO, 1983 (EURO report 84).
15 Naismith LD, Robinson JF, Shaw GB, MacIntyre MMJ. Psychosocial rehabilitation after myocardial infarction. *BMJ* 1979; 1: 439–46.
16 Mayou R, Macmahon D, Sleight P, Florencio MJ. Early rehabilitation after myocardial infarction. *Lancet* 1981; **ii**: 1399–1401.
17 Friedman M, Thorenson CE, Gill JJ, *et al*. Alteration of type A behaviour and reduction in cardiac recurrences in post-myocardial infarction patients. *Am Heart J* 1984; **108**: 237–48.
18 Frasure-Smith N, Prince R. Long-term follow-up of the ischaemic heart disease life stress monitoring program. *Psychosom Med* 1989; **51**: 485–513.
19 Patel C, Marmot MC, Terry DJ, *et al*. Trial of relaxation in reducing coronary risk: four year follow-up. *BMJ* 1985; **290**: 1103–6.
20 Steptoe A. Process underlying long-term blood pressure reductions in essential hypertensives following behavioural therapy. In: Elbert T, Langosch A, Steptoe A, Vaitl D, editors. *Behavioural medicine and cardiovascular disorder*. Chichester: John Wiley & Sons, 1988.
21 Bundy BC, Carroll D, Wallace LM, Nagle RE. Psychological treatment of chronic stable angina. *Psych Health Issue* 1994; **95**: in press.

225

22 Norris RM, Caughey OE, Merilees CJ, Scott PJ. Prognosis after myocardial infarction: six year follow-up. *Br Heart J* 1974; **36**: 786–90.

23 Townsend P. Poverty in the United Kingdom: a survey of household resources and standards of living. London: Penguin, 1983.

24 Rose GA. Ischaemic heart disease: chest pain questionnaire. *Millbank Mem Fund Q* 1965; **43**: 32–9.

25 Bedford A, Foulds GA, Sheffield BF. A new personal disturbance scale. DSSI/sAD. *Br J Soc Clin Psychol* 1976; **15**: 387–91.

26 Spielberger RL, Lushene R, Vagg PR, Jacobs GA. *Manual for the state–trait anxiety inventory form (Form Y) ("Self-evaluation Questionnaire")*. Palo Alto: Consulting Psychologists Press, 1983.

27 Office of Population Censuses and Surveys. *General household survey 1972*, London: HMSO, 1975.

28 Office of Population Censuses and Surveys. *General household survey 1978*. London: HMSO, 1980.

29 Yarnell JWG, Fehily AM, Milbank JE, *et al*. Short dietary questionnaire for use in epidemiological survey: comparison with weighted dietary records. *Hum Nutr Appl Nutr* 1983; **37a**: 103–12.

30 Taylor HL, Jacobs DR, Schucker B, *et al*. A questionnaire for the assessment of leisure time physical activities. *J Chronic Dis* 1978; **31**: 741–55.

31 Platt S, Weyman A, Hirsch S, Hewett S. The social behaviour assessment schedule: rationale, contents, scoring and reliability of a new interview schedule. *Soc Psychiatry* 1980; **15**: 43–55.

32 Anonymous. World congress of cardiac rehabilitation. Bordeaux, France 1992.

33 Mulchay R. Twenty years of cardiac rehabilitation in Europe: a reappraisal. *Eur Heart J* 1991; **12**: 92–3.

34 American College of Cardiology. Recommendations on cardiovascular rehabilitation. *J Am Coll Cardiol* 1986; **7**: 451–3.

35 Dixhoorn J van, Duivenvoorden HJ, Stahl HA, Pool J. Physical training and relaxation therapy in cardiac rehabilitation assessed through a composite criterion for training outcome. *Am Heart J* 1989; **118**: 545–52.

36 Dickersin K, Yuan IM, Curtis LM. Factors influencing publication of research results: follow-up of applications submitted to two institutional review boards. *JAMA* 1992; **267**: 389–98.

37 Coursol A, Wagner EE. Effect of positive findings on submission and acceptance rates: a note on meta analysis bias. *Prof Psychol Res Pract* 1986; **17**: 136–7.

38 Rahe RH, Ward HW, Hayes V. Brief group therapy in myocardial infarction rehabilitation: three-to-four-year follow-up of a controlled trial. *Psychosom Med* 1979; **41**: 229–41.

39 Stern MJ, Gorman PA, Kaslow L. The group counselling vs exercise therapy study: a controlled intervention with subjects following myocardial infarction *Arch Intern Med* 1983; **143**: 1719–25.

40 Thompson DL, Meddis R. Prospective evaluation of in-hospital counselling for first time myocardial infarction. *J Psychosom Res* 1990; **34**: 237–48.

41 Oldridge N, Guyatt G, Jones N, *et al*. Effects on quality of life with comprehensive rehabilitation after acute myocardial infarction. *Am J Cardiol* 1991; **67**: 1084–9.

42 Pocock SJ. *Clinical trials: a practical approach*. Chichester: John Wiley, 1983.

11 Influence on spouses and influence of spouses

DEE JONES

Introduction

The experience of a serious illness, particularly if it is a sudden and life threatening event, is a crisis not only for the individual sufferer but also for the spouse and wider family. These events threaten the spouse's stability, security, adaptability, beliefs, assumptions, and even resources.[1] Leahey and Wright[1] described six basic assumptions about families faced with life threatening illness:

- The diagnosis of life threatening illness is a social contract between the patient, family, and health care system
- A life threatening diagnosis changes the family's life trajectory
- Families need to review a life threatening event
- Family members' reactions influence the course of a life threatening illness
- Family function is often altered by a life threatening illness
- Family members' beliefs about life threatening illness influence how they and the patient cope with the situation.

The main objectives of spouses, faced with a life threatening cardiac illness, is to reorganise and stabilise as the sufferer moves through the acute, transitional, and rehabilitation stages. Ability to cope effectively takes time and may require professional input and support. A spouse's ability to cope with the initial crisis and subsequent recovery period may also influence positively or negatively, the patient's rehabilitation.

This chapter discusses the impact of cardiac illness upon spouses' quality of life, their needs, their influence upon patients, their rehabilitation, and finally their role in the rehabilitation of patients.

As most published studies of rehabilitation following myocardial infarction include only male patients, most of the studies of spouses, to date, are of wives. It needs to be recognised that a substantial proportion of patients are women and therefore many spouses are husbands.

The impact of patients' myocardial infarction on spouses

Psychological impact

It is well documented that myocardial infarction causes severe physical, emotional, and psychological distress to sufferers. The effect of a member of the family having a myocardial infarction upon spouses/partners or principal carers is probably of equal importance. Husbands and wives merit attention as carers and as patients in their own right.

Due to the suddenness of their partner's illness, spouses report considerable distress in the immediate aftermath of a myocardial infarction, following admission to coronary care unit; this often takes the form of a feeling of numbness, panic, unreality, and a sense of loss.[2-4] In our study of over 1700 spouses, 97% reported moderate or severe distress immediately after the infarction; the same rates were reported for men and women. After discharge, 69% of spouses were still moderately or severely distressed; older spouses were less distressed than younger ones.

Fear of a recurrence, permanent incapacity, and death is prevalent among spouses, particularly in the early days after the patient's myocardial infarction.[2,5,6] Many spouses report feelings of guilt and blame themselves for the myocardial infarction in their desire to find a cause (they "allowed the husband to work too hard", "encouraged decorating", "caused stress"). These feelings often lead to overprotective responses in women towards their husbands during the convalescence period.[2]

Feelings of depression and anxiety are also commonly experienced and have been documented in both qualitative and quantitative studies. In our study of unselected men and women 17% of husbands and 34% of wives were significantly anxious soon after discharge; older (aged over 65 years) spouses tended to be less anxious. Seven per cent of husbands and 17% of wives were significantly depressed soon after discharge. Some studies have reported anxiety as being higher among spouses than among patients.[4,6] Furthermore, some spouses develop new psychosomatic symptoms, including sleep, appetite, and bowel disturbance, headaches, stomach pains, faintness, sickness, chest pain, and palpitations.[2,7-10]

For some but not all spouses such feelings of distress continue through the convalescent period, most commonly exacerbated by guilt, fear of upsetting the patient, and fear of another heart attack. By 12 months the majority have adjusted well and feel that they are restored to their previous mood, but a minority are still severely emotionally disturbed—causing distress not only to themselves but also to the patients and other members of the family.[2] Severe psychological reactions appear to be more prevalent among younger wives (aged under 45 years), in those with a previous psychiatric history, and in women who have always been dependent on their husbands.

There is only a minimal amount of literature available documenting the problems experienced by spouses of patients undergoing coronary artery bypass grafts; the little there is indicates that such surgery is a disorganising experience for the entire family.[11] Spouses fear not only the surgery itself but also the responsibility of caring for a newly discharged patient; furthermore, they felt anger at patients for causing their stress.[12] After surgery, husbands and wives also seem to experience very similar psychosomatic symptoms to those of spouses of myocardial infarction patients.[13]

Marital relationship

Wives tend to relate their experience of their husbands' myocardial infarction to the context and meaning to them of their marital relationship and the potential losses involved, fearing the effect of the illness on their relationship and the possible consequent changes in the nature and quality of the interpersonal relationship.[14,15]

The crisis of a myocardial infarction occurs within a wide variety of marital contexts—nature of relationship, length of marriage, communication, roles, etc. Many couples will have had problems in their relationship before the crisis and the impact of the illness will, to an extent, depend on the quality of the relationship before onset.[2] From their research, Skelton and Dominian[2] reported in 1973 that within the first three months almost half of their sample of patients experienced an appreciable change in their relationship; increased tension and irritability. This was exacerbated more by the inability of some husbands to express their feelings than by their health status. At twelve months after onset, one in six wives of healthy patients felt that their marital relationship had remained noticeably impaired; these wives tended to remain anxious and overprotective.

Some wives describe their husbands as becoming more depressed, irritable, frustrated, demanding, impatient, easily upset, and difficult to please.[16] In 1973, Tyzenhouse considered that one in five wives experienced problems of such severity that they require professional counselling.[16]

At 12 months after their husband's myocardial infarction, the mental wellbeing of wives is usually related to the state of their marriage.[17] A minority of wives report that their marriage has deteriorated directly as a consequence of the infarction.[17] Those wives who have made a successful adjustment after a year tend to be those who have continued employment, enjoy their occupation, maintained leisure activities, and have satisfactory family life and marriages.[17] Some marriages, however, appear to benefit from such a crisis, with an increase in warmth, mutual evaluation, and appreciation as a consequence of being able to spend more time together. Such couples (one in four) seem to have made positive efforts to improve their relationship. Good marriages have a tendency to improve but poor marriages cope less satisfactorily and are characterised by tension and strain.[17]

During the rehabilitation phase after myocardial infarction a reversal of roles often takes place, with wives taking on more household chores and house maintenance. Also, acting as the primary support person in the relationship can be a form of role reversal for some, if the husbands, before the illness, played a strong supportive role in the relationship.[3] The accompanying ambiguity of roles, within traditional partnerships in particular, can lead to confusion and frustration.[18] Such tensions and strains tend to increase if communication is poor and if there have been significant pre-existing marital problems.[3]

Sexual activity is an aspect of marriage that can be affected by a myocardial infarction and be the source of much anxiety and fear.[17–19] There is usually a temporary reduction in sexual activity and satisfaction, but a substantial minority seem to experience a long term deleterious effect on their sexual relationship.[19] For many of course, owing to medical history, medication, or quality of their relationship, sexual relations were unsatisfactory prior to the myocardial infarction or cardiac surgery—as many as half of the wives of myocardial infarction patients are unsatisfied with their sexual activity and a quarter of these report that this is directly due to the myocardial infarction or surgery. A reduction in sexual activity and consequent satisfaction is mostly as a consequence of spouses' or patients' fear of a recurrent myocardial infarction.[19] In the early days of recovery, 54% of our sample of male and female spouses indicated that their sexual activity was the same as before the infarction and 37% that it was less frequent than before.

A minority (about one in 10) report an improvement in their sexual relations, because of the overall improvement in their relationship.[19–21] Not surprisingly, there is a strong association between the emotional relationship between the husband and wife and the successful resumption of sexual activity.[19]

Much of the dissatisfaction reported is a consequence of sexual dysfunction in their partners. It is generally accepted that at least some of those problems may be caused by drug treatment but it is difficult, of course, to assess in individual patients whether the sexual problems are due to the disease or to medication. There is far more literature on drug-related male sexual dysfunction than for females, although it is clear that female sexual dysfunction may be caused by drug therapy; the extent of this has, in all likelihood, been under-estimated.

Evidence indicates that hypertensive agents, diuretics and β blockers are associated with sexual dysfunction in men. A few studies have indicated that anti-hypertensives and diuretics have an effect on vaginal lubrication and loss of libido in women.

Family

Tensions can arise within the family as a whole; conflicts can develop between patients and their children, particularly teenage boys, during the recovery phase. Patients can become very anxious about noise, emotional tensions, and family arguments.[18,22] Consequently, wives often find themselves in the role of buffers between their husbands and their children or grandchildren, trying to protect their husbands from any emotional upset or stress, fearing that stress might cause a recurrence of a myocardial infarction or an angina attack. Middle aged women often find themselves as "women in the middle", torn between the interests of their husbands and their children or grandchildren.

Social life

Studies of patients and their spouses indicate that their social life can be deleteriously affected by the illness; friends change and their social activities decrease.[18,23] Patients may be advised to give up long term hobbies and leisure pursuits. Those wives who acknowledge that their sources of network support have reduced tend to have poorer quality of life outcomes.[24] Those patients temporarily or permanently not returning to work are most likely to experience a significant change in their social network.

In contrast to myocardial infarction sufferers, those who had undergone coronary artery bypass grafts seem to experience a decrease in their level of dependence, thus enabling them to be less dependent on their spouses, which in turn enables spouses to maintain their social activities.

Employment

Currently, in the United Kingdom, two thirds of women of working age are in part-time or full-time employment, and there is every indication that this proportion will continue to rise. The desire to care for an ill husband obviously can conflict with a woman's commitment to her occupation and is likely to have an impact upon it and cause further conflicts of interest and loyalties.

Of the 41 working wives whom Skelton and Dominian[2] interviewed in 1973, a quarter stopped work temporarily and one abandoned work altogether. Most working women find their occupation helpful but wives of self-employed husbands, in their study, were forced to take on much of their husband's business responsibilities, workload, and strain at a time of emotional stress and found that this had a negative effect upon them.

Finances

A reduction in husbands' and/or wives' income can cause an added burden and strain; almost a third of Skelton and Dominian's sample of wives expressed financial anxiety. American studies indicate a higher prevalence of such anxieties, but this probably indicates a difference in health service and social security arrangements.

Some men may suffer a reduction in salary as a consequence of their myocardial infarction or surgery; they may have to retire on disability pensions, some may have to reduce their responsibilities, level of physical effort or their hours, or any combination of these. Men in the lower income groups are less likely to be employed full-time after having a myocardial infarction and so they and their spouses are more likely to be subject to the added stress of financial uncertainty.[16]

The needs of spouses

Several studies have examined the needs of spouses of myocardial infarction patients both in terms of their needs during the crisis period and later during the convalescent period. Many studies have reported on the particular needs, expressed by spouses retrospectively, that were experienced whilst the patient was hospitalised. Most express the desire to be considered and included by the staff and not excluded from the patient's care. Wives would not only like to be present with the husband whenever possible but would like to be accepted and involved in his care—to be informed of his treatment and reasons for it.[25–27] They also feel the need to receive support from the staff: to be able to express their emotions to staff and in turn to be supported and comforted by staff. Of primary importance is spouses' need to be reassured that patients are receiving the best care possible, in order to maintain their own hope.[26,28]

Information about heart disease

Consistently, when asked, spouses report their strongest need as being for educational information, during both the crisis period and the recovery period.[15,29] In our study the most frequently reported causes of distress while patients were hospitalised was a lack of information. Just over half the spouses reported discussing the illness with a hospital physician, less than half with a nurse, a third with a general practitioner, a quarter with relatives, and a tenth with friends. Men were more likely to have talked with physicians than were women, wives being more likely to talk to nurses, general practitioners, relatives, and friends. Initially wives desire to know as much as possible about the illness and how it will affect their husbands—to have specific facts about the patient's condition, treatment, and disease process explained frankly in terms that they could understand. Also, during patients' hospitalisation, spouses would like to receive information about what to do in an emergency should reinfarction occur. After the initial crisis has been overcome, spouses then desire to know in some detail how the illness will affect patients and to be provided with guidelines and instructions on how they can assist them to achieve the best regimen—level and type of permitted physical activity, how to change diet appropriately, safe sexual activity, and smoking cessation.[15,29] Spouses play a crucial role in controlling the level and nature of sexual activity regained following myocardial infarction and may fear recurrence of a myocardial infarction; they therefore require clear confirmation of when it is safe to engage in sexual relations.[30]

Prevention of recurrence

The second strongest area of need is in the area of prevention; spouses are generally very strongly motivated towards doing everything possible to prevent a recurrence of the illness. Wives feel responsible for managing the changes that have been precipitated by the illness (in family dynamics, marital relationship, etc), managing their own anxiety, and assisting husbands to maintain their prescribed rehabilitation regimen. They perceive their role as changing with passage of time from the initial crisis; as their concern with managing their own anxiety decreases so it increases with assisting husbands to manage their stress—stress is seen by the majority as a cause of initial and recurrent myocardial infarctions.

Support services

A third category of needs could be labelled as support services. Although this category was rated overall least highly in the study by Doherty and Power,[15] elements within it were rated very highly and were reinforced by other findings; wives expressed a desire to talk to another wife of a myocardial infarction patient, to meet with a support group of wives in order to share fears, anxieties, and feelings, and to benefit from spiritual support. These three aspects seem to remain important throughout the recovery period. Wives wanted to discuss their fears and feelings with health professionals and to discuss the cardiac event's psychological impact on their husbands.

Some wives report needing assistance from formal services—more often those who are younger, who are working outside the home, and who are professional women. This need is particularly acute in the early days of recovery.[15]

Discrepant feelings

Moser, Dracup and Marsden[29] in their study of cardiac patients and their spouses reported that spouses ranked nearly all their needs higher than did patients. Patients ranked lowest needs that were generally related to emotional concerns—information related to the psychological impact of the cardiac event on both patient and spouse. It must be borne in mind that because, in all these studies, most if not all spouses were female and patients male, the findings may reflect the different responses to (illness) crises of men and women.

Unmet needs

Many needs that were highly ranked by spouses seem not to have been met satisfactorily. In one study it was reported that more than 70% of cardiac patients and their spouses had not received information concerning appropriate action to be taken should an emergency arise.[29] Forty to seventy per cent of patients and spouses reported not receiving information about lifestyle changes, appropriate care, expected physical and psychological course of the illness, and sexual activity. In particular, wives expressed a desire for more information on diet—how to prepare more appropriate meals for their families—and about the level and nature of physical activity that their husbands should be taking.[9,31,32] Also, many spouses felt that their emotional needs had not been met—that is, they did not have adequate opportunity to discuss their fears and feelings. Inadequate information and communication at such a time of crisis can cause anxiety and further problems to spouses, as can a lack of communication with patients themselves.[32]

Spouses' impact on patients

Hospitalisation

Sullivan[3] developed many years ago the concept of empathic anxiety and anxiety contagion. He stated that during periods of severe physical illness empathic anxiety or anxiety contagion emerges. Laughlin[34] defined anxiety contagion as anxiety that arises by intuitive communication from one person to another. Families become extremely sensitised to the verbal and non-verbal cues transmitted by each other, and non-verbal communication becomes more important in times of distress. Through these intimate forms of communication, anxiety is transmitted from one family member to another.

During such stressful times as the occurrence of a myocardial infarction, family members are more receptive to anxiety contagion than they would normally be. Family members transmit anxiety to patients and create stress and consequent harmful responses in patients (including raised blood pressure) when visiting patients in hospital.[35] Our findings, like those of Frederickson,[35] indicate that family members' anxiety and distress are closely correlated with those of patients. That such visits precipitate anxiety and related symptoms places health professionals in a difficult dilemma. Despite this stressful situation, both patient and spouse value visits highly.[27] However, studies have shown significantly lower anxiety among patients when family members are prepared by nurses before visiting patients in coronary care units than among patients whose visiting family have not been so prepared.[36,37]

Recovery period

Attitudes and reactions of family, particularly spouses, have a profound effect on a patient's adaptation to an illness and rehabilitation during the recovery period.[5] A large study of 2320 male survivors demonstrated that those who were socially isolated and without family support were four times more likely to die after an acute myocardial infarction, even when other physiological factors were controlled for.[38] On the other hand, better recovery is positively associated with patients having good family support and a close relationship with significant others with whom they can confide and who themselves have a substantial network of support.[39,40]

Marriage can be a mediator between external stressors and their negative effects.[41,42] A spouse's ability to respond optimally to his or her partner has a significant impact on the patient's physical and emotional adjustment to cardiac illness.[5,10,43] Specific aspects of the marriage relationship have been demonstrated to influence the recovery of patients after myocardial infarction. Waltz studied 521 myocardial infarction couples longitudinally and reported in 1986[44] that patients' long term subjective feeling of wellbeing was strongly associated with the presence of an "intimate attachment", and that positive feeling states at 12 months after infarction were associated with the presence of an emotionally close conjugal bond. He concluded that such "love resources" were, in his sample, a major determinant of effective coping with the sequelae of illness and long term successful adaptation. Being emotionally integrated within a marriage seems to enable greater satisfaction with life and better long term health outcomes.

Waltz speculated, on the other hand, that negative social resources, lack of "love resources", and lack of intimacy may increase the risk of development of cardiac invalidism or chronic "illbeing" consequent upon a myocardial infarction. Such factors may enable health professionals to predict poor prognosis, survival rates, and quality of life—a speculation that is supported by other research within cardiac and cancer contexts.

An emotionally close relationship, by affirming social identity and maintenance of a positive self image, provides individuals with a secure

235

environment in which to adapt to a new situation. Being valued as a person improves self esteem and self worth and hence facilitates the adaptive process. Such interpersonal relationships may compensate for loss of previous health and socially prized roles.

Rehabilitation and support of spouses

We have seen that a myocardial infarction, cardiac event, or cardiac surgery has a major impact on spouses, which in turn can impede or accelerate the successful recovery of patients. Furthermore it is well documented that spouses have specific needs themselves which are not being satisfactorily met during hospitalisation and subsequently during the recovery phase. Some have seen such suppport as being the role of social workers and others as that of nurses; in the United Kingdom initial support is likely to be provided by coronary care nursing staff.

Assessment

In order to minimise the impact of stress upon the family and consequent family dysfunction, health professionals need to view the family, particularly the spouse, as well as the patient as recipients of care.[45] Some partners, however, do not perceive assessment and support of health professionals as therapeutic but rather as intrusive.[46] It is therefore of paramount importance that health professionals assess the needs of partners with great sensitivity and flexibility, bearing in mind that needs of families will differ and also that the needs and reactions of each family will vary and change over time.

A thorough assessment of each family unit or diad is required as soon as possible after the hospital admission. This assessment can of itself prove to be therapeutic, as it can convey care and concern for the partners, and demonstrate their inclusion in the patient's treatment.[47] Doherty and Power[15] described three aspects to a thorough assessment: the needs of the spouse, spouse's level of skill, and the degree of burden the illness will represent to the spouse. Each spouse possesses different abilities and skills that he or she can employ to cope with the trauma. A health professional will need to assess spouses' awareness of their own needs, determine if they are able to ask for help and support, the extent and adequacy of their support network, and their ability or skill at accessing that support system.

Additionally, the nurse will need to identify the person who will be most able to assist the patient with treatment and rehabilitation goals. The partner's expectations for the recovery and rehabilitation of the patient can be assessed at this time; some will expect the patient to remain a chronic invalid with a poor quality of life.[48] Obstacles to optimum outpatient care can also usefully be identified at this time to facilitate the

236

appropriate referrals and to enable the development of an appropriate discharge plan. A thorough assessment of this nature also enables health professionals to identify indicators of role insufficiency—that is, the disparity between the caring role requirements and the ability of the partner to fulfil them.[49] Nursing staff will then better be able to plan their appropriate intervention in terms of role supplementation, providing the necessary knowledge and information and enabling spouses to perceive the situation as the patient perceives it to be.[49] It should be borne in mind that many patients will not have spouses, in which case it is recommended that a principal carer be identified (daughter, son, or friend) for the benefit of the patient.

Education and information

Evidence consistently indicates that the first requirement of partners is for information and education. As mentioned earlier, patients in coronary care units whose families are provided with written and verbal information and time with a "resource nurse" prior to visiting have been demonstrated to have lower anxiety than those in a control group.[36] Similarly, Chatham[43] demonstrated that candidates for cardiotomy whose wives received instruction on how best to provide support to their husbands during the perioperative period were better oriented, more appropriately behaved, less confused, slept for longer periods, and had fewer delusions than the control group. Furthermore, Chatham observed that although wives in the control group were very motivated to help and support their husbands, they lacked purposeful direction.

The plans based on the information gleaned at assessment of care and rehabilitation of patients need to be negotiated and discussed with spouses. Spouses are important factors in the maintenance of rehabilitation regimes; the most frequent reason given for non-attendance at a cardiac rehabilitation exercise programme among post-myocardial infarction patients has been reported as being a lack of support from the spouse.[50]

Information about the illness, treatment, and rehabilitation needs to be clearly communicated, in easily understood language, to the spouse. High anxiety at this time will inevitably be a barrier to comprehension and retention; written, easily digestible backup material may help to overcome this problem.

Support

A programme of support should be designed that is suited to the particular needs, skills, and resources of the couple; some will need to acquire skills in relaxation and stress management and others strategies and skills in lifestyle changes.

Most spouses will require counselling and advice on the emotional

237

effects of the cardiac event on both patients and spouses—depression, anxiety, anger, frustration, loss of control, and loss of libido. Many wives have indicated a desire to talk to other spouses and couples who have undergone similar experiences.

It is important that marital problems, and in particular difficulties with communication and sharing of emotional responses, should be identified and, where necessary, such communication and sharing facilitated.[15] It is well documented that anxiety and fear exist concerning sexual activity, and many myths abound regarding the impact of sexual activity on the heart and the consequent dangers. Care is necessary in the way in which advice is provided—evidence has been provided of situations where information had a deleterious effect.[19] Cooper[51] recommended that a physician should give full factual information and advice in an "authoritative" manner to allay anxiety and facilitate optimum rehabilitation.

Throughout the time that patients are in hospital many nursing skills are required—provision of social support, assessment, education, counselling, and discharge planning—and these activities need to be undertaken in an appropriate sequence in response to the changing needs of spouses. The initial task during the crisis phase is to provide emotional support in order to prevent or reduce anxiety, by assisting spouses to cope with psychological reactions to the crisis event: grief, fear of environment, loss of control, etc. Immediate concerns about the patient need to be alleviated, treatment and machinery explained, spouses involved in patient care, and confidence given concerning patient care. Many spouses will, at this time, need an opportunity to express their feelings and/or require spiritual support—perhaps from a chaplain.[10,52] Continued support should be provided or changed as the support network is identified and evaluated. Evidence indicates that spouses from higher socioeconomic groups have more extensive social networks and are consequently more able to access support from non-kin sources. Other families may benefit from intervention to mobilise or supplement social networks.[23] The mere availability of support has been shown to buffer families from situational stress.[53]

Discharge and aftercare

Appropriate and timely discharge planning should ameliorate the spouse's anxiety about leaving the protective environment of the hospital and the stress of taking over responsibility for patient care, thus enabling the patient to transfer smoothly from hospital back into the community. When family needs have been identified, it is desirable to ensure that they are documented and communicated to the appropriate community based services: general practitioners, primary care teams, community nurses, outpatient departments, and cardiac rehabilitation programmes. Such referrals will require effective channels of communication between the ward staff and health and social services in the community.

Dhooper[23] suggested that, for some families, the need for and ability to benefit from education and information may not become apparent until after the patients have been discharged from hospital and are in the rehabilitation phase. Not all families can benefit from material and information provided in the acute phase[54]; also, their need or desire for such information may not come to light until they have returned home.[23]

After the immediate crisis of admission is past, spouses are more receptive to cognitive support, including need for education and information. It has been recommended that certain goals should be achieved before patients return to the community (see box).[47]

Recommended goals in helping patients' spouses at discharge

- Explanation of the cardiac event
- Description of risk factors
- Discussion of therapeutic plan
- Explanation of medication regime and possible side effects
- Explanation of exercise regime and limitations
- Advice on sexual activity
- Provision of information on sources of advice and support
- Provision of information regarding cardiac rehabilitation programmes

---

The immediate period after discharge from hospital is a time of distress and anxiety to most spouses. Spouses have often reported that they would like further information about a myocardial infarction, its immediate treatment, long-term management, prognosis, rehabilitation, diet, exercise, sexual activity and medication. Much of the information provided in hospital is not successfully absorbed and needs reinforcing or elaborating upon after discharge. This can be done by the provision of easily read written information, discussion with primary health care team, attendance at a rehabilitation programme, or any combination of these strategies.

Some spouses benefit during the initial post-discharge period from being offered a telephone number that they can ring if they are anxious. At least some spouses require some form of support to compensate for their lack of informal support during the early months after patients have been discharged.

Until relatively recently, if support and counselling advice were provided, it was patient oriented and did not include spouses. However, more recently, spouses have been included in counselling and information programmes—both in hospital and in outpatient/community based cardiac rehabilitation programmes.

Inpatient education/counselling groups are designed to (a) provide spouses with information regarding anatomy and pathophysiology of the heart, risk factors; (b) encourage sharing of fears and anxieties; and (c) provide information about post-discharge rehabilitation (changes in lifestyle, etc).

Outpatient groups have tended to (a) provide information about the heart, treatment, medication, and post-myocardial infarction recovery; (b) provide information about lifestyle changes and how to achieve them; (c) train in relaxation techniques, and stress management; (d) discuss appropriate sexual activity; (e) enable the spouses to share fears, anxieties, anger, psychosomatic symptoms, and mood changes in self and patient; and (f) provide social support.

In some programmes spouses attend all sessions and in some they attend specific ones. It seems to be important that spouses have an opportunity to talk with each other.

In our study we asked spouses their opinion of the rehabilitation programmes attended in six centres; three quarters found them helpful, and they appreciated receiving information about infarctions, talking with other people, and having the opportunity to meet others in similar situations. Two thirds thought them useful to the patients; they mentioned benefits as being relaxation of the patient, provision of information, and sharing with others in the same position.

It may be that such programmes are not essential to all spouses; some may benefit from written information alone. At present there is inadequate information about the predictors of those spouses (or patients) who are at risk of poor outcome and would benefit from which type of support, if any. As some patients and/or spouses can become chronically affected by their experience of a myocardial infarction, it is important to establish the predictors, identify those needing support, establishing appropriate means of helping them and meeting their needs, and evaluating those new programmes or strategies.

The role of spouses in rehabilitation of patients

Overall, the literature supports the view that spouses are an important factor to be considered when examining recovery after a myocardial infarction or other cardiac event. They can be a valuable resource during the rehabilitation process because they can support patients during the adjustment phase and assist and encourage them in lifestyle changes and health promoting behaviours.[8,17,32,44]

Wives' perceptions of their husbands' physical capabilities can either assist or impede the recovery process. At worst spouses can create dependency and encourage cardiac invalidism, but at best they can influence patients' successful adaptation to their "new life",[55] which in turn results in a better long term recovery.[39,40] Spouses have a significant impact not only on the health and functioning of the family but also on patients' physical and emotional adaptation to the cardiac illness.[5]

Evidence indicates that wives are almost invariably involved in the long term care of patients after myocardial infarction, trying to control the long term consequences of an infarction; they monitor diet, activity, prescribed treatment, and medication.[10] Wives play a key role in supporting husbands in their lifestyle changes, encouraging them to change their diet, quit smoking, and maintain a regular exercise schedule. Wives feel responsible for creating a calm and stress-free environment by themselves avoiding nagging and by preventing family and friends from upsetting their husbands.[10] Most wives soon discover that nagging and being overprotective are counterproductive.

In order to provide optimal support, spouses need not only adequate and appropriate information about improving diets and exercise but also detailed information regarding cooking instructions and the type and nature of exercise that is appropriate and safe.

Summary

Since evidence indicates that a myocardial infarction can have a major impact on the quality of life of spouses, and they in turn can affect the long term outcome of post-myocardial infarction patients, it is crucial that they are considered and involved appropriately at all stages of treatment and rehabilitation.

References

1 Leahey M, Wright L. *Families and life-threatening illness: assumptions, assessment and intervention.* Springhouse, PA: Springhouse Corporation, 1987.

2 Skelton M, Dominian J. Psychological stress in wives of patients with myocardial infarction. *BMJ* 1973; 2: 101–3.

3 Bramwell L, Whall AL. The effect of role clarity and empathy on support role performance and anxiety. *Nurse Res* 1986; 35: 282–7.

4 Hilbert GA. Family satisfaction and affect of men and their wives after myocardial infarction. *Heart Lung* 1993; 22: 200–5.

5 Bedsworth JA, Molen MT. Psychological stress in spouses of patients with myocardial infarction. *Heart Lung* 1982; 11: 450–6.

6 Thompson DR, Meddis R. Wives' responses to counselling early after myocardial infarction. *J Psychosom Res* 1989; 34: 249–58.

7 Mayou R, Williamson B, Foster A. Attitudes and advice after myocardial infarction. *BMJ* 1976; **1**: 1577–9.

8 Stern MJ, Pascale L. Psychosocial adaption post-myocardial infarction: the spouse's dilemma. *J Psychosom Res* 1979; **23**: 83–7.

9 Hentinen M. Need for instruction and support of the wives of patients with myocardial infarction. *J Adv Nurs* 1983; 8:519–24.

10 Nymathi AM. The coping responses of female spouses of patients with myocardial infarction. *Heart Lung* 1987; **16**: 86–92.

11 Gillis C. Reducing family stress during and after coronary artery bypass surgery. *Nurs Clin North Am* 1984; **19**: 103–12.

12 O'Connor A. Factors related to the early phase of rehabilitation following aorto-coronary bypass surgery. *Res Nurse Health* 1983; **6**: 107–16.

13 Benson Stanley MJ, Frantz RA. Adjustment problems of spouses of patients undergoing coronary artery bypass graft surgery during early convalescence. *Heart Lung* 1988; **17**: 677–82.

14 Michela JL. Interpersonal and individual impacts of a husband's heart attack. In: Baun A, Singer J, editors. *Handbook of psychology and health: Vol 5. Stress and coping*. Hillsdale NJ: Lawrence Erlbaum, 1987.

15 Doherty ES, Power PW. Identifying the needs of coronary patient wife-caregivers: implications for social workers. *Health Soc Work* 1990; **15(4)**: 291–9.

16 Tyzenhouse PS. Myocardial infarction: its effect on the family. *Am J Nurs* 1973; **73**: 1012–13.

17 Mayou R, Foster A, Williamson B. The psychological and social effects of myocardial infarction on wives. *BMJ* 1978; **1**: 699–701.

18 Segev U, Schlesinger Z. Rehabilitation of patient after acute myocardial infarction—an interdisciplinary, family-oriented program. *Heart Lung* 1981; **10**: 841–7.

19 Papadopoulos C, Larrimore P, Cardin S, Shelley S. Sexual concerns and needs of the postcoronary patient's wife. *Arch Intern Med* 1980; **140**: 38–41.

20 Hellerstein HK, Friedman EH. Sexual activity and the postcoronary patient. *Arch Intern Med* 1970; **125**: 987–99.

21 Stern M, Pascale L, Ackerman A. Life adjustment post myocardial infarction: determining predictive variables. *Arch Intern Med* 1977; **137**: 1680–5.

22 Doehrman SR. Psycho-social aspects of recovery from coronary heart disease: a review. *Soc Sci Med* 1977; **11**: 199–218.

23 Dhooper S. Social networks and support during the crisis of heart attack. *Health Soc Work* 1983; **9**: 294–303.

24 Finlayson A. Social networks as coping resources. Lay help and consultation patterns used by women in husband's post-infarction career. *Soc Sci Med* 1976; **10**: 97–103.

25 Stillwell SB. Importance of visiting needs as perceived by family members of patients in the intensive care unit. *Heart Lung* 1984; **13**: 238–42.

26 Leske JS. Needs of relatives of critically ill patients: a follow-up. *Heart Lung* 1986; **15**: 194–9.

27 Norris LO, Grove SK. Investigation of selected psychosocial needs of family members of critically ill adult patients. *Heart Lung* 1986; **15**: 194–9.

28 Molter NC. Needs of relatives of critically ill patients: a descriptive study. *Heart Lung* 1979; **8**: 332–9.

29 Moser DK, Dracup KA, Marsden C. Needs of recovering cardiac patients and their spouses: compared views. *Int J Nurs Stud* 1993; **30**: 105–14.

30 Block AR, Boyer SL, Imes C. Personal impact of myocardial infarction: a model for coping with physical disability in middle age. In: Eisenberg MG, Sutkin LC, Jansen MA, editors. *Chronic illness and disability through the life span: effects on self and family*. New York: Springer, 1984: 209.

31 Wishnie H, Hackett R, Cassem N. Psychological hazards of convalescence following myocardial infarction patients. *JAMA* 1971; **215**: 1292–6.

32 Bramwell L. Wives' experiences in the support role after husbands' first myocardial infarction. *Heart Lung* 1986; **15**: 578–84.

33 Sullivan HS. *The interpersonal theory of psychiatry*. New York: WW Norton, 1953

34 Laughlin HP. *The neuroses*.Woburn, Massachusetts: Long Butterworth and Co, 1967.

35 Frederickson K. Anxiety transmission in the patient with myocardial infarction. *Heart Lung* 1989; **18**: 617–22.

36 Doerr B, Jones J. Effects of family preparation on the state anxiety level of the CCU patient. *Nurs Res* 1979; **28**: 315–16.

37 Norheim RN. Family needs of patients having coronary artery bypass graft surgery during the intraoperative period. *Heart Lung* 1989; **18**: 622–6.

38 Ruberman W, Weinblatt E, Goldberg JD, Chaudbury BS. Psychosocial influences on mortality after myocardial infarction. *N Engl J Med* 1984; **311**: 552–9.

39 Ell KO, Haywood LJ. Social support and recovery from myocardial infarction: a panel study. *J Soc Serv Res* 1984; **4**: 1–19.

40 Croog SH, Levine S. *The heart patient recovers*. New York: Human Sciences Press, 1977.

41 Pearlin L, Johnson JS. Marital status, life-strains and depression. *Am Soc Rev* 1977; **42**: 704–15.

42 Broadhead WE, Kaplan BH, James SA, *et al.* The epidemiologic evidence for a relationship between social support and health. *Am J Epidemiol* 1983; **117**: 521–37.

43 Chatham MA. The effect of family involvement on patient's manifestations of postcardiotomy psychosis. *Heart Lung* 1978; **7**: 995–9.

44 Waltz M. Marital context and post-infarction quality of life: is it social support or something else? *Soc Sci Med* 1986; **22**: 791–805.

45 Gillis CL. Reducing family stress during and after coronary artery bypass surgery. *Nurs Clin North Am* 1984; **19**: 103–12.

46 Hopps J. The catch in social support. *Soc Work* 1986; **31**: 419–20.

47 Sirles AT, Selleck CS. Cardiac disease and the family: impact, assessment, and implications. *J Cardiovasc Nurs* 1989; **3(2)**: 23–32.

48 Power PW, Dell Orto AE. Families, illness and disability: the roles of the rehabilitation counsellor. *J Appl Rehabil Counselling* 1986; **17(2)**: 41–4.

49 Meleis AI. Role sufficiency and role supplementation: a conceptual framework. *Nurse Res* 1975; **24**: 264–71.

50 Andrew GM, Oldridge NB, Parker JO, Cunningham RA, Reichnitzer PA, Jones NJ, *et al.* Reasons for dropout from coronary exercise programs in postcoronary patients. *Med Sci Sports Exerc* 1981; **13**: 164–8.

51 Cooper A. Myocardial infarction and advice on sexual activity. *Practitioner* 1985; **229**: 575–9.

52 Stern M, Pascale L, McLoone J. Psychological adaptation following an acute myocardial. *J Chronic Dis* 1979; **29**: 513–26.

53 Wethington E, Kessler R. Perceived support, received support, and adjustment to stressful life events. *J Health Soc Behav* 1986; **27**: 78–9.

54 Dimond M, Jones SL. Social support. In: Dimond M. editor. *Chronic illness across the life span*. New York: Appleton-Century-Crofts, 1983.

55 Beach EK, *et al.* The spouse: a factor in recovery after acute myocardial infarction. *Heart Lung* 1992; **21**: 30–8.

12 Cardiac rehabilitation: future directions

JOHN HORGAN AND HANNAH M McGEE

Introduction

Cardiac rehabilitation faces many challenges which traverse its scientific basis, mode of delivery and professional direction in the coming decades. Four key challenges can be identified. Firstly, there is the issue of outcomes: what are to be the end points for an evaluation of the effectiveness of cardiac rehabilitation? The structure and mode of delivery of cardiac rehabilitation services, for example, whether they are hospital or community based, is a second major question to be resolved. Associated with this is the third question, that of the changing nature of the cardiac population. The population to be served is increasingly diverse—more female patients and more older patients, with various cardiac problems beyond myocardial infarction (MI) and bypass graft surgery, and undergoing an expanding range of procedures such as complex angioplasty or transplantation. Finally, in order for rehabilitation to develop optimally as a specialty within cardiology, issues such as training standards and audit must be developed, preferably via supportive structures within rather than imposed from outside. These four challenges are considered further in the following sections.

Appropriate outcomes for cardiac rehabilitation

Mortality

Previously the scientific community demanded "hard" end points, such as reduction in death and re-infarction rate, as indices of the effectiveness of the rehabilitation process. Meta-analysis of available randomised trials has indeed shown a significant reduction in cardiovascular mortality in the

244

early years following MI for patients undertaking a structured cardiac rehabilitation programme.[1,2] A trial of sufficient power to evaluate this finding further, while timely, may prove difficult—partly because of the expense but also because of the ethical difficulty of withholding a treatment in those centres already providing cardiac rehabilitation as a standard service. Furthermore, because of the increasing age and medical complexity of the population being served, difficulties in trial management, such as cross over between treatment groups and non-compliance are likely to make evaluation complex. This chapter accepts the collective findings of previous research as reviewed in earlier chapters and moves the focus of discussion from the question of "whether cardiac rehabilitation?" to "what format of cardiac rehabilitation?" and "what outcomes from cardiac rehabilitation?"

Quality of life

The spectrum of health benefit can be identified as ranging from mortality through morbidity to quality of life. These must be considered as a continuum rather than as separate entities. Thus the published meta-analyses[1,2] document a 20–25% reduction in mortality with structured cardiac rehabilitation, with no difference in the number of non-fatal cardiac events experienced by rehabilitation and control groups. While the latter finding has often been cited to suggest that cardiac rehabilitation is ineffective, there is implicit in this interpretation an assumption that a particular segment of the cardiac population does not benefit from cardiac rehabilitation. However, the findings instead indicate that the proportion of the population having a recurrence does not change but that, since a significant reduction in mortality has been achieved, many of those documented as having recurrent non-fatal events are presumably individuals who would have died without intervention. It follows that a similar proportion who would have had a recurrent event, were they in the control group, actually have an event-free recovery in the medium term if they are in the rehabilitation group. This positive effect may be better measured by health status or quality of life measures.

In the future, quality of life indicators will become increasingly important end points for cardiac rehabilitation. As with other medical areas, progress in preventive and treatment strategies mean that the life extending outcomes already achieved in cardiology are becoming more difficult to surpass. Life enhancement, always a legitimate clinical goal, thus increasingly comes to the fore as a target for intervention. From the patient's perspective, long term management of a chronic disorder such as heart disease may involve considerable disruption to vocational, family, and social activities, and overall quality of life achieved is likely to be considerably more important to patients than clinical markers traditionally emphasised by clinicians. Indeed, evaluation of cardiac rehabilitation using quality of life end points would complement trends in current evaluation strategies with well-accepted procedures such as coronary artery bypass grafting (CABG) and angioplasty (DB Mark *et al*, Canadian–US GUSTO substudy, unpublished). Quality of life methodologies have advanced dramatically in the past decade, and we are now at a point where quality of life can be reliably and validly assessed.[3] Decisions about assessment can increasingly focus on what dimensions of quality of life to measure rather than whether assessment is possible. Assessment procedures should have the possibility to measure issues such as the reduction or absence of health difficulties, as well as positive aspects of wellbeing such as increased self efficacy and life satisfaction. Fries *et al*[4] describe the challenge of the "compression of morbidity"—that is, to reduce the individual and collective burden of disability and ill health which accumulates towards the end of life—as the major challenge for the coming decades. Just as mortality has become outmoded as the only end point given the current nature of cardiac populations, a previously used intermediate variable—vocational status—has also become redundant because of the changing demography of the population and the meaning of employment status in economies unable to support a full workforce.

Quality of life is now considered a legitimate end point in a wide range of disorders, be they cancer, acquired immune deficiency syndrome, or hypertension. It should be adopted enthusiastically as a major outcome measure for cardiac rehabilitation. There will be few to argue with its legitimacy as an outcome measure; rather, the challenge will be to identify assessment tools which have sound psychometric properties, can be used routinely in clinical (as distinct from research) settings, and will provide a valid representation of the range of influences of cardiac rehabilitation on patient functioning.

Research concerns

The challenge for future research studies will be to incorporate a range of suitable end points, from mortality to quality of life, and to demonstrate the effectiveness of cardiac rehabilitation services as deliverable in a regular clinical context with a range of patients representing the clinical spectrum of disease. To date, work has focused primarily on specialist centres and on younger (< 65 years) male myocardial infarction patients. Large scale studies are now required to demonstrate the effectiveness of cardiac rehabilitation services in the 1990s. This evidence will be crucial to the wider acceptance of cardiac rehabilitation in what is probably now a well-disposed but substantially cautious cardiology community. The evidence will also be essential to justify ongoing funding of these services.

Clinical outcomes and cost

Quality of life as an outcome is patient focused. Two other forms of outcome are important for cardiac rehabilitation. From the clinical perspective, management of known risk factors for heart disease (such as cholesterol, cigarette smoking, and hypertension) is an important intermediate level between quality of life and mortality. From a societal perspective, the cost of achievement of risk factor management and patients' quality of life is important.

Costs are relevant from two stand points. Firstly with respect to other services, it will be increasingly important to determine the *net*, rather than *gross*, costs of cardiac rehabilitation services. Secondly, information to date suggests that cardiac rehabilitation has significant secondary preventive benefits, which can be documented at the level of cost savings in subsequent health and social service use.[5,6] Because of its impact on wide-ranging aspects of functioning (such as diet, exercise, and psychosocial factors), the full financial benefits of cardiac rehabilitation may be difficult to fully assess. However, it is likely that it represents good value for money or, in economic terms, is associated with a low cost per quality adjusted life year (QALY) gained.[7] For cardiac rehabilitation services in the future, it will be important to determine service costs alongside benefits in quality of life across different programmes. Such exercises constitute necessary research tasks. Alongside this is the more routine task of ongoing audit of established services.

Audit

Audit must become an integral part of rehabilitation services. Data reflecting access to and coverage of the general clinical population in a cardiac service are important, as are figures on time to treatment. Indicators of patient satisfaction such as attendance and drop-out rates are one dimension of service relevance and effectiveness, while outcomes such as maintenance of smoking cessation and regular exercise are another. Audit can challenge services to focus ever more specifically on the aspects requiring improvement. In developing systems of audit, it will be important that they reflect qualitative aspects of cardiac rehabilitation

---

Factors by which outcomes will be judged in evaluating future cardiac rehabilitation programmes

- Are they worthwhile—for the patient? Patient participation will depend significantly on whether patients perceive benefits in quality of life, in exchange for their efforts

- *Are they effective*—for the clinician? Do they positively influence risk profiles?

- *Are they efficient*—from the point of view of administrators and ultimately society at large? Do they represent good value for health spending?

247

outcome as distinct from a series of process variables describing only use of the service. The latter, although important, should be seen as necessary but insufficient data to reflect the nature of cardiac rehabilitation.

The structure of cardiac rehabilitation services

Cardiac rehabilitation is structured in a wide variety of ways both within and across countries. The structure of future services must be that which most effectively facilitates the goals of these services. Cardiac rehabilitation should serve

- to develop patients' lifestyle management skills safely and effectively
- to encourage generalisation of these skills during the programme, and ultimately
- to promote long-term maintenance of these skills.

The increasing costs relating to all aspects of medical endeavour make it unlikely that residential cardiac rehabilitation will be established in those countries where it is not already the norm and so it can be expected that much rehabilitation will take place in an outpatient setting. Ideally, the early phases of outpatient cardiac rehabilitation should take place in conjunction with the hospital where patients receive their specialist investigation. Perhaps more importantly, the optimal centre would be that closest to the patient's home. Such outpatient facilities should offer a programme of sufficient length to provide the patient with the appropriate skills of self management on conclusion. There is no general agreement as to how long such programmes should last, and programme durations may vary from 6 to 12 weeks depending on the availability of facilities. Similarly, programmes vary in intensity from one to three organised sessions per week. However, some programmes continue indefinitely and offer the patient a weekly, or even more frequent, facility for continuing exercise and the use of supportive services at the original centre. In other settings, the development of rehabilitation support services in community centres associated with varying sporting activities has been espoused as a satisfactory step-down mechanism for patients who have completed hospital-based cardiac rehabilitation programmes.

Time-limited v ongoing programmes, and their location

The variety of rehabilitation approaches reflects the varying goals of developing, generalising, and maintaining healthy lifestyles for cardiac patients. However, this seemingly unstructured system of service delivery does little to raise the profile of cardiac rehabilitation as a scientifically based, systematic healthcare intervention. An agreed service structure, with clear guidelines about access to or transfer from one component of the service to another, is needed. This may take the form of an outpatient, hospital-based, structured multidimensional course with a focus on health restoration, followed by a community-based unstructured (that is, ongoing) facility with a focus on health maintenance activities. A clear separation of these services, with encouragement for cardiac patients to undertake maintenance activities in the community, following completion of an outpatient programme, is likely to best encourage both professional and financial support for cardiac rehabilitation. (Indeed, it may be more helpful to reserve the phrase "cardiac rehabilitation" for the former process of restoring a patient's functioning and "secondary prevention" for the latter maintenance phase of service delivery.)

Community "maintenance" strategies can and should extend beyond exercise, because patients may need support in aspects of health maintenance such as stress management. The financing of hospital-based and community services may also be different, in that the latter may be seen as one to be supported through social services, community development funds, or other sources depending on the particular local government system in place.

Structured maintenance activities

Transfer of patients from hospital-based programmes to step-down systems will need to be tempered by the condition of the individual patient. While a large cohort of patients with ischaemic syndromes may be transferred in a relatively routine manner, patients with more complex problems such as heart failure or transplantation will require detailed and individualised guidelines on maintenance. This also raises the consideration of training standards *vis-à-vis* supervision of discharged patients by staff in community settings. A balance must be struck between permanently maintaining an increasing population of complex cardiac patients within hospital-based programmes and releasing them to enthusiastic but less supervised programmes of exercise and other lifestyle management strategies in community settings. Otherwise cardiac rehabilitation programmes will become saturated or community maintenance will be seen as being less than optimal so that non-medicalised "secondary prevention" is discouraged. It must be made possible to develop clear lines of communication, between medical specialists and those in community settings, on recommendations for a particular patient's activities in step-down programmes.

Variations in the mode of delivery

In this discussion, we have considered hospital-based programmes as equating with hospital-based scheduled courses attended periodically over a number of weeks and directly supervised by cardiology staff. However, a number of other mechanisms of service delivery have been developed, involving self-instruction manuals and telephone-directed counselling.[8-10] Such approaches reduce costs and provide support to patients who are unable to attend institution-based courses because of distance, access to transport, or other factors. More complete evaluation of these options is needed to determine what proportion of patients can safely and effectively start on these programmes.

One concern would be that such systems are developed *instead of*, rather than *as a complement to*, institutional courses, because of their lower cost. Such programmes are likely to be suitable only for the low risk patient. In one series, for instance, of 378 consecutive male MI patients aged $\leqslant 70$ years,[8] 175 were excluded because of conditions precluding a symptom-limited treadmill test three weeks after MI and a further five because of symptoms at stress testing—that is, 48% of an already low risk group were excluded. Thus the danger would be that high risk patients, those in most need of support to attain an acceptable quality of life, would be excluded in the interests of cost containment.

Future structures

It will be useful in future to consider patient lifestyle management following cardiac events as comprising two separate although complementary components—that is, early cardiac rehabilitation in conjunction with specialist cardiac services followed by a step-down community system of secondary prevention. There are many unanswered questions about the specific format of cardiac rehabilitation services, from variations in duration and intensity to site of programme delivery. These (coupled with considerations of appropriate strategies for differing clinical populations as considered next) constitute the primary research agenda for the remainder of this century.

The population requiring cardiac rehabilitation

Changes in the cardiac population

The emphasis to date in terms of provision of cardiac rehabilitation has been on patients recovering from MI and CABG. Rehabilitation programmes cater less often for heart failure patients or those who have undergone coronary angioplasty, heart valve replacement, or pacemaker implantation. Furthermore, for cardiac transplantation patients, rehabilitation requires a high degree of expertise and more sophisticated forms of exercise testing than are currently available in many centres. In terms of demography, patients are increasingly likely to present at an older age, and a focus on older populations brings with it a larger proportion of female patients than was previously enrolled in structured programmes.

While the population requiring cardiac rehabilitation is broadly expected to be older over the coming years, a subgroup—children with complex congenital heart disease requiring reconstructive surgery—requires particular mention. These children need comprehensive rehabilitation to promote physical capabilities, healthy lifestyle, and good psychosocial functioning if they are to attain the potential offered by surgery.[11] Rehabilitation needs to actively involve the parents and to target the children with interventions suitable to their level of cognitive development. In this regard, the knowledge base developed from other areas of childhood illness and disability will be particularly useful in the development of programmes.

Implications for programme delivery

At the level of service delivery, the changing profile of the cardiac population will provide a new challenge to those involved. With an increasingly complex case mix of cardiac disease, the present focus of most rehabilitation centres on traditional end points such as exercise testing will be more modest if not precluded altogether. It will be increasingly evident that cardiac rehabilitation is a secondary preventive rather than a curative strategy. From being satisfied with training systems (and health-care systems) focused on cure as the prime outcome, the challenge facing us will be to become equally satisfied with the more modest but equally significant rehabilitation achievements of the more complex of our patients. Indeed, it is possible that these moderate improvements in patients with complex cardiac problems will yield substantial health-care savings in terms of decreased dependency in terms of both activities of daily living and medical interventions. Work in cardiac rehabilitation in older populations may complement a range of interventions in other areas (such as promoting adequate nutrition and alleviating carer burden) which serve to maintain older people in a relatively healthy and independent state in community settings for as long as possible. As cardiac rehabilitation services become more firmly established, they will be able to focus on and include these more complex patient groups.

Programme access and acceptability will be an increasingly pertinent issue, given the changing profile of the population for consideration. These factors will mean that individualisation of programme content, with patients opting for and/or being advised on a "menu" of components from a multidisciplinary rehabilitation package, is likely to be a format for the future. Screening instruments—for exercise, dietary, or psychological components of the programme, for example—will be used to determine whether patients require and/or are suited to various components.

The experience of the previous three decades has been a learning curve from which to consolidate our skills for new cardiac populations. Cardiac rehabilitation will join an increasing array of secondary preventive and supportive services targeted at maintaining health and independent living for older populations with chronic disease.

Professional roles in the delivery of cardiac rehabilitation services

The cardiologist

The role of cardiologists in initiating cardiac rehabilitation programmes in those countries where it is well developed is quite clear. The cardiologist is in a unique position to recommend rehabilitation to patients in a positive way and is also in a pivotal position within the medical institution and health service, acting as an advocate for the establishment and financial support of the rehabilitation service. However, the increasingly interventional nature of modern cardiology has diverted the attention of a new generation of cardiologists from lifestyle management towards more technological areas of endeavour. Consequently, in most countries, only a minority of cardiologists or associated physicians have espoused an interest in cardiac rehabilitation, while those who acknowledge its benefits but cannot find time to develop and deliver programmes are increasing in numbers. The British Cardiac Society's working party report on cardiac rehabilitation[12] recommended the involvement of an interested physician, preferably a cardiologist, as being one of the most important requirements for the establishment of a programme. Undoubtedly this involvement is a most important one. For a generation of cardiologists, most of whom have trained without significant exposure to the delivery of a structured cardiac rehabilitation programme in their places of work, the prospect of developing such a service *de novo* is naturally daunting. Coupled with this is the increasing specialisation of the research literature and fraternities even within the discipline of cardiology. Thus the scientific issues and developments in cardiac rehabilitation are likely to remain unfamiliar to a wide audience within cardiology. The training requirements for cardiologists recently drafted by the Royal College of Physicians joint committee on higher medical training (unpublished) is to be welcomed in that it makes provision for some introduction to the process of cardiac rehabilitation during the training period in the United Kingdom. However, it does not make this a mandatory requirement.

The vacuum created by the non-participation of cardiologists and physicians with an interest in cardiology in the rehabilitative process has led to the involvement of a number of other health professionals in the development and management of rehabilitation programmes. While the working party of the British Cardiac Society recommended cardiologist involvement at a significant management level, it acknowledged the reality of current circumstances within the British Isles and appreciated that, if significant progress was to be made in the immediate future, it would happen with the development of many programmes that have only peripheral input from the medical profession.

Other health professionals

In those countries with an established tradition of cardiac rehabilitation, an increasing trend whereby management of cardiac rehabilitation services is developing among non-cardiologists has been viewed with concern, and cogent arguments have been put forward for the retention of management by cardiologists. Where this view is espoused there is no shortage of interventional cardiologists, and a career in rehabilitative cardiology is feasible. In those countries with developing cardiac rehabilitation services, it would be unfortunate if a dichotomy were to develop between programmes supervised by cardiologists or physicians and those coordinated by other health professionals. The multifactorial nature of cardiac rehabilitation demands skills of physiotherapists, occupational therapists, physical educationalists, nurses, psychologists, nutritionists, vocational counsellors, and pharmacists. The disparate skills of these various specialties are of relevance to some if not all of those patients undergoing cardiac rehabilitation. The continuing treatment of cardiac patients is within the ambit of some or all of these groups independently of one another.

The continuing *medical* management of patients with established cardiac disease is properly the province of the cardiologist, who ideally should have a global view of the optimal management strategy for the various manifestations of cardiac disease. It makes sense, both pragmatically and from the perspective of advocating a long course of rehabilitation and prevention with maximum credibility to the individual patient, that the cardiac rehabilitation service should be accessed via, and overseen by, the cardiologist. After all, many if not all of the staff involved in the delivery of cardiac rehabilitation will already be part of the team of professionals working with the cardiologist in other aspects of patient care.

Training in cardiac rehabilitation

In most centres in the British Isles, intensive involvement in the day to day running of services by cardiologists and physicians is not feasible. Thus it becomes necessary to provide education about the holistic approach of cardiac rehabilitation for those related specialties that are to be involved in the provision of the cardiac rehabilitation service. General educational activities for all staff involved should be separated from a more detailed training required to coordinate the various services required for a multidisciplinary programme. We reiterate the recommendation of the working party on cardiac rehabilitation,[12] that there be systematic training of professionals to coordinate rehabilitation programmes. Such training is feasible where collaboration is achieved between academic centres, health authorities, and a clinical centre, as has been the case at Beaumont Hospital, Dublin, since 1992 (JH Horgan, unpublished report).

At Beaumont Hospital, a 6 month training programme was constructed in conjunction with teaching input from a masters course in sports medicine (exercise physiology and testing) and a coronary care nursing course (basic cardiology), alongside tailored lectures in applied cardiology, in dietary, psychosocial, and vocational counselling, in pharmacology, and in programme administration. The teaching component (120 hours) is complemented by on-site training and experience of the work of each member of the programme team. Training in small groups (four to six students) is made possible by making use of the teaching opportunities in other courses, and in this way the balance of costs and trainee management within a busy clinical context is achieved. Trainees, all experienced cardiology prersonnel, are seconded for the duration of the training programme.

This is but one mechanism to achieve such training. Resources and constraints in different regions will determine the structure of training offered. Whatever the structure of training offered in different regions, however, it is clear that some uniformity of expertise and minimum standard of training will be required in the coming decade if the specialty is to acquire both credibility and resources. The rapid growth of societies such as the British Association for Cardiac Rehabilitation, with well-attended conferences and a working party on training guidelines, is reflective of an active interest in training and accreditation among those working in the area. In this vein, recommendations for training ("core competencies") have been prepared by the American Association for Cardiovascular and Pulmonary Rehabilitation (unpublished report).

Fully trained, any one of the forementioned specialties can undertake coordination of a cardiac rehabilitation programme, effectively incorporating the skills of associated professionals but without assuming any of the many roles required beyond that of their own professional training and competency. This concept of skill coordination allows the optimal utilisation of individual specialist services available from within the multidisciplinary team associated with cardiology. In turn, this helps to develop a rehabilitation perspective throughout the cardiology system.

Professional and organisational developments

Until relatively recently, cardiologists and physicians interested in cardiac rehabilitation interrelated by holding small local meetings relating to the subject or by organising symposia as part of national cardiac society or heart foundation meetings. On an international scale similar symposia and scientific sessions were included in the larger meetings, such as those sponsored by the American College of Cardiology, the American Heart Association, and the European Cardiac Society. A world congress on cardiac rehabilitation has been established under the auspices of the International Societies and Federations of Cardiology. This now has a large attendance and meets every four years. At present, this group forms the most international forum.

The increasing involvement of non-medical specialists in cardiac rehabilitation has created a need for organisational structures. The American Association for Cardiopulmonary Rehabilitation, founded in the '80s, has proved a most successful organisation and organises a very well-attended annual meeting in various parts of the USA. As a consequence of its success, similar organisations have now been founded in Britain (1992) and are planned for some other European countries. The European Association for Cardiovascular Rehabilitation was also established in 1992. The primary aim of each of these organisations, whether meeting independently or in conjunction with major meetings on cardiovascular medicine, is to promote the development of the concept of cardiac rehabilitation and to advance knowledge and provide education for new practitioners. At present, non-medical rehabilitation specialists may attend the meetings of the cardiac societies and associations but normally do not have a role in the organisation of the scientific sessions and are not members of the various subcommittees. Conversely, however, membership of other (cardiovascular rehabilitation) societies are open to any involved profession, including cardiologists and relevant physicians. It seems clear that in the future most of the work in the area of cardiac rehabilitation will be carried out by health professionals other than physicians. Therefore optimal working relationships among the various organisations are mandatory in the interest of patients.

The quality of patient therapy is driven forward by scientific research and therapaeutic application of the most available therapies in best meeting the requirements of the various manifestations of cardiovascular disease. The cardiologist, in a dual role as scientist-practitioner, is in a unique position to observe and distil changing trends in patient presentation and treatment in cardiology generally, and to consider their implications for the delivery of cardiac rehabilitation services. With respect to the cardiac rehabilitation service associated with his or her clinical practice, this is likely to be the most useful "consultative" role for the cardiologist. In a complementary way, other professionals involved in cardiac rehabilitation can identify theoretical or methodological developments in those aspects of service delivery which are likely to improve outcome for patients. These may be disseminated via the programme coordinator and via systematic periodic review of service performance by the team. In the future, it will be necessary for organisations to ensure that

255

Professional and organisational aspects of cardiac rehabilitation services

- The involvement of a variety of professionals is required to make cardiac rehabilitation a viable and expanding service

- The role of the cardiologist is significant in guaranteeing and protecting resource allocation and in incorporating cardiac rehabilitation as a standard aspect of the care of cardiac patients

- The role of a designated coordinator for individual programmes is important for the cohesion, standard and continuity of the programme offered

- Inter-professional difficulties must not be allowed to jeopardise the success of cardiac rehabilitation

- The resources of everyone involved are required to represent the service maximally in the current climate of health service evaluation and accountability

---

the dissemination of the knowledge referred to is optimal, through the periodic meeting of rehabilitation specialists. Such a development can only expedite the optimisation of cardiac rehabilitation services, expand knowledge, and promote the goals that such a cohesive approach will clearly assist.

The professional developments referred to here are important in signalling a growing interest in cardiac rehabilitation and serve to provide the "critical mass" of professionals and service delivery which can make cardiac rehabilitation an established and well-supported service in the coming decades. As evidence of this increased visibility and credibility, the NHS Executive has supported an initiative to investigate current formats of cardiac service delivery and to advise on the nature of services to be funded by the NHS in the future. The report from this investigation is due in 1995. It will be complemented by a document from the British Association for Cardiac Rehabilitation, which is also to be published in 1995, which will provide guidelines for good practice in the range of services to be offered in a cardiac rehabilitation programme. Thus there is evidence of a forum developing whereby purchasers (or commissioners) and service providers are moving to make their parameters explicit. This should serve to increase the range and the quality of service delivery to patients.

Conclusions on the future of cardiac rehabilitation

- Research and clinical activities have reached the point where a critical mass of evidence, clinical practice, and professional experience has developed

- Key challenges are the appropriate end points of rehabilitation, how services are to be delivered, the response to a changing cardiac population profile, and how the various professionals must contribute to these developments

- The challenges will be met by the initiatives of the many professionals involved in the development and support of organisational structures for the promotion of cardiac rehabilitation in a variety of countries and across continents

- Increasingly, the challenges will be met *because of* the driving forces of accountability and management within the health services: it will be up to professionals in cardiac rehabilitation to document the outcomes of their endeavours

- The next decade will be one of considerable responsibility and opportunity, being the foundation for cardiac rehabilitation services into the second millennium

References

1 Oldridge NB, Guyatt GH, Fischer ME, Rimm AA. Cardiac rehabilitation after myocardial infarction: continued experience of randomised clinical trials. *JAMA* 1988; **260**: 945–50.
2 O'Connor GT, Buring JE, Yusuf S, *et al*. Overview of randomised controlled trials of rehabilitation with exercise after myocardial infarction. *Circulation* 1989; **80**: 234–44.
3 Spilker B (editor) *Quality of life assessment in clinical trials.* New York: Raven, 1990.
4 Fries JF, Green LW, Levine S. Health promotion and the compression of morbidity. *Lancet* 1989; **i**: 481–3.
5 Levin L, Perk J, Hedback B. Cardiac rehabilitation—a cost analysis. *J Intern Med* 1991; **230**: 427–35.
6 Oldridge N, Furlong W, Feeling D, *et al*. Economic evaluation of cardiac rehabilitation soon after myocardial infarction. *Am J Cardiol* 1993; **72**: 154–61.
7 Hopkins A (editor) *Measures of the quality of life and the uses to which such measures may be put.* London: Royal College of Physicians, 1992.
8 DeBusk F, Haskell WL, Mill NN, *et al*. Medically directed at-home rehabilitation soon after clinically uncomplicated acute myocardial infarction: a new model for patient care. *Am J Cardiol* 1985; **55**: 251–7.
9 Lewin B, Robertson IH, Cay EL, Irving JB, Campbell M. Effects of self-help post-myocardial-infarction rehabilitation on psychological adjustment and use of health services. *Lancet* 1992; **339**: 1036–40.
10 DeBusk RF, Miller NH, Superko R, *et al*. A case management system for coronary risk factor modification after acute myocardial infarction. *Ann Intern Med* 1994; **120**: 721–9.
11 Balfour IC, Drimmer AM, Nouri S, Pennington DC, Heinkens CL, Harvey LL. Pediatric cardiac rehabilitation. *Am J Dis Child* 1991; **145**: 627–30.
12 Horgan JH, Bethell H, Carson P, *et al*. British Cardiac Society Working Party report on cardiac rehabilitation. *Br Heart J* 1992; **67**: 412–18.

Index

INDEX

Related titles

CLINICAL ECHOCARDIOGRAPHY

John B Chambers

Perhaps the first book to put this major diagnostic tool into its clinical context, *Clinical Echocardiography* begins with a brief introduction on the technology followed by chapters on all the different disease patterns. Each one discusses the indications and gives many examples of echocardiograms showing the diseases. This concise text atlas is at the same time a cardiology text and an introduction to echocardiography, containing over 400 illlustrations.

Readership: clinical cardiologists, general physicians, trainees, technicians

ISBN 0 7279 0810 3   260 pages approx   April 1995

EXPLAINING CARDIAC SURGERY:
Patient Assesment and Care

Russell Millner, Tom Treasure

There are 15000 coronary surgery patients in the UK every year. The implications for management pre and post surgery go far beyond the sphere of the surgeon. This book is directed specifically at the non-surgical staff managing those patients. As well as describing the indications for the different surgical procedures, the authors discuss the practical issues involved in preparation, immediate and longterm aftercare.

Readership: trainee cardiologists, general physicians, junior doctors, GPs, intensive care staff

ISBN 0 7279 0853 7   250 pages approx   May 1995

For further details of these books and our full range of titles write to Marketing Department, BMJ Publishing Group, BMA House, Tavistock Square, London WC1H 9JR or telephone Diana Chapple on 0171 383 6541.